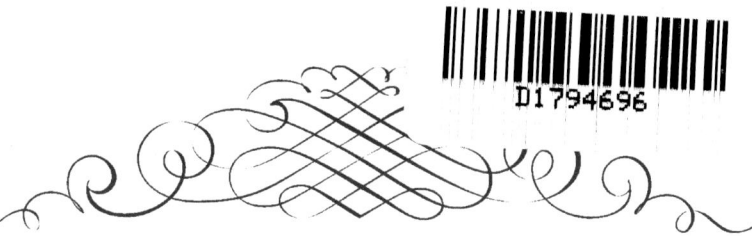
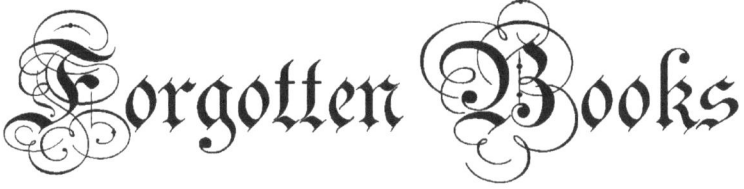

ISBN 978-1-332-74859-4
PIBN 10278424

This book is a reproduction of an important historical work. Forgotten Books uses
state-of-the-art technology to digitally reconstruct the work, preserving the original format
whilst repairing imperfections present in the aged copy. In rare cases, an imperfection in
the original, such as a blemish or missing page, may be replicated in our edition. We do,
however, repair the vast majority of imperfections successfully; any imperfections that
remain are intentionally left to preserve the state of such historical works.

OBSTETRICS.

A MANUAL FOR STUDENTS AND PRACTITIONERS.

BY

DAVID JAMES EVANS, M.D.,

Lecturer on Obstetrics and Diseases of Infancy, McGill University, Montreal, Canada,
Assistant Obstetric Physician to the Montreal Maternity, etc.

SECOND EDITION, REVISED AND ENLARGED.

ILLUSTRATED WITH ONE HUNDRED AND SEVENTY-TWO ENGRAVINGS.

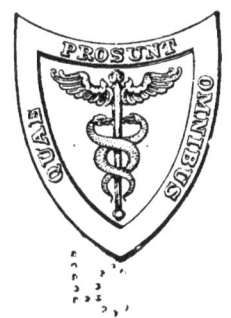

LEA & FEBIGER,

PHILADELPHIA AND NEW YORK.

1909.

PREFACE TO THE SECOND EDITION.

In this edition the sections dealing with the Implantation of the Ovum, the Development of the Placenta, and Toxæmia have been entirely rewritten. Accouchement Forcé has been discussed and the newer obstetric operations introduced, while Symphysiotomy is merely referred to, having fallen into disuse. The entire book has been revised and numerous changes and additions introduced. Several new illustrations have been added, and some of the old cuts replaced with newer and better ones.

D. J. E.

McGill University,
Montreal.

CONTENTS.

MENSTRUATION.

PREGNANCY (Normal).

CONTENTS.

MANAGEMENT OF NORMAL LABOR.

THE PUERPERAL STATE.

PATHOLOGY OF PREGNANCY.

PATHOLOGY OF LABOR.

PATHOLOGY OF THE PUERPERAL PERIOD.

OBSTETRIC OPERATIONS.

OBSTETRICS.

MENSTRUATION.

MENSTRUATION is a periodic discharge of blood and mucus from the uterus and the Fallopian tubes of the woman during the period of sexual activity—*i. e.*, from puberty to the menopause.

The **cause** of menstruation is unknown. Many theories have been advanced; but all that can be said is that *nervous influences* proceeding from the sympathetic nerve-ganglia in the lower abdomen and pelvis periodically bring about a condition of congestion of the sexual organs.

It is presumed that the function is analogous to "rut" in the lower animals, and that from the erect posture of the woman, the pelvic congestion results in bloody discharge.

Structural changes: According to Leopold, the intra-uterine *mucous membrane* becomes thickened and softened almost to liquefaction, but remains practically intact throughout, while it is quite distinct from the *paler* muscular tissue of the uterus. The *uterine glands* are swollen and lengthened. In the superficial portion of the endometrium is an enormously distended *network of capillaries.* As the venous return is slower than the arterial supply, there occurs a *diapedesis of blood.* This blood, along with an excess of mucus from increased activity of the uterine glands, forms the *menstrual discharge.*

The **onset** of menstruation, or puberty, varies in different countries, occurring earlier in southern than in northern climates. Generally in temperate climates it appears about the fourteenth year. It is more likely to come on earlier in city-bred than in country-bred girls.

Character of the flow: The flow is chiefly composed of blood, but also contains mucus and epithelial detritus.

It has a peculiar odor, which is more marked in brunettes

2—Obst.   17 than in blondes, and is caused by secretions from the sebaceous glands at the vaginal outlet.

The discharge is dark in color, as a rule does not clot, and is alkaline in reaction.

Duration and quantity: Menstruation lasts from three to seven days. As a rule, it occurs every twenty-eight days.

The actual quantity of the discharge is from four to six ounces.

Menopause: Menstruation ceases in the forty-fourth year usually; but there are many exceptions. As a rule, a woman menstruates during a period of about thirty years.

The cessation of menstruation is termed the *menopause* or *climacteric.*

Ovulation: By this term we designate the process of formation, development, and discharge of a mature ovum from its Graafian follicle in the ovary.

The **Graafian follicle** is derived from the germinal epithelium on the surface of the ovary. These cells, becoming isolated in the stroma of the ovary, develop a special containing membrane from the theca folliculi, which becomes divided into two layers, the *tunica externa,* and the *tunica interna.* The epithelial cells develop and line this membrane, forming the *membrana granulosa,* and a fluid, the liquor folliculi, distends the cavity.

This fluid pushes the primordial ovum to one side, where it is surrounded by a mass of cells, the *discus proligerus.*

It has been calculated that at birth each ovary contains 35,000 immature follicles. These do not develop till about the time of puberty, when one or more rapidly mature and rupture.

As the follicle matures it approaches the surface of the ovary, the liquor folliculi increases till it points at the surface, ruptures the tunica externa and washes out the ovum surrounded by its discus proligerus.

The ovum is then swept into the fimbriated extremity of the Fallopian tube, through which it passes into the cavity of the uterus. This process is repeated every four weeks during a period of about thirty years.

The ovum: The *immature ovum* is a simple epithelial cell without a cell-wall, but having cell-contents—*i. e.,* the yolk, a nucleus termed the germinal vesicle, and a nucleolus called the germinal spot (Fig. 2). It early develops two walls, the outer, termed the vitelline membrane; the inner, the cell-membrane. Between these walls is a clear area, termed the zona pellucida.

As the *ovum matures* previous to its escape from the Graafian follicle its germinal spot approaches the cell-membrane, where

FIG. 1.

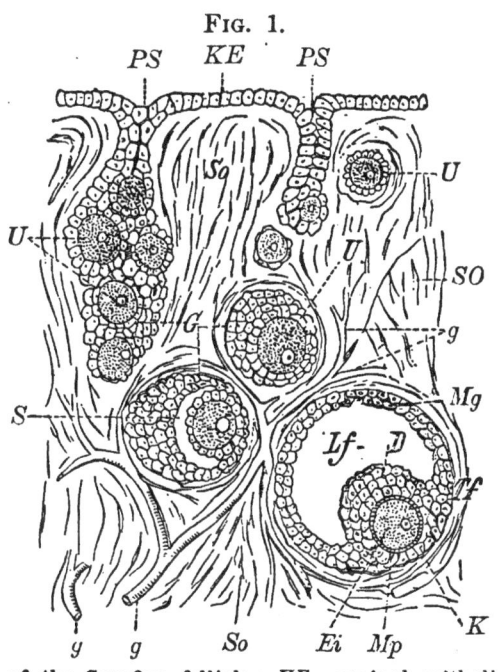

Development of the Graafian follicle: *KE*, germinal epithelium, from which Pflüger's tubes, *PS*, in ovarian stroma are developed; *So*, ovarian stroma; *g, g*, small vessels; *U, U,* primitive ova; *S*, space between membrana granulosa and ovum; *Lf*, liquor folliculi; *D*, discus proligerus; *Ei*, ripe ovum, with germ-vesicle and germinal spot (*K*); *Mp*, membrana pellucida; *Tf*, muscular sheath of follicle; *Mg*, membrana granulosa. (Wiedersheim)

it seems to disappear, and a portion of the ovum is extruded, known as the *first polar body*. After a stage of quiescence the process is repeated, and a *second polar body* is extruded.

Then appears a new and smaller germinal spot, termed the *pronucleus*.

When these phenomena have taken place the ovum is mature and the Graafian follicle ruptures.

The **corpus luteum** is formed at the site of the ruptured Graafian follicle. On the escape of the ovum the walls of the follicle collapse, and blood, derived in part from the vessels at the point of rupture and from those of the theca interna, escapes into its cavity.

Proliferation of the yellow-tinged cells of the theca interna takes place, forming a festooned layer about the central clot, gradually compressing it into a very small space.

The *mature corpus luteum* becomes larger than the original Graafian follicle, and may occupy one-third of the ovary.

FIG. 2.

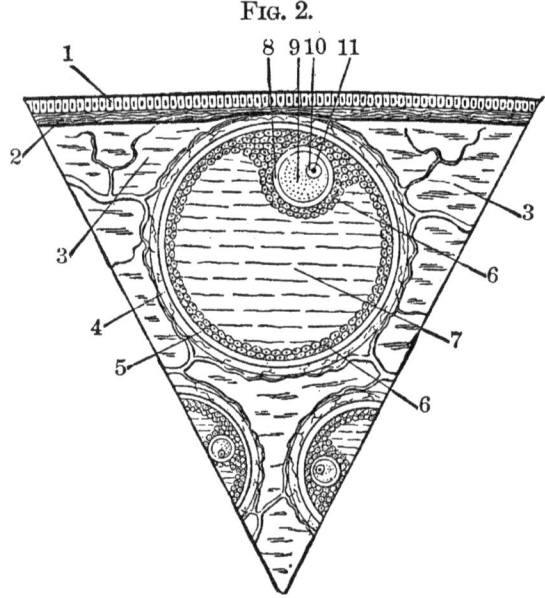

Triangular bit of ovarian stroma cut from ovary : Magnified to show Graafian follicle and ovule : 1, epithelial covering of ovary ; 2, tunica albuginea (fibrous); 3, 3, different parts of stroma ; 4, Graafian follicle (tunica fibrosa) ; 5, Graafian vesicle or ovisac ; 6, 6, tunica granulosa ; 7, liquor folliculi ; 8, vitelline membrane, or zona pellucida ; 9, granular vitellus, or yolk ; 10, germinal vesicle ; 11, germinal spot.

The cavity of the follicle is obliterated by this ingrowth of lutein cells and organization of the blood-clot into connective tissue. The lutein cells then degenerate, and ultimately a punctured scar marks the site of the follicle.

The corpus luteum of pregnancy differs from that found at other times in its more definite character.

Ovulation and menstruation : Neither ovulation nor menstruation is dependent on the other.

Both depend on the same cause, a periodic nervous excitation and congestion. As a rule, they do occur synchronously; but Leopold has proved that ovulation has taken place in the intermenstrual period.

Pregnancy has been known to take place before the onset of menstruation and after the climacteric.

PREGNANCY (Normal).

EMBRYOLOGY.

Impregnation and Conception.

The propagation of the species requires the union of the vital elements of the two sexes.

In the act of *copulation* the male deposits within the female a fluid, the *semen*, which contains the vitalizing element.

The **semen** is a white, viscid, dense fluid having a peculiar odor, secreted by the testicles of the male. It consists of water, albuminous matter, salts of lime and sodium, and contains numerous peculiar organisms called *spermatozoids*.

These spermatozoids form the essential fecundating part of the semen, are about $\frac{1}{600}$ inch in length, and resemble the tadpole of the frog. Each one is made up of three parts; head, middle piece, and tail, and is capable of very rapid vibratory movement (Fig. 3).

After emission, if in proper surroundings, the organisms retain their vitality for a considerable time. Excessively acid or alkaline fluids destroy them.

While pregnancy has been known to follow the deposition of semen on the external genitals of the female, as a rule, the acid mucus of the lower vagina proves fatal to the spermatozoids.

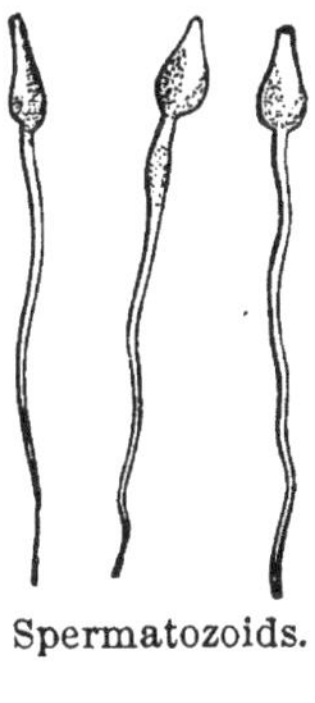

At the crisis of the sexual act the semen is usually deposited in the upper portion of the vagina, into which the cervix projects. Hence the spermatozoids find their way into

Fig. 3.

Spermatozoids.

the cavity of the uterus, and ultimately reach the Fallopian tubes. They have been found on the surface of the ovary.

As a rule, the **meeting-place** of the spermatozoids and ovum is in the Fallopian tube. Many claim that the normal place of meeting is the upper portion of the uterine cavity; and it is not infrequent that they come in contact on the surface of the ovary or in the abdominal cavity (ectopic gestation). If the ovum is discharged at the height of the menstrual conges-tion, it probably does not reach the cavity of the uterus for some days. Hyrtle found the ovum in the uterine extremity of the tube in a girl who had died on the fourth day of men-struation.

Pregnancy is *more likely to occur* after copulation during the first eight days succeeding the cessation of menstruation.

Fertilization of the ovum: Of the large number of sper-matozoids deposited in the vagina, but few probably come into

FIG. 4.

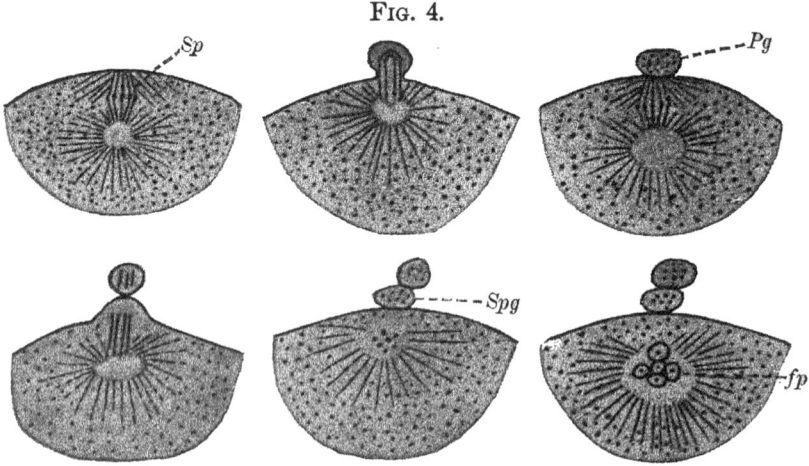

Formation of polar globules in arteria glacialis: *Sp,* nuclear spindle; *Pg,* first polar globule; *Spg,* second polar globule; *fp,* female pronucleus. (After O. Hert-wig.)

contact with the ovum; and of these, but a single spermatozoid actually takes part in the fertilization of the ovum.

By friction with the walls of the tube the cells of the discus proligerus disappear and the zona pellucida becomes surrounded with an albuminous covering which seems to attract the sper-matozoid.

The successful spermatozoid, after penetrating the zona pel-lucida, comes in contact with a projection of the protoplasm of the ovum and its tail disappears. The head then penetrates the cell-contents and disappears, to reappear subsequently as a small round body, the *male pronucleus* (Fig. 4). Finally, the male pronucleus and the female pronucleus unite, and conception has occurred. Thus the life-history of the embryo, fœtus, and infant begins.

Changes in the Ovum; Development of the Fœtus.

The impregnated ovum is at first a **simple cell.**

Its wall is the *vitelline membrane ;* its contents, the *granular vitellus,* or *yolk,* and a *nucleus ;* which latter is a complex structure, formed, as we have seen, of the male and female pronuclei.

Segmentation : Mitotic changes take place in the newly-formed nucleus, a dyaster is formed, and segmentation of the vitellus into two parts follows, still within the vitelline membrane. These two cells then divide into four, and so division proceeds till the whole ovum becomes converted into a mass of cells, and it is then designated the *Morula* or mulberry mass.

The first division results in two cells, which differ somewhat both in size and appearance. This difference is perpetuated, so that as a result of their further division two groups of cells differing in size and appearance are formed.

The larger are termed *epiblastic cells,* and the smaller *hypoblastic cells.*

The blastodermic vesicle : These two sets of cells then arrange themselves in a special manner ; the epiblastic cells completely surrounding the hypoblastic cells, which collect in a roughly spherical mass (Fig. 6). Between these two layers of cells a little albuminous fluid begins to accumulate, separating them from one another except at one spot. The fluid rapidly collects, and the ovum now forms a distended vesicle, termed the *blastodermic vesicle.*

At this stage the epiblastic cells completely line the blastodermic vesicle, while the mass of hypoblastic cells having become distended by the accumulation of fluid is flattened and pressed out over a small area of the epiblastic cell-lining, the central portion being thicker than the periphery (Fig. 7). This thicker part is the commencement of the **embryonic area.**

It is only this part of the blastodermic vesicle which is concerned in the formation of the embryo ; the remaining portion being the non-embryonic part, and concerned only in the for-

FIG. 5.

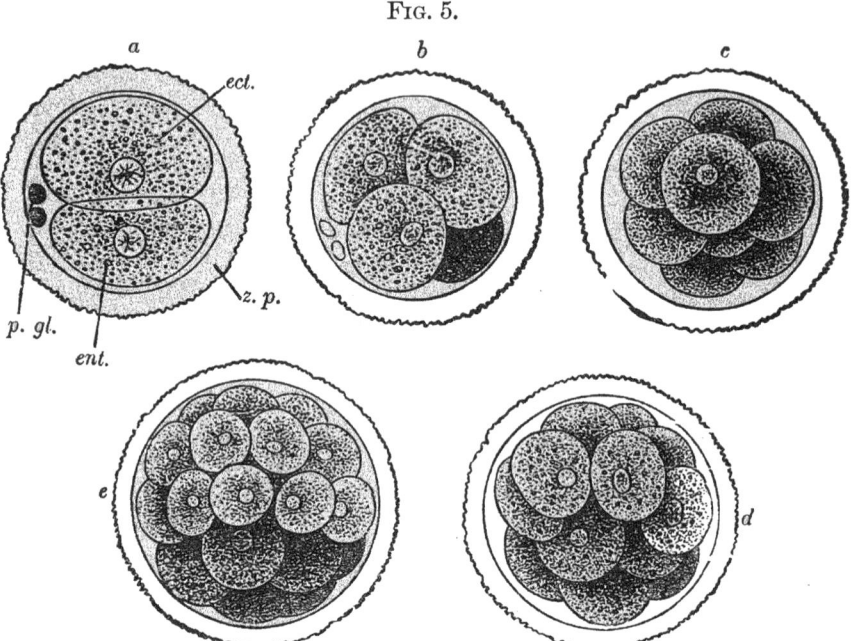

Diagram showing first stages of segmentation in a mammalian ovum. (Allen Thompson, after E van Beneden)

FIG. 6.

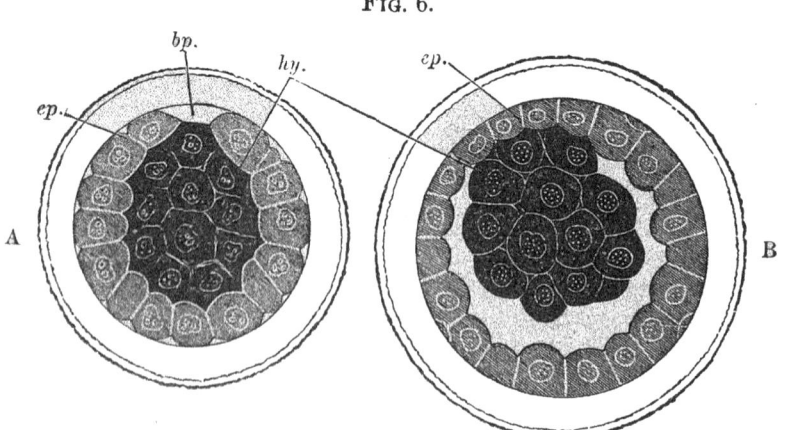

Two further stages following segmentation (rabbit's ovum) . *ep*, epiblast ; *hy*, hypoblast ; *bp*, opening in epiblast (blastopore) not yet closed ; in B, this opening has closed.

mation of the amnion and the umbilical vesicle, as we shall see later.

The *primitive* epiblastic cells peripheral to the thickened layer

FIG. 7.

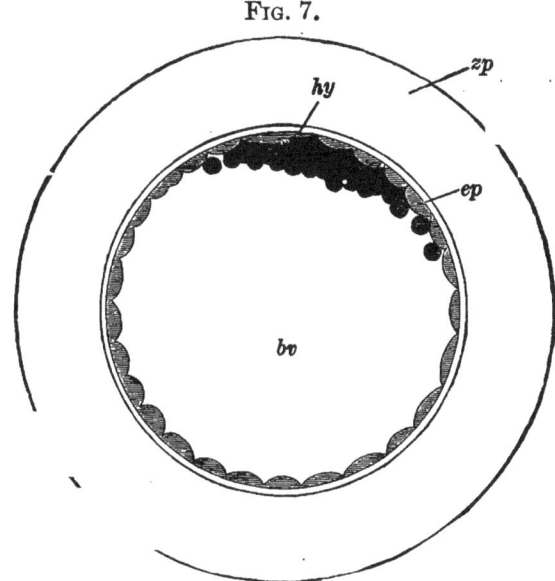

zp, zona pellucida; *ep*, epiblast; *hy*, hypoblast; *bv*, cavity of blastodermic vesicle.

FIG. 8.

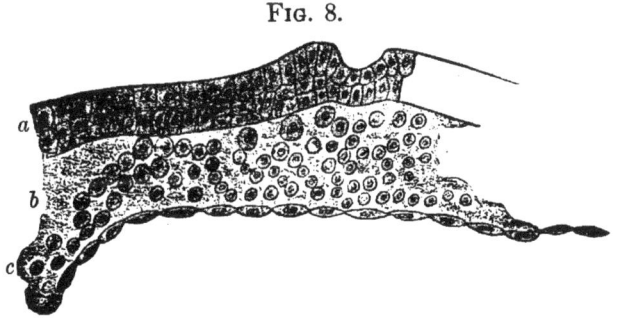

Transection of eighteen-hour chick embryo, showing beginning of medullary groove and the three layers: *a*, ectoderm; *b*, mesoderm; *c*, entoderm. (Manton collection.)

of hypoblastic cells now disappear, leaving this portion of the wall (if one could look, as it were through the vitelline membrane) somewhat clearer (**area pellucida**).

The hypoblastic cells now appear as a darker streak in the area pellucida, termed the **primitive streak**; which then develops with a groove known as the **primitive groove**, which is the first evidence of the formation of the embryo, indicating, approximately, the position of the future vertebræ.

Cleavage of the hypoblastic cells: If a section be made through this streak, or groove, at this period (Fig. 10), the hypoblastic cells will be found to have separated into two layers, termed respectively the *ectoderm* (permanent epiblast) and the *entoderm* (permanent hypoblast); while between them another layer has formed, derived in part from both, termed the *mesoderm* (mesoblast).

Cleavage of the mesoderm: In the course of time this mesoderm develops lateral reduplications and divides into two layers, the parietal and the visceral layers, inclosing spaces. The parietal layer unites with the ectoderm to form the *somatopleure;* and the visceral layer unites with the entoderm to form the *splanchnopleure.*

The space included between the two leaves of the cleft mesoderm is the primitive body-cavity, or cœlom, which afterward becomes the pleuroperitoneal cavity.

FORMATION OF THE DECIDUA.

The mucous membrane lining the uterine cavity undergoes certain changes of a preparatory nature as the result of the pregnancy stimulus. The altered mucous membrane is then termed the *decidua*, from the fact that it is largely cast off after labor.

Shortly after impregnation of the ovum, and consequent upon the pregnancy stimulus, the endometrium becomes thickened, and as a result its surface indented by furrows of some depth. The mouths of the uterine glands may still be distinguished without difficulty.

The formation of decidua is limited to the lining of the uterus, that of the cervix not being affected.

Certain terms are employed to designate various portions of the decidua. These originated with William Hunter, who first described the decidua, and, though our understanding of the anatomical conditions of the pregnant uterus have altered, these terms have been retained.

The decidua, as a whole, is called the *decidua vera ;* that portion immediately beneath the ovum is termed the *decidua serotina ;* while the portion forming a capsule around the ovum is called the *decidua reflexa.*

Fig. 9.

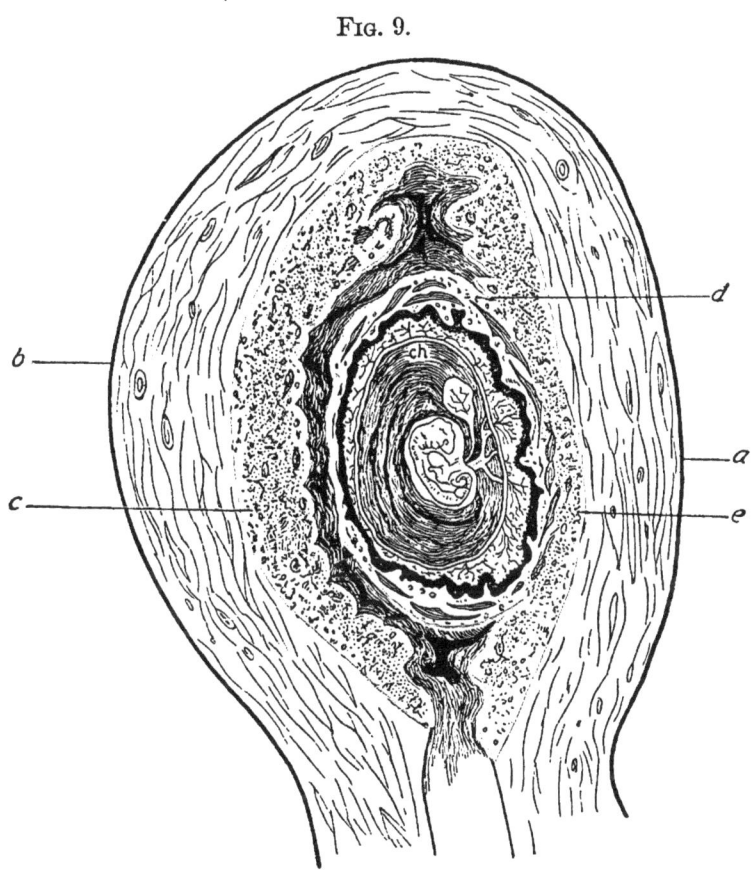

Semi-diagrammatic outline of an anteroposterior section of the gravid uterus and ovum of five weeks: *a,* anterior uterine wall; *b,* posterior uterine wall; *c,* decidua vera; *d,* decidua reflexa; *e,* decidua serotina; *ch,* chorion with its villi. (Modified from Allen Thomson.)

Decidua vera : This is composed of two portions, the upper *compact layer* of large round or polygonal cells with large nuclei, epithelial in appearance, the *decidual cells ;* and a lower *spongy layer,* composed of dilated and hyperplastic uterine glands, mainly forming the thickness of the membrane.

The vera increases during the first four months of pregnancy to finally measure 1 cm. in thickness, then it gradually becomes reduced to 2 mm. at term.

The result of the pregnancy changes in the mucous membrane is that stroma cells are markedly increased in size,

FIG. 10.

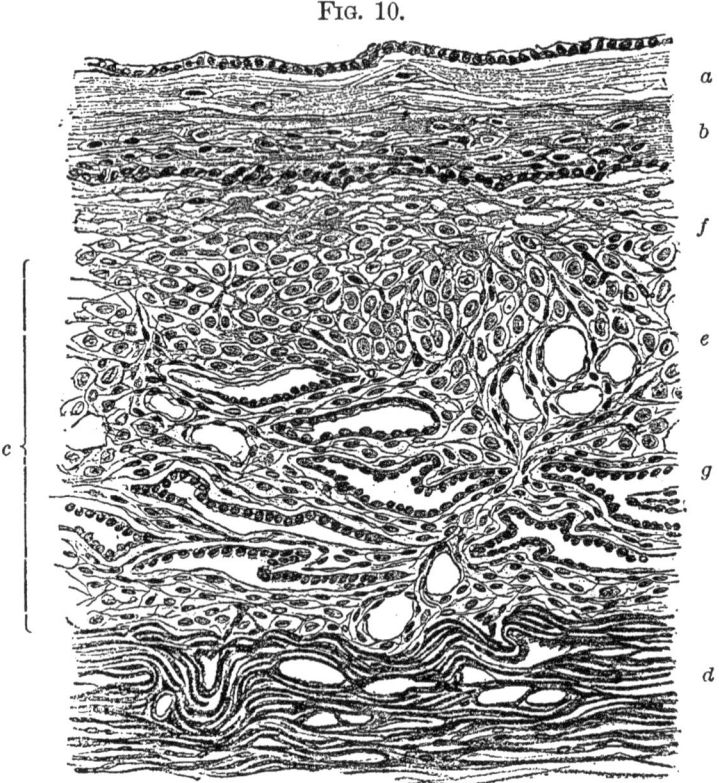

Section through the decidua: *a*, amnion; *b*, chorion; *c*, decidua; *d*, uterine muscle; *e*, line of separation in the cellular layer; *f*, cellular layer; *g*, glandular layer. (Friedlander.)

while there is a marked decrease in size of the epithelial cells.

The decidual cells are derived from the stroma cells of the endometrium (connective tissue), which have undergone marked increase in size. They finally closely resemble sarcoma cells in appearance.

Decidua reflexa or capsularis: The ovum is shut off from the uterine cavity by a capsule of decidual tissue. At first a space exists between the reflexa and vera, which becomes gradually obliterated as the ovum enlarges. By the fourth month of pregnancy the reflexa and vera are in contact throughout, and as a result of pressure from the growing ovum the reflexa disappears. The decidua reflexa thus has but a brief existence.

Decidua serotina or basalis: This term is applied to that portion of the decidua lying immediately beneath the ovum, and from which the placenta is developed. It is the same in structure as the vera, but it has been invaded by fœtal tissue with certain hereafter described results.

In the serotina large numbers of bloodvessels are observed; the arteries pursue a spiral course penetrating the entire thickness of the membranes, while the veins become markedly dilated and form large sinuses.

IMPLANTATION OF THE OVUM AND DEVELOPMENT OF THE PLACENTA AND MEMBRANES.

The ovum in its passage along the Fallopian tube to the uterine cavity acquires a capsule of varying thickness, derived, in part, from fœtal elements, and, possibly, in some part, from maternal. The majority of cells composing this capsule, which is termed the **trophoblast,** are epithelial in appearance, having a rounded or cuboid outline and vesicular nuclei. Scattered among these are masses of protoplasm without cell-walls, but containing numerous darkly staining nuclei.

The trophoblast possesses distinct phagocytic qualities, which enables it to eat its way through the epithelial layer of the decidua and penetrate the subjacent connective tissue, thus bringing about the burial of the ovum in the decidua (Fig. 11).

The trophoblast cells then invade the surrounding decidual tissue and open up numerous capillary bloodvessels, so that small lacunæ or blood-spaces are formed, which are lined with trophoblast cells derived from the outer layer of the ovum, and contain maternal blood from which is derived the nourishment of the ovum. The whole trophoblast becomes rapidly honeycombed by these spaces, leaving bands or columns of trophoblast between them.

Development of the chorionic villi: The chorion or outer membrane of the ovum is probably in its earliest stages composed of a single layer of epiblastic cells, forming the capsule of the blastodermic vesicle or early ovum. This is soon lined by a mesodermic layer. After the implantation of the ovum and the honeycombing of the trophoblast by the maternal blood, the mesoblastic connective-tissue layer begins to send up little bud-like processes which project into the columns and bands remaining between the blood-spaces. Thus are formed

Fig. 11.

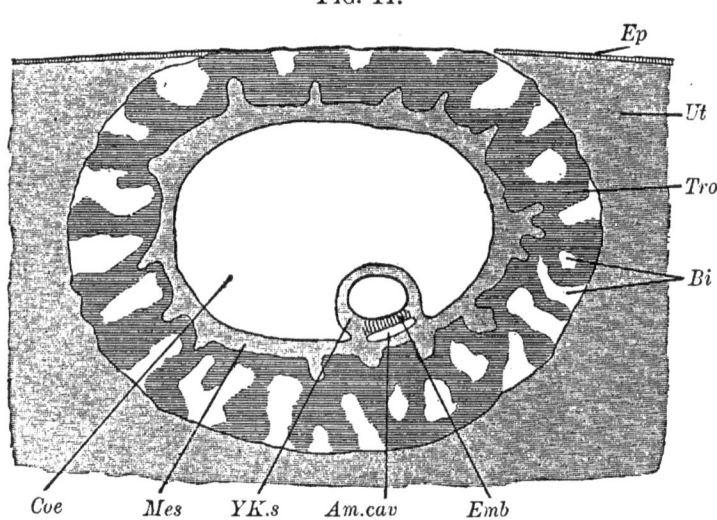

Diagram based on Peter's ovum: *Ep,* uterine epithelium; *Ut,* mucous membrane (decidua) of uterus. *Tro,* trophoderm; *Bi,* spaces formed by degeneration of trophoderm, maternal blood enters these spaces from the decidual bloodvessels; *Emb,* embryonic shield; *Am. cav,* amniotic cavity; *YK.s,* yolk sac, the entodermal lining of which is indicated by a heavy black line; *Mes,* chorionic mesoderm; *Coe,* extra-embryonic celom.

the primary villi, each being composed thus of a mesoblastic core and epiblastic outer layer.

The epithelium derived from the epiblast covering each villus becomes arranged in two layers, the inner, adjoining the connective-tissue core, is formed by well-marked cuboidal or roundish cells with clear protoplasm and vesicular nuclei, while the outer layer is made up of coarsely granular protoplasm without cell formation, containing numerous irregularly shaped nuclei.

The inner layer is called after the man who first described it, *Langhan's layer*, while the outer layer is designated *syncytium*. Both are, it is generally conceded, derived from the fœtal epiblast.

The early chorionic villi soon branch out in every direction ; some float free in the maternal blood in the intervillous spaces, while others become attached by their ends to the neighboring decidual tissue (fastening villi), serving to firmly fasten the ovum to the uterine wall.

The villi are composed of a stroma, mucoid and thread-like in character, with a double layer of epithelial cells on the surface. At first they are entirely devoid of bloodvessels, and it is probable that at this stage the ovum receives its nourishment by osmosis from the maternal blood in the primary intervillous spaces.

Vascularization of the chorion: The early embryo is joined to the connective-tissue layer of the chorion by a mesoblastic pedicle, called the *abdominal pedicle*. In it is a small process of the entoblast, being an extension of the hind gut. Thus entoblastic tissue gives rise to the fœtal bloodvessels, and fine fœtal capillaries are formed which extend along the abdominal stalk to the interior of the chorion and lead to the vascularization of the villi. By the fourth week there can be noted in each villus an arterial and a venous vessel united by a fine capillary network.

Formerly, it was taught that the allantois produced the fœtal bloodvessels, but it has nothing to do with the formation of connective tissue or bloodvessels in the somatopleure. In the human embryo the allantois presents itself as a rudiment, which in the form of a fine canal is enclosed in the connective tissues at the base of the abdominal stalk.

At first the villi are equally distributed over the outer surface of the whole chorion. Later, they become more abundant over that portion in connection with the decidua serotina or basalis, the site of the future placenta. This portion of the chorion is called the *chorion ƒrondosum.* The balance of the villi, in contact with the decidua reflexa or capsularis, is termed the *chorian læve*, as they later completely atrophy.

Formation of the amnion: The amnion was formerly described as being, in the human ovum as in that of the chick,

derived from the somatopleure. Later investigators have
demonstrated that it is derived from the epiblast at a very

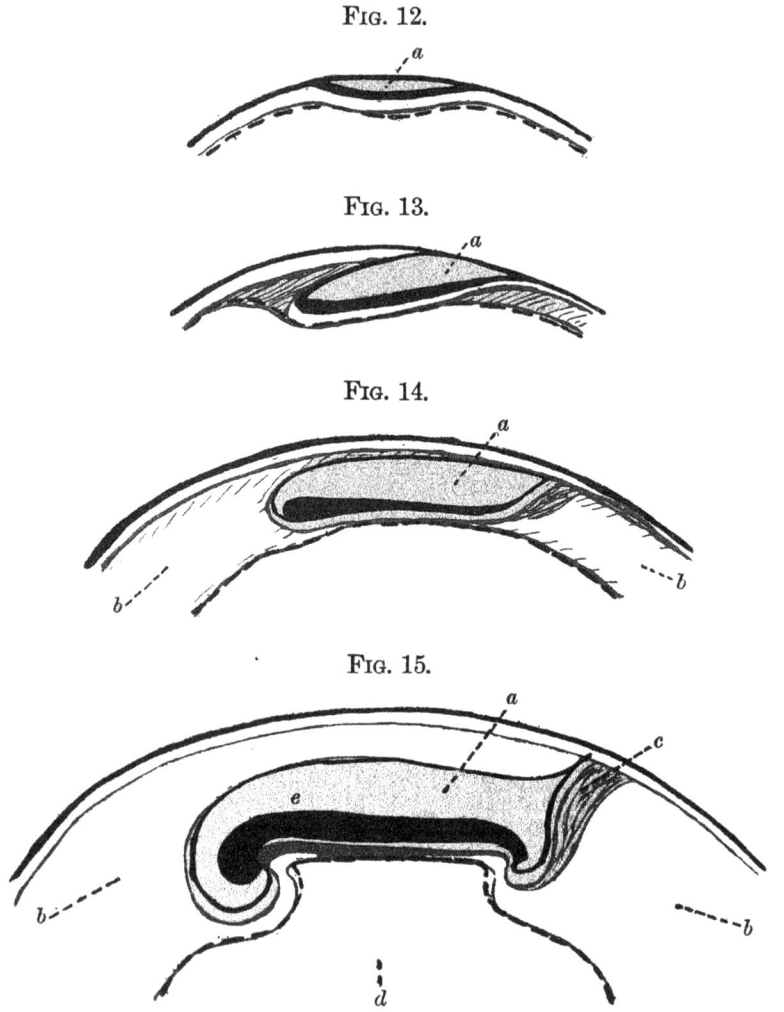

FIG. 12.

FIG. 13.

FIG. 14.

FIG. 15.

Diagram of the formation of the amnion. ▬▬▬ Ectoblast. ══════ Mesoblast.
·········· Entoblast   *a*, amniotic cavity; *b*, exocelom, splitting of mesoblast; *c*, precursor of abdominal stalk; *d*, yolk-sac; *e*, embryo

early stage of development. There forms longitudinally (Fig.
12) in the epiblast, just above the embryonic site, a little slit-
like opening, the *amniotic cavity*. Its formation tends to dis-

place the forming embryo downward in the direction of the yolk-sac.

The rapid growth of mesoblast about the embryo results in a splitting off or separation of the newly formed amniotic cavity from the epiblast, the separation beginning at the cephalic end of the embryo and extending downward to the caudal (Fig. 13). Thus the epiblastic amnion becomes covered with a thin layer of mesoblast. The mesoblast at this time splits

FIG. 16.

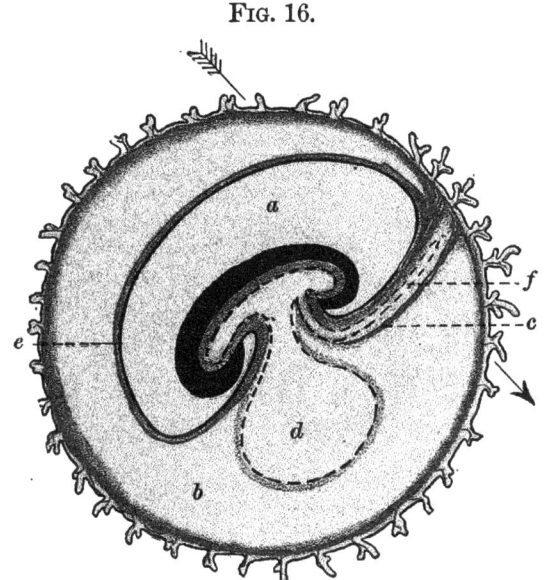

Formation of abdominal stalk and the allantois. ▬▬▬ Epiblast. ≡≡≡≡ Mesoblast. ········ Endoblast. *a,* amniotic cavity; *b,* exocelom; *c,* abdominal stalk; *d,* yolk-sac; *e,* amnion ; *f,* allantois.

into two layers, forming the somatopleure and splancnopleure, as previously described (Fig. 14).

The further development of the somatopleure advances the separation of the amniotic sac from the peripheral epiblast, leaving only one point of attachment situated close to the caudal end of the embryo, the so-called abdominal stalk, the precursor of the umbilical cord (Fig. 15). Thus the amnion is from its commencement a closed space, its inner surface composed of epiblast, directly derived from the embryonic epiblast, surrounded and covered by a thin mesoblastic layer.

3—Obst.

Through the increase of fluid in the cavity of the amnion, the liquor amnii, the sac is greatly enlarged. In its enlargement the amnion gradually surrounds the embryo, pushing the somatopleure in front of it, thus closing off the abdominal cavity except at the umbilical opening, till finally the amnion is in direct contact throughout with the chorion, with which it becomes loosely united (Figs. 16 and 17).

FIG. 17.

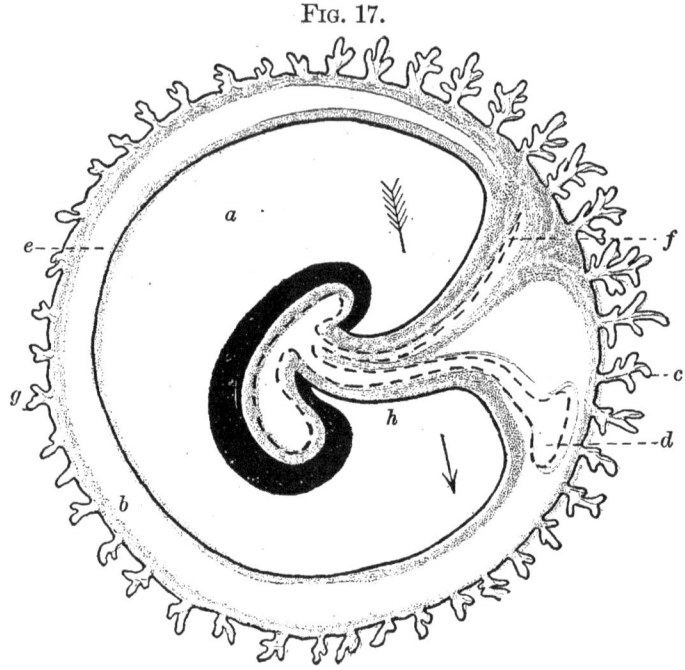

Formation of the umbilical cord. ━━━ Epiblast. ------- Mesoblast. · · · · Entoblast. *a*, amniotic cavity : *b*, exocelom ; *c*, chorion frondosum ; *d*, yolk-sac ; *e*, amnion , *f*, allantois , *g*, chorion læve ; *h*, amniotic sheath.

Structure of the amnion : The mesodermic layer of the amnion becomes converted into mucoid-like tissue, and does not contain bloodvessels ; while the epiblastic layer changes to a single layer of small cuboidal epithelial cells.

The *amniotic fluid*, which increases in quantity as pregnancy advances, varies largely in amount, but averages about 600 c.c. at term.

Development of the placenta : The fertilized ovum on reaching the uterine cavity becomes attached to the decidua vera,

usually on the upper part of the anterior wall.   The erosive
action of the outer covering of the ovum, the trophoblast,

Fig. 18.

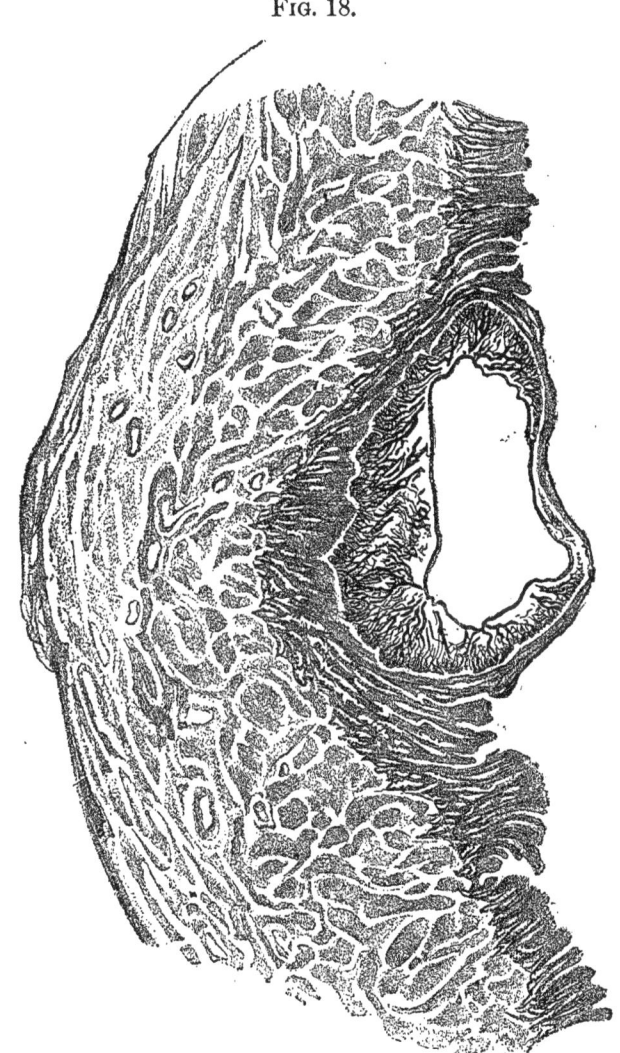

Cross-section of uterine wall with ovum attached (the fourth week).

causes it to penetrate into the decidua, as previously related.
The trophoblast penetrates the capillaries in the decidua, and
so the primary blood-spaces are formed, which are the pre-

cursors of the intervillous blood-spaces of the future placenta.
The villi are now formed on the chorion and project from its
entire periphery, coming in contact alike with both the decidua serotina and reflexa.   The blood-supply of the serotina,

Fig. 19.

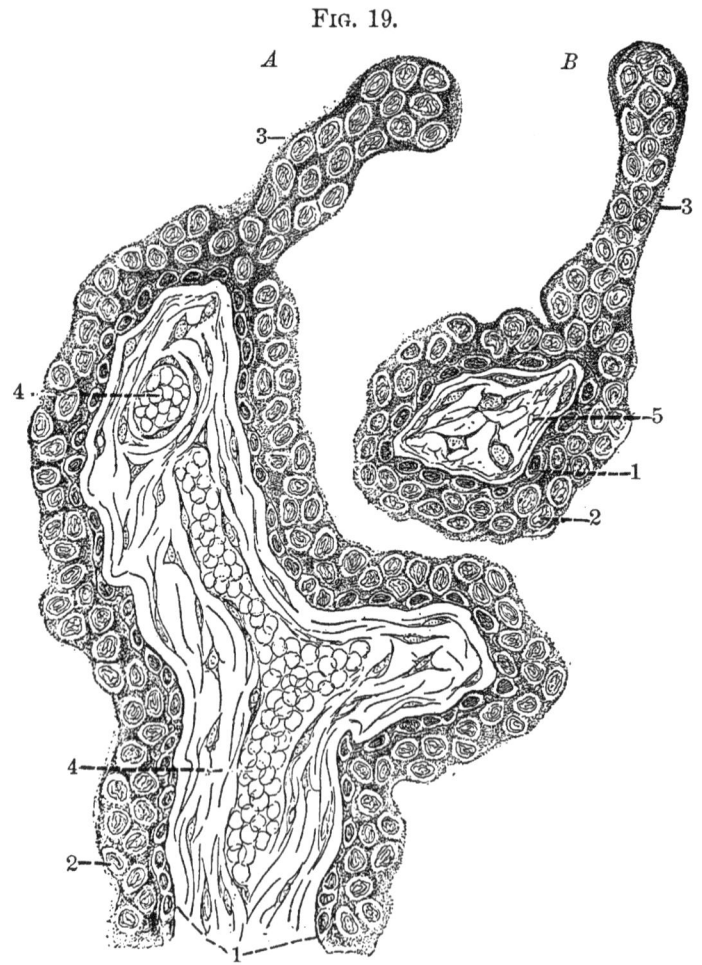

Chorionic villus of a four-weeks' ovum: *A*, Longitudinal section; *B*, tranverse
section; 1, Langhans' cell-layer: 2, syncytium; 3, club-like knot of syncytium;
4, fœtal capillary vessel; 5, connective tissue (stroma) (Bumm).

becoming more abundant as pregnancy advances, the villi in
contact with it become more rapidly developed, and thus form
the *chorion frondosum*.   The chorion læve in contact with the

reflexa being poorly supplied with blood, develop slowly, and finally disappear when the expanding ovum compresses the reflexa against the vera, thus obliterating the uterine cavity about the fourth month.

The placenta is formed by the union of the chorion frondosum and the decidua serotina; thus both fœtal and maternal tissues contribute to its formation. It is completely formed by the end of the fourth month of pregnancy.

As the chorionic villi proliferate, the intervillous blood-spaces, containing maternal blood in which they are bathed, increase in size chiefly at the expense of the veins opening into them. The free or unattached villi are driven by the blood current away from the arteries, and thus tend more easily to penetrate the veins. The exit of the blood current extends itself progressively by the degeneration and absorption of the intervening connective tissue by the action of the syncytium. The veins thus contribute chiefly to the permanent intervillous spaces. Of the intervening connective tissue, nothing remains but the column-like portions around the arteries and island-like masses, together forming the septa of the placental cotyledons (Figs. 20 and 21).

In the early stages the placental formation proceeds along the contiguous vera. The projection of the chorion frondosum into the lower portion of the reflexa gives the early placenta a cup-like form, but as soon as the reflexa becomes united with the vera the peripheral edge of the placenta becomes compressed owing to the atrophy of the læve, the serotinal villi develop further and penetrate the venous vessels under the edge of the adjoining vera, thus forming a decidual ring at the margin of the placenta.

The circulation of blood in the maternal portion of the placenta is so arranged that each cotyledon has its own special blood-supply. The arteries enter along the decidual septa, and open high up into the intervillous spaces. The blood leaves the spaces by fine openings leading from them into the maternal veins or *sinuses* lying parallel to the base, and by the circular vein or sinus at the margin of the placenta.

The fœtal and maternal circulation are self-contained, there being no communication between the fœtal blood contained in the chorionic villi and the maternal blood in the intervillous spaces.

The umbilical arteries from the cord branch out to individual stems going to little bundles of villi, and terminate at the end villi in sharply bent capillaries lying close under the epithelial coats. From these capillaries the veins spring, and

FIG. 20.

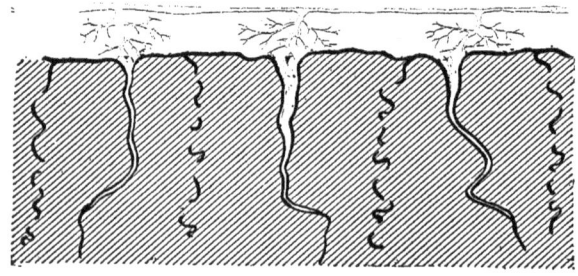

Scheme of placental attachments.

ultimately unite into larger vessels emptying into the umbilical vein in the cord.

The transmission of substances from the mother to child and vice versâ is accomplished partly by osmosis and partly by direct selective activity of the syncytium.

FIG. 21.

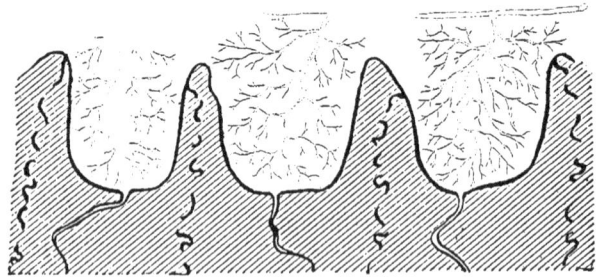

Scheme of placental attachments.

In the later months of pregnancy characteristic changes take place in the placenta. The stroma of the villi becomes thicker as the result of the formation of connective tissue. After the twelfth week the cell-layer of Langhans gradually disappears, leaving the villi with a single epithelial layer composed of syncytial cells, which remains till term.

Fibrin formation characterizes the senile placenta. The favorite positions of this fibrin formation being the superficial layer of the decidua basalis (the fibrin layer of Nitabuch) and the chorionic surface of the placenta, especially at the margins.

This fibrin formation in the decidual basalis, probably resulting from degeneration of fœtal and decidual cells where they come in contact, suggests that one function of the decidual formation is to protect the maternal organism from invasion by fœtal tissues.

PLACENTA AND MEMBRANES AT TERM.

At the end of pregnancy the placenta is a flattened circular mass, 15 to 18 cm. in diameter, and from 2 to 3 cm. thick. From its margins the membranes extend. It averages from 500 to 600 gm. in weight, about one-sixth that of the fœtus.

Maternal aspect—that in contact with the serotina—is covered with a thin layer of decidua, the superficial layer of the serotina, grayish in color and ragged in appearance. It is divided by deep sulci into lobules of irregular outline, termed *cotyledons*. With a lens the torn openings of bloodvessels can be seen in the decidual layer.

Fœtal aspect: The fœtal aspect of the placenta, being covered by amnion, presents a glistening appearance. Through this can be seen the vessels connected with the umbilical cord, branching out in all directions. The cord is usually attached to the placenta somewhat centrally.

Circular sinus: At the margin of the placenta the circular sinus or marginal vein, which returns a portion of the maternal blood, may be seen.

The placenta is at once the respiratory, alimentary, and excretory organ of the fœtus. In it the fœtal blood parts with its carbonic acid and other waste products, receiving in return, from the maternal blood, the materials necessary for the nutrition of the unborn child.

The **fœtal membranes**, consisting of the amnion, chorion, and a thin layer of decidua, extend from the margin of the placenta. The innermost membrane, the *amnion*, is a tough glistening structure, quite transparent. It is loosely attached to the chorion and surface of the placenta.

The **chorion**: The external membrane is a friable opaque structure; thicker than the amnion and much more easily torn. On its outer surface can be seen attached thin sheets of decidua torn from the lining of the uterus.

The **umbilical cord** extends from the navel of the child to the fœtal surface of the placenta. It averages 50 to 55 cm. in length and from 1 to 1.5 cm. in thickness. It is dull, bluish-white in color, and contains two arteries and a vein. It is usually spiral in appearance, the twists being from left to right. The cord is covered by epithelium in direct continuation with the skin of the fœtus. Within, surrounding the bloodvessels, is a mucoid connective tissue, termed *Wharton's jelly.*

The Ovum at Different Periods of Pregnancy.

First month: At the end of the fourth week the ovum measures about 1 inch in diameter, and the straightened-out embryo about $\frac{1}{2}$ inch. The chorion is covered with villi, and the amnion does not quite fill the cavity of the chorion, the space separating them containing a clear fluid.

Second month: At the end of this month the ovum is nearly 2 inches in diameter, and the embryo $\frac{3}{4}$ inch long. The amnion fills the chorion. The chorion læve is atrophying, but the cord is not yet twisted and contains a loop of intestine at its base.

Third month: By the twelfth week the ovum is 4 inches in the long diameter, and the fœtus, as it is now called, is about $3\frac{1}{2}$ inches (7–9 cm.) in length. The placenta is completely formed and the rest of the chorion is quite free from villi. The cord is twisted and the loop of intestine has been withdrawn into the abdominal cavity.

Fourth month: At the end of the sixteenth week the fœtus measures about 6 inches (17 cm.) in length. The head is proportionally very large. The sex can be distinguished. Lanugo is present.

Sixth month: The average length of the fœtus is now about 12 inches (28–34 cm.), and it weighs about $23\frac{1}{2}$ ounces (676 gm.). The testicles in males are still in the abdominal cavity.

Seventh month: At the end of this month the fœtus measures in length 13.75 to 15 inches (35–38 cm.), and weighs 41½ ounces (1170 gm.). The whole body is covered with lanugo, except the palms of the hands and the soles of the feet. The pupillary membrane disappears.

Eighth month: The fœtus now measures 15 to 16 inches (39 to 41 cm.) in length and weighs 3½ pounds (1571 gm.) Lanugo is disappearing from the face, and the left testicle is in the scrotum. Ossific centres are present in the lower epiphyses of the femurs. The child if born is viable.

Ninth month: At the end of this month, the thirty-sixth week, the fœtus averages about 5½ pounds (2504 gm.) in weight. At this period, if the infant should be born, Hirst considers that with ordinary care it should certainly live. The length of the embryo in centimeters may be approximated during the first five months by squaring the number of the month to which pregnancy has advanced. Thus, at four months, $4 \times 4 = 16$ cm. In the second half of pregnancy by multiplying the month by 5. Thus, at six months, $6 \times 5 = 30$ cm.

The consideration of the infant at full term, the fortieth week, will be taken up under the heading *Labor;* but it is convenient at this point to refer to the peculiarities of fœtal circulation.

Fœtal Circulation (Fig. 22).

The fœtal blood, having been oxygenated in the terminal villi in the placenta, is returned by various branches to the **umbilical vein.** This is carried along the cord to the fœtal body, which it enters at the umbilicus. It runs thence along the anterior abdominal wall to the under surface of the liver, where it branches, the larger branch emptying into the portal vein, while the smaller, called the **ductus venosus,** empties directly into the ascending vena cava.

Thus the largest quantity of the "arterial" blood from the placenta must pass through the fœtal liver, where it probably undergoes some changes before entering the general circulation.

Hence is poured into the **right auricle** of the heart, from the **ascending vena cava,** a stream of blood derived from (1) the

FIG. 22.

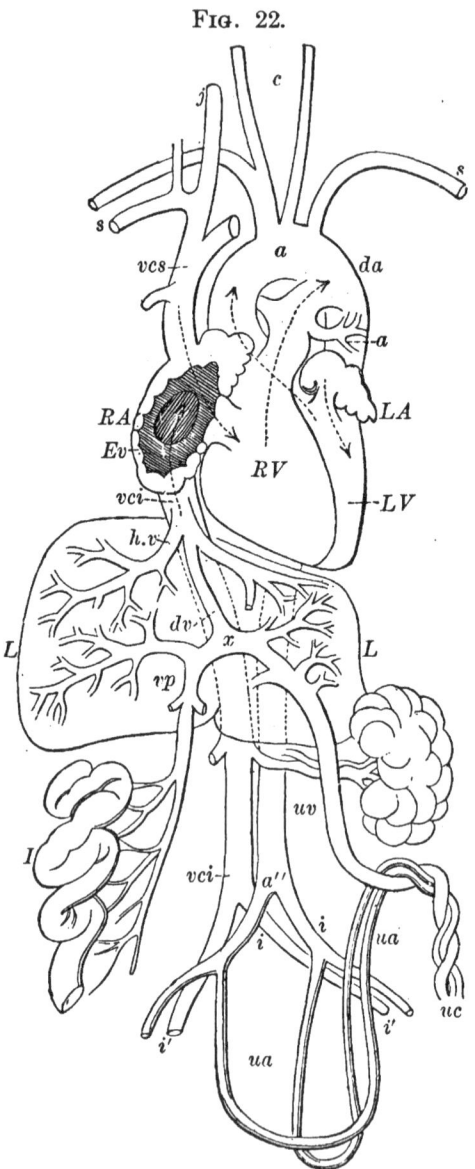

hepatic veins; (2) the ductus venosus; and (3) the lower extremities of the fœtus along the *iliac veins.*

This mixed stream enters the right auricle posteriorly, is guided across it by a fold of membrane, termed the **Eustachian valve**, through the **foramen ovale**, an opening in the inter-auricular septum, and thus enters the left auricle.

The Eustachian valve, by directing the blood-current from the right ventricle, thus "short-circuits" the s t r e a m from the undeveloped fœtal lungs, which in their unexpanded condition could not contain such a large quantity of blood.

From the **left auricle** the blood enters the **left ventricle**, passing thence

Diagram of the circulatory organs of the human fœtus at six months: *RA*, right auricle; *RV*, right ventricle; *LA*, left auricle; *Ev*, Eustachian valve: *L*, liver; *K*, left kidney; *I*, part of small intestine; *a*, aortic arch; *a'*, its dorsal part; *a''*, posterior end of abdominal aorta; *vcs*, superior vena cava; *vci*, inferior vena cava near its junction with the right auricle; *vci'*, posterior part of inferior cava; *s*, subclavian vessels; *j*, right jugular vein; *c*, common carotid arteries: the four dotted arrow-lines indicate the course of the circulation; *da*, ductus arteriosus· an arrow-line starting at *vci* indicates the course of blood-flow from the inferior cava through the foramen ovale; *hv*, hepatic veins; *vp*, vena portæ; *x* to *vci*, the ductus venosus; *uv*, umbilical vein; *ua*, umbilical arteries; *uc*, umbilical cord; *i, i*, iliac vessels. (Allen Thomson.)

to the **aorta.** The greater part of the stream is then directed through the carotids to the head, a small quantity only continuing along the aorta.

The venous blood returning from the **head** is collected in the **descending vena cava,** and passing thence into the right auricle anteriorly, it finds its way into the **right ventricle.** It is then forced into the **pulmonary artery,** whence it passes by another "short circuit," termed the **ductus arteriosus,** emptying into the aorta just beyond where the carotids branch to the head ; only a sufficient quantity for their nutrition being directed to the *lungs.*

This venous blood then descends along the aorta, the larger quantity passing thence to the iliac arteries, from the internal pair of which two arteries pass directly to the umbilicus, and thence along the cord to the placenta. These arteries within the body are termed the **hypogastric arteries.**

Thus the **lower limbs** of the fœtus receive but a poor supply of what is practically venous blood ; hence their poor development at birth as compared with the head, which receives a rich supply of fairly freshly oxygenated blood. With the expansion of the lungs at birth the whole course of the circulation changes to that which persists throughout life.

CHANGES IN THE MATERNAL ORGANISM RESULTING FROM PREGNANCY.

Uterus.

The **increase in the size** of the uterus takes place chiefly in the body of that organ.

The *cavity* of the body increases in length from $1\frac{1}{2}$ inches (3.7 cm.) in the unimpregnated state, to 12 inches (30.5 cm.) ; the width, from $1\frac{1}{4}$ inches (3.2 cm) to 9 inches (23 cm.) ; the depth (anteroposterior), from nothing to between 8 and 9 inches (20–23 cm.). The capacity is increased from nothing to about 500 cubic inches (8300 c.cm.).

The *weight* of the organ increases from 1 ounce (30 gm.) to about 24 ounces (720 gm.).

These measurements vary with the size of the fœtus, the quantity of liquor amnii, and in multiple pregnancy.

This increase in size is a growth, and not a mere distention, for in ectopic gestation the uterus is found to go on growing, up to and beyond the fourth month.

The **changes in shape** are characteristic. In the non-pregnant condition the uterus is pyriform, the large end being uppermost; and flattened anteroposteriorly.

In the earlier months of pregnancy the lower part seems to increase in capacity faster than the upper, so that the shape of the uterus becomes roughly spherical; while at the fifth month, according to Webster, the organ is once more pyriform in shape, but the widest part is lowermost.

At the end of pregnancy the uterus assumes very much the shape of the non-pregnant organ, the roomiest part being again uppermost.

Thus up to the fifth month the increase in the capacity of the uterus is chiefly in its lower part; and from then till term mainly in its upper portion.

Muscle-fibres : The marked increase in the bulk of the uterine wall during pregnancy is mainly due to *hypertrophy of the muscle-cells.* Helme states that there is no hyperplasia, but that the existing fibres increase from seven to eleven times in length and from three to five times in breadth.

The arrangement of these muscle-fibres will be discussed later under the heading of *anatomy of labor.*

The **connective tissue** of the uterus increases in proportion to the muscular. There exists a true hyperplasia of the connective tissue, which begins in the neighborhood of the blood-vessels.

The **arteries** of the uterus become markedly increased in calibre and length. At the placental site there is a spiral arrangement of the arterial twigs, as they penetrate the uterine decidua and empty into the lacunæ. The **veins** become correspondingly increased in size. In fact, the uterus may be regarded as a huge venous plexus during pregnancy, as the blood-supply is so great. The walls of these veins are reduced to the intima, so that after labor the mere contraction of the uterine muscle-fibres is sufficient to obliterate their lumen.

The **lymphatics** of the uterus become increased both by hypertrophy and hyperplasia. Beneath the decidua enormous lymph-spaces develop, the tubes or vessels leading from these to the lymphatic plexus beneath the peritoneal layer of the uterus reaching the size of goose-quills. This condition of the uterine lymphatic system explains the remarkably rapid absorption of the uterus after labor, as well as that of septic material from the uterine cavity.

The **nerves** of the uterus take part in the general development, the increase being chiefly in the primitive sheath, and not in the nerve-substance.

The **ligaments** of the uterus hypertrophy during pregnancy, and their relationships become altered with the elevation of the fundus in the abdominal cavity.

The **connective tissue** throughout the pelvis becomes succnlent and distensible.

Uterine contractions : Throughout pregnancy the uterus is in a state of alternate contraction and relaxation. This condition favors the circulation of the maternal blood in the uterine wall and placental sinuses. These contractions may be noted as soon as the fundus becomes accessible to examination from the abdominal surface.

Relation to Pelvis and Abdomen.

Up to the third month, while the uterus has increased in size and become quite globular in form, its level in the pelvis has undergone no marked change. It has become somewhat more anteflexed, and from its weight has sunk down somewhat into the pelvis, the cervix being carried backward, so that on making a vaginal examination at this period, the anterior uterine wall can be readily felt and seems to bulge forward.

By the end of the third month the fundus uteri has risen to the brim of the pelvis, and may be felt on moderately deep pressure just above the symphysis pubis.

By the end of the fourth month the fundus is in contact with the anterior abdominal wall.

At the sixth month it reaches the level of the umbilicus.

At the seventh month it is half-way between the umbilicus and the xiphoid cartilage.

At the ninth month it is up to the level of the lower ribs ; but within about *two weeks of labor* it falls forward somewhat, and seems to be on a slightly lower level, on account of the descent of the presenting part of the fœtus into the brim of the pelvis.

The **intestines** are displaced upward by the uterus as it

ascends, so that on percussion a dull note is obtained over the whole central part of the abdomen.

There is a certain amount of **dextro-rotation** of the uterus retained throughout pregnancy, so that the organ leans somewhat to the right as a rule. This right obliquity of the uterus may be accounted for by its relation to the sigmoid flexure and descending colon, the left side of the organ being pushed forward by these structures.

Alterations in the Cervix.

There are two conditions of the cervix during pregnancy which are peculiarly characteristic. Both are due to a partial obstruction in the venous return which leads to softening and a marked blue or violet discoloration.

The **softening of the cervix** begins, as a rule, about the second month. It is first apparent about the tip, but spreads upward as pregnancy advances, so that in the later months the whole cervix becomes so soft that the finger, if unaccustomed to vaginal examination, may have difficulty in finding the os uteri. The cervix in pregnancy has been likened in feel to that of the pouted lips.

The **violet discoloration** is due simply to the venous engorgement, and it may be present even in the first few weeks of pregnancy. The **canal** of the cervix remains throughout pregnancy unaltered in length. Its mucous glands secrete a peculiarly tough mucus, which stops up the canal like a cork throughout pregnancy (mucous plug).

Vagina, Vulva, and Breasts.

The **vagina** and **vulva** become somewhat hypertrophied during pregnancy. The color of the mucous membrane becomes bluish. There is a slightly increased secretion of mucus, and the parts become lax and soft.

Changes in the Breasts.

With the onset of pregnancy there is an **increased determination** of blood to the breasts; and certain alterations preparatory to the function of lactation begin.

These glands attain complete development in the first pregnancy.

The **lobules** enlarge and become distinct from one another.

The **epithelium** lining the acini becomes active, leading to a certain amount of desquamation of the upper layers.

These cells undergo fatty degeneration and are set free, constituting **colostrum-corpuscles.**

Very early in pregnancy a small quantity of **serum** may be expressed from the nipples.

The **fat** and **connective tissue** surrounding the lobules hypertrophy, and the breasts become enlarged and more prominent.

Coincident with these changes there is increased **tenderness** on pressure.

The **skin** becomes stretched and striæ develop, having a radial distribution and direction. The veins on the surface become more obvious.

The **areola** becomes darker from deposit of pigment, this being more marked in brunettes than in blondes (Fig. 23).

FIG. 23.

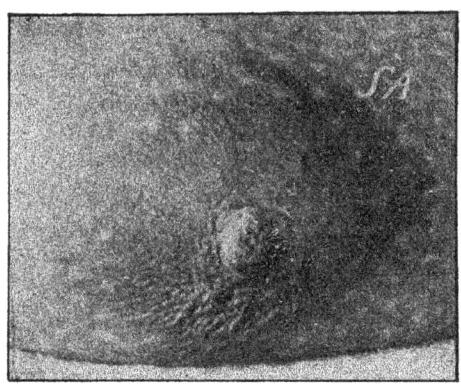

Brunette: Wrinkling of primary areola; *S. A.,* well-defined secondary areola.
(Dickinson.)

The *sebaceous follicles* of the areola, ten or twenty in number, become more prominent, being of lighter color. These follicles at the margin of the areola being uncolored, stand out prominently as white spots, forming the so-called *secondary areola.*

The **nipples** become more prominent as a rule, and are softer than in the non-pregnant state. In the later months of pregnancy dried flakes of secretion may be found encrusted on their surface.

Alterations in Other than the Generative Organs.

Nervous system: There is present during pregnancy a condition of *exalted nerve-tension.* Hence there is an increased tendency to nervous instability. The woman is more prone to hysterical attacks. There are often present perversions of taste, smell, etc.; also neuralgia, especially of the face and teeth. Mental affections are apt to develop during this period.

This condition of increased nerve-tension causes about two-thirds of all pregnant women to suffer from *vomiting* at some time or another of their pregnancy.

This so-called *vomiting of pregnancy* begins, in a large majority of cases, early in the second month; it usually persists during the second and third months, but may last throughout pregnancy. It may be looked upon as one of the symptoms of the pregnant condition.

It usually *occurs* on first rising in the morning, and may be mild or sufficiently severe to endanger the woman's life.

The essential *exciting cause* of the vomiting probably originates in the physiological uterine contractions occurring throughout pregnancy (see *Pernicious Vomiting*).

Circulatory system: The blood undergoes little change in pregnancy. The amount of hæmoglobin and of red corpuscles is slightly increased, and there exists a definite increase in the number of white cells.

The *heart,* from increase in the work it has to do, undergoes some hypertrophy. Both *spleen* and *thyroid gland* increase in size.

Respiratory system: As the range of movement of the diaphragm becomes interfered with by the uterus the thorax widens to a slight extent. Owing to increased oxidation-processes, the work of the lungs is augmented.

Alimentary system: There is but little change in the alimentary system. The digestive processes are somewhat more active, and, as a rule, the appetite is increased. Digestive disturbance is common.

THE LIVER: Recent work on toxæmia of pregnancy has established that during pregnancy the functions of this organ are in a state of unstable equilibrium.

The frequency of symptoms of indigestion associated with pregnancy is probably due to this fact.

Urinary system: The KIDNEYS, during pregnancy, are subjected to increased work, and frequently give clinical evidence of this fact.

The ureters are not infrequently compressed by the enlarging uterus, and the result is an impairment of the renal function.

The urine output is, roughly, about 1500 cc. per diem. The daily output of *urea* during the latter part of pregnancy is reduced, varying between 16 and 24 gm.

The BLADDER in the early months of pregnancy is compressed by the enlarging uterus, giving rise to frequency of micturition.

Cutaneous system: The functions of the skin are increased during pregnancy.

Pigmentation is increased. There is, as a rule, a marked deposit of pigment over the linea alba, so much so as to constitute one of the signs of pregnancy; it may reach from the pubes to the ensiform cartilage. The skin around the eyes is darkened, and frequently irregular spots of pigment appear on the surface of the body, chiefly in the face.

Lineæ albicantes: Certain skin-cracks are to be noticed, chiefly as a result of over-stretching. They are termed *striæ, lineæ albicantes, lineæ maternæ,* or *lineæ gravidarum,* and appear usually on the skin of the abdomen and breasts. They run usually in the lines of tension, and are due to yielding of the corium in stretching, the epidermis being continuous over them without any change in structure. They vary in length up to two or more inches, and when recent are red in color. Later on, as a result of scar-formation, they become white, and form strong presumptive evidence when present of previous pregnancy.

DURATION; DIAGNOSIS; HYGIENE AND MANAGEMENT OF PREGNANCY.

Duration of Pregnancy.

As a rule, it is impossible to predict exactly the date when labor will take place.

If the **date of fruitful coitus** can be fixed, then labor will most likely set in two hundred and seventy-one days later, according to Ahlfeld.

4—Obst.

The **common rule** is that labor will occur on the day of the tenth menstrual period—*i. e.*, two hundred and eighty days after the first day of the last menstruation. Allowance must always be made for the short month February.

As a rule, one seldom predicts the exact day of labor, and the variation of a week or two is far from common.

When pregnancy occurs during a period of amenorrhœa, as lactation; or if the date of the last menstruation cannot be ascertained, then the probable date of labor may be fixed by **noting the height of the fundus.** The *measurement* is made by placing one tip of a pair of calipers on the symphysis pubis and the other on the fundus uteri. The height of the fundus in centimeters, divided by $3\frac{1}{2}$, gives, fairly accurately, the duration of pregnancy in lunar months. At the tenth lunar month the fundus is 35 cm. above the symphysis pubis.

The **date of quickening**—*i. e.*, the first occasion on which the mother feels the movements of the fœtus—is of some value in estimating the duration of pregnancy. Quickening occurs in the twentieth week as a rule in primiparæ; and in the twenty-first or twenty-second week in multiparæ.

Diagnosis of Pregnancy.

The **recognition of pregnancy** is not always an easy matter, especially in the earlier months of gestation.

Careful, systematic, and, if necessary, repeated examination cannot fail to permit a certain diagnosis being made.

Failure in diagnosis is nearly always the result of careless and unsystematic examination.

For **convenience of study** the nine calendar months of pregnancy may be divided into *trimesters;* and a classification of the symptoms and signs as to these three periods be made.

First Trimester—Subjective Symptoms.

The **suppression of menstruation** constitutes, as a rule, the first evidence of pregnancy. This function is usually suspended throughout gestation; but this is not invariable. Some women menstruate at least once, and occasionally several times after the occurrence of pregnancy. The value of this sign as evidence is less in women who are very irregular in menstruating.

Causes : Suppression may result from exposure to cold ; from the presence of debilitating disease, as tuberculosis, anæmia, etc. ; over-anxiety or marked fear of pregnancy may produce this result, as may also sudden mental shock ; change of climate or surroundings occasionally act in the same way. These exceptions should be held in mind ; but suppression of menstruation in a healthy woman of regular habit usually means pregnancy.

Nausea and vomiting, occurring in the morning especially, form one of the most common symptoms of pregnancy.

The sensation usually comes on when the woman first assumes the erect position in the morning, hence the term *" morning sickness "* commonly applied to it.

These symptoms, as a rule, appear in the fourth or fifth week ; but may occur even earlier. They cease, as a rule, about the fourth month ; but may persist throughout pregnancy. The *causation* has already been referred to.

The **mammary changes** begin as early as the second month, the congestion of the parts causing a sensation of fulness, with tingling and tenderness. Increase of pigmentation about the areolæ and the presence of serum in the lacteal ducts become apparent during the third month.

Vesical irritation is often complained of very early in pregnancy. As a result of the increase in the normal anteversion of the uterus, the bladder is pressed upon and its functions interfered with ; this usually persists till the fourth month.

Frequently **digestive disturbances** arise early in pregnancy, having a reflex origin. The appetite becomes capricious, and acidity is common.

Nervous disorders, which are purely functional, are not infrequent. *Ptyalism* is not uncommon, and may persist throughout gestation. *Neuralgias,* cardiac disturbances, mental perturbation and irritability frequently manifest themselves very early and are often very persistent.

First Trimester—Objective Signs.

These are confined chiefly to the *uterus* and the *breasts.*

The **softening of the cervix** uteri begins in the first month of pregnancy. The whole cervix, beginning first at the external os, gradually softens as a result of the physiological uterine congestion. This change is most marked in the primipara, but is also present in the multipara. The cervix becomes plugged with mucus as a result of the increase in the activity of the cervical mucous membrane.

A **violet discoloration** of the mucous membrane of the cervix, vagina, and vulva may be noted on inspection of these parts, beginning as early as the fifth week in many cases. This discoloration, being due to a certain degree of venous stasis, becomes more marked as pregnancy advances; it shades from a pale violet tinge to a dusky bluish hue.

The **softening and enlargement of the body of the uterus** consequent upon pregnancy may be readily made out by careful combined examination. *Hegar's sign* (see below) of early pregnancy depends upon the presence of these changes, and may be obtained as early as the eighth week. As a result of the presence of the ovum in the upper segment of the uterus, all the diameters of the latter become increased, while the empty lower segment simply becomes softened and perhaps rather thinned out.

On **bimanual examination** the bulky, partly softened cervix can be felt; just above this is a very soft compressible area; and

Fig. 24.

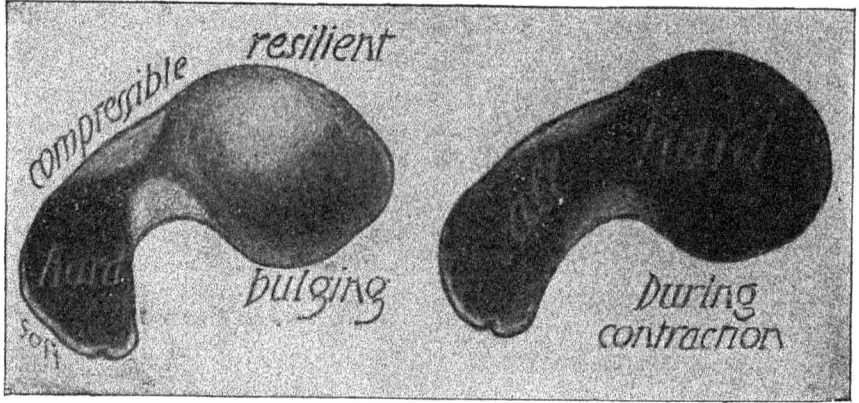

Changes in the pregnant uterus of the sixth week · on the left when relaxed, on the right when contracting. (Dickinson)

above this again the boggy rounded fundus uteri may be distinguished (Fig. 24). The sensation conveyed to the examiner's finger is that the cervix is joined to the body of the uterus by two longitudinal bands (*Hegar's sign*). This is best obtained by placing the thumb of the right hand in the anterior vaginal fornix and introducing the forefinger of the same hand into the rectum, then the left hand placed over the pubis presses the uterus downward so that the cervix and

Fig. 25.

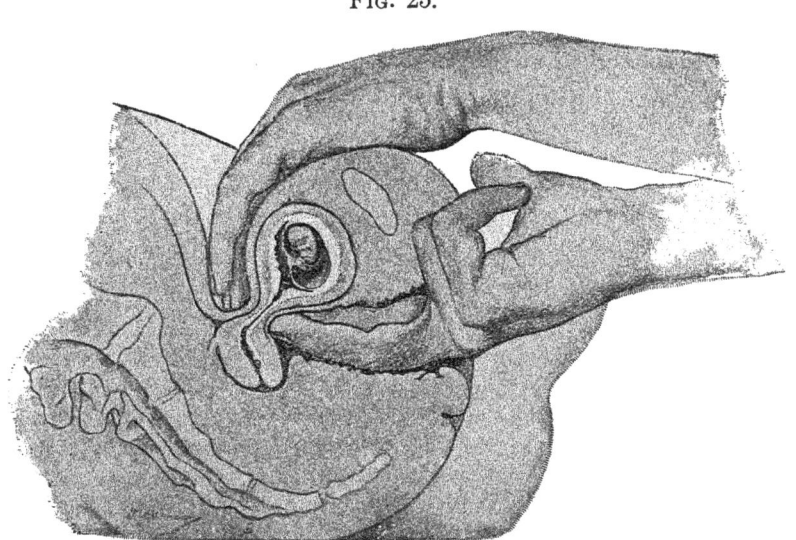

Bimanual examination for compressibility of the isthmus at the sixth week. (Dickinson.)

lower part of the body may be grasped between the thumb and forefinger of the right hand ; or as shown in Fig. 25.

In the *third month* the body of the uterus is felt to be enlarged and rounded as well as softened ; while the whole organ, which pretty well fills the pelvic cavity, is in a position of marked anteversion as a rule.

Second Trimester.

In this period the **subjective symptoms** are : (1) continued absence of menses ; (2) the passing away of the troublesome nausea and vesical irritation ; (3) the sensation of " quickening "—*i. e.*, fœtal movement.

The **objective signs** are: (1) enlargement of the abdomen; (2) progressive changes in the mammæ; (3) progressive changes in the uterus; (4) the *feeling* of *uterine contractions* and of the *foetal movements* by the examiner; (5) *auscultation* of *foetal heart-sounds;* (6) *ballottement.*

In the fourth month the fundus becomes easily accessible from the anterior abdominal wall; hence at this period for the first time may be felt the **irregular intermittent uterine contractions** which continue throughout pregnancy. These contractions take place at intervals of from ten to twenty minutes, and lead to marked hardening of the whole uterine tumor.

Fœtal movements, or **quickening**, are usually first noticed by the mother about the twentieth week. As pregnancy advances these movements become more marked and constant, and may be best obtained by the physician by suddenly placing his cold hand on the mother's abdomen over the uterus.

On *auscultation* a loud *bruit* may be heard over some portion of the uterus as early as the fourth month. This sound has been termed the "**uterine souffle.**" It is synchronous with the maternal pulse, and is very uncertain in its duration and place. It is heard not only during pregnancy, but it is occasionally associated with the presence of interstitial fibroids and with ovarian tumors.

The **fœtal heart-sounds** may be heard as early as the twentieth week by skilled examiners. They are heard best while the patient is in the dorsal position with the abdominal wall relaxed, and with the bell of the stethoscope resting lightly in contact with it. If pressure be made on the bell, or even if it be held in place by the hand, the sounds cannot be heard so well.

The *rate of pulsation* varies from 120 to 150 per minute, being slower in males than in females. The sounds are *double*, the first being somewhat clearer than the second. The sounds of the fœtal heart have been very aptly compared to those of a watch ticking under a pillow. The fœtal heart-sounds bear no relation to, and are quite distinct from, the maternal pulsations.

By the sixth month, the fundus having reached the level of the umbilicus, which has become flattened out, the **abdomen** has become **quite prominent.**

At this time also a **brownish pigmentation** may be noted extending from the pubes up to and beyond the umbilicus.

Ballottement, one of the most valuable signs of pregnancy, becomes available late in the fourth month. It is a passive movement of the fœtus obtained by its sudden displacement from below by the examiner (Fig. 26). While placing the

FIG. 26.

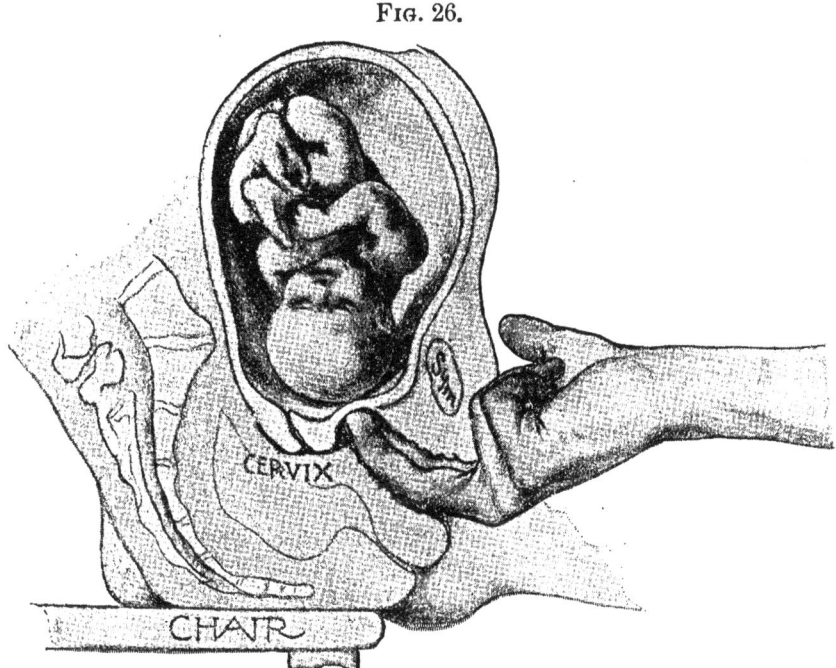

Internal ballottement, semi-recumbent posture, at sixth month. (Dickinson.)

forefinger of the right hand in the anterior vaginal fornix, one may by a brisk impulse displace the fœtus upward, which, as it resumes its original position, conveys a gentle tap to the finger-tip held in the vagina. Ballottement can only be *simulated* by a small cystic ovarian tumor having a long pedicle.

Third Trimester.

The **subjective symptoms** in this period are: (1) continued absence of menstruation; (2) fœtal movements; (3) pressure-symptoms.

The **objective signs** are: (1) continued enlargement of the abdomen; (2) continued mammary and uterine changes; (3) development of striæ on abdomen and breasts.

Owing to the great enlargement of the uterus **pressure-symptoms** become very marked in many cases. *Varices* of the lower limbs and vulva, often accompanied by *œdema*, become more or less marked. *Constipation* from pressure on the rectum, and *vesical irritation* from displacement of the bladder upward, are common.

Disturbances of digestion and of *respiration* are common, both resulting from the great abdominal distention.

The **movements of the fœtus** can be plainly seen through the abdominal wall.

The skin on the abdomen frequently shows linear markings, which appear as **red radiating striæ,** chiefly on the lower quadrants.

The **umbilicus** becomes prominent, and there is an increase in the deposit of pigment in the middle line.

"**Settling**": Within two weeks of labor the presenting part of the fœtus partially enters the brim of the pelvis, becoming more accessible to the examining finger. The cervix also becomes somewhat thinned out and feels shortened. At this time the prominence of the abdomen becomes less marked.

To these changes occurring in the last two weeks preparatory to labor the term "*settling*" has been applied.

The **mammary changes** continue to become more marked, and *colostrum* can be expressed from the nipples.

Summary of Diagnosis.

The **presumptive evidences** *of pregnancy* are: (1) menstrual suppression; (2) morning sickness; (3) irritable bladder; (4) mental and emotional phenomena.

The **probable evidences** are: (1) mammary changes; (2) abdominal changes (*e. g.*, size, shape, markings); (3) uterine changes (size, shape, color, and consistency of cervix); (4) uterine contractions and bruit.

The only **positive** signs are *fœtal:* (1) fœtal heart-sounds; (2) fœtal movements; (3) ballottement.

Differential Diagnosis of Pregnancy.

The physician is not infrequently called upon to make an examination where the patient either feigns, desires, or, more commonly, conceals the condition of pregnancy. The difficulties of diagnosis are much greater before the fourth month of gestation; but careful systematic examination will scarcely fail to establish a certainty in the majority of cases. Care must be taken not to express an opinion until a reasonable certainty of the condition present is obtained.

First Trimester.

In this period the following conditions may resemble pregnancy: amenorrhœa; subinvolution; metritis; uterine fibroid; retained menses; malignant disease; tumors in the neighborhood of the uterus, as ovarian growths; salpingitis; and ectopic gestation.

Simple amenorrhœa accompanied by symptoms of gastric irritation may very closely resemble pregnancy; but a careful bimanual examination will demonstrate the absence of uterine changes.

In **subinvolution** the uterus does not increase in size, and it is not globular; while its texture is harder than that of the organ in pregnancy.

In **metritis** the uterus, while enlarged, is sensitive to the touch, and is hard and dense. Its shape is that of the unimpregnated organ simply increased in size.

An **interstitial fibroid** of the uterus may be distinguished by its denseness and by the irregular contour. Menstruation, instead of being absent, is, as a rule, increased.

Retained menses may cause an enlargement of the uterus; but in such cases the fact that menstruation has never been established, and a history of abdominal pains occurring at monthly intervals, will indicate the nature of the case.

In **malignant disease** of the uterus the menstruation is, as a rule, increased, and intermenstrual hemorrhages occur.

In **ovarian tumors** the uterus is not affected and menstruation persists as a rule. The tumor is usually situated to one side of the uterus and causes some displacement of that organ.

Ectopic gestation may simulate uterine pregnancy ; but careful examination will reveal the presence of a tumor outside the uterus.

In the Later Months of Pregnancy

the following conditions may lead to an error of diagnosis : obesity, ascites, tympanites, phantom tumor, and large ovarian or fibroid tumors.

In **obese women** with irregular menstruation it is not infrequently difficult to establish a diagnosis of pregnancy ; but the absence of mammary changes and auscultatory signs will clear up the case.

In **ascites** a diagnosis may be made by placing the patient in the dorsal decubitus and percussing the abdomen. Both flanks will give a dull note, while the middle area of the abdomen will be clear. Fluctuation may be obtained ; and on changing the position of the patient the area of dulness will alter.

In **tympanites**, the whole abdomen, while enlarged, gives a clear note on percussion. The bimanual examination in both the above conditions will reveal the unimpregnated condition of the uterus.

Phantom tumors, which are occasionally met with in hysterical women, can be recognized on applying the usual tests of auscultation, percussion, etc.

Pseudocyesis, or *spurious pregnancy*, is a very interesting condition met with usually in women about the time of the menopause. The woman imagines herself to be pregnant, and develops many of the characteristic symptoms of that condition. Enlargement of the abdomen, fulness and tenderness of the breasts, may mislead the careless examiner ; but in both the above classes of cases the administration of an anæsthetic, to permit of a thorough examination, will clear up the diagnosis:

Ovarian and **fibroid tumors**, if large, may cause distention of the abdomen ; but in these cases the absence of all signs of a fœtus will suffice to distinguish the conditions from pregnancy.

Diagnosis of Parity or Nulliparity.

Certain mechanical effects are produced on the abdominal wall and birth-canal of a woman who has previously borne a full-term child, which time fails quite to eradicate. On these depends the diagnosis of parity or nulliparity.

If the ovum has been discharged before it was sufficiently large to produce these changes, then it is practically impossible to be certain as to parity.

These signs consist of changes in the breasts, perineum, vagina, and cervix, as well as laxity and striæ of the abdominal wall.

In the **parous woman** the *breasts* are apt to be well developed and somewhat pendulous, the nipples being large and prominent. Occasionally striæ may be noticed.

The *abdominal wall* is lax and yielding, the skin being marked with white striæ.

The *perineum* may show marks of laceration and be somewhat lax; the fourchette being absent.

The *vagina* is capacious and lax, the walls being somewhat smooth. The remains of the hymen may be noticed as forming numerous small caruncles (carunculæ myrtiformes).

The *cervix* is short and broad; very often it is lacerated, generally on the left side.

Diagnosis of Life or Death of Child.

It is not always easy to decide that the child is dead. The woman may suspect this to be the case because of certain vague sensations of coldness about the pubes, and because of a feeling of weight or dragging. She may cease to feel the movements of the fœtus.

The matter can only be settled if after repeated examination the physician fails to hear the fœtal heart or feel fœtal movements. If at the same time the uterus ceases to grow, and the breasts become flabby, it may be inferred that the child has perished.

Hygiene and Management of Pregnancy.

While the condition of the pregnant woman is a purely physiological one, it must be borne in mind that the borderline between health and disease may be very easily passed. Hence it is the duty of the physician to give every woman engaging his services for her confinement such hygienic instruction as she may require. In fact, a certain degree of professional attention should be given to all women throughout the whole period of pregnancy.

Diet: The diet during pregnancy should be plain. Simple, easily digestible, and highly nutritious food should be taken at regular intervals. Overeating, especially in the later months, should be guarded against. Meat should be eaten but once daily, and fruit, both cooked and fresh, should form a principal part of all meals.

Exercise: All violent exercise should be avoided. Walks in the open air and simple gymnastics within doors should be indulged in daily. All lifting and straining should be avoided. Motoring may be permitted in moderation, but not over rough roads. The same applies also to carriage-driving.

Clothing should be worn in such a manner as to avoid undue pressure upon either chest or abdomen. The corset, if worn at all, should be a short one and should be very loose. Women with lax abdominal walls should wear an abdominal support so arranged that the pressure is exerted upward.

Bathing should be indulged in daily, especially since the function of the skin is increased during pregnancy. If the woman is in the habit of taking cold baths daily, they may be continued, but the initial shock may be avoided by having the bath warm at first, and then adding cold water to it. In the later months at least two warm baths per week should be taken. Very hot and very cold baths should be avoided.

The care of the breasts: Attention should be given the breasts preparatory to nursing. As these organs enlarge, the clothing must be arranged so as to avoid undue pressure upon them. The nipples, if retracted, should be drawn out and gently manipulated for a few minutes daily. In the last few weeks daily inunctions of the nipples with fresh cocoa-butter or white vaseline may be recommended as a prophylactic against fissures during nursing. The use of astringent lotions, such as tea, brandy, etc., commonly employed, should be proscribed.

Should **vaginal discharge** be present, daily injections of boric-acid solution at the temperature of the body may be employed, the fountain-syringe only being used.

Sexual intercourse must be restricted, and should not be indulged in at the menstrual dates, especially by women who have previously aborted.

Digestive irregularities should. be controlled. The regular action of the bowel must be maintained. Woman seems to be a naturally constipated organism, and is especially so during pregnancy. All violent purgatives should be avoided; the best laxatives are aloin and cascara sagrada. The mineral waters prove very useful, such as salines, etc.

The **urinary excretion** requires careful attention throughout pregnancy. Chemical and microscopical examination of the urine should be made every month at first; and in the later months every week. The total amount voided in the twenty-four hours should be noted.

The **nervous condition** of the pregnant woman should always be noted. All undue excitement should be avoided, and any depression of spirits combated. Plenty of sleep—at least eight hours each night—should be obtained. Daily naps should be encouraged.

The **use of drugs** should be avoided as much as possible during pregnancy. Large doses of quinine and calomel should not be administered. The all too common habit of taking drugs of the coal-tar series by women, to relieve headache, etc., should be especially discouraged during pregnancy, on account of their deleterious action on the heart. Many of the cases of severe cardiac failure following labor may be set down to this pernicious habit.

The physician should make a careful **general examination** of every pregnant woman under his care about the eighth month of the pregnancy. A careful external and, if thought necessary, an internal examination should be made. The pelvis should be measured and the attitude of the fœtus noted. The breasts and nipples should also be examined. Inquiry should also be made as regards the presence or absence of vaginal discharge. If present, its character should be noted and a bacteriological examination made.

OBSTETRIC ANATOMY.

For *detailed anatomy* of the female pelvic structures the student is referred to special works; or to obstetric systems, such as Jewett's " Practice of Obstetrics."

The **chief anatomical elements** concerned in labor are three in number, namely: (1) the uterus; (2) the pelvi-genital canal ; (3) the fœtus.

In the **act of parturition** the mutual reaction of these elements is concerned.

The *uterus* may be conceived of as a muscular sac opening into a curved tube, the upper part of which is bony, therefore rigid ; and the lower part yielding, being formed of muscle and other soft structures. This *curved tube* is the pelvi-genital canal, which includes the distensible vagina, the upper part being intrapelvic, while the lower, in the pelvic floor, is subpelvic.

The *fœtus* is the passenger, and consists of two ovoids, the trunk and the head ; the former plastic, the latter more or less rigid, and therefore the more important as regards its relations to the birth-canal.

The Uterus.

At term the uterus is an ovate viscus ; it is less part of the birth-canal than it is the engine by which the passenger—the fœtus—is expelled.

The **cavity** of the uterus at term has been stated as measuring 12 inches in length, 9 inches in breadth, and 8 inches in depth.

The **walls** of the uterus vary in thickness from one-fourth to one-fifth of an inch ; the posterior being thicker than the anterior.

The **muscle-fibres** of the uterus may be distinguished at term as forming roughly three layers : an outer, a middle, and an inner layer :

In the **outer layer** there are two sets of fibres : (1) longitudinal and (2) transverse (Fig. 27).

The *longitudinal fibres,* posteriorly from the junction of the body with the cervix, pass in the form of a broad band vertically upward over the fundus and down the middle line anteriorly to the cervix ; the marginal fibres toward the fundus branching off to interlace with those of the round and broad ligaments.

The *transverse fibres* arranged at right angles to these pass across the uterus from side to side ; at the fundus passing from one cornu to the other. These fibres interlace in great part at the sides of the uterus, but some of them are prolonged along the broad and the round ligaments as well as along the tubes.

Fig. 27.

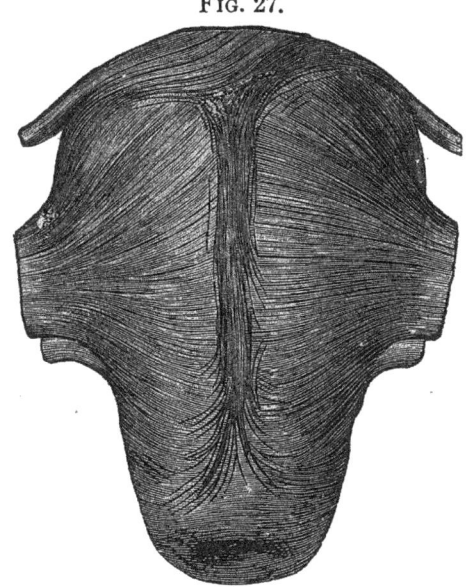

External muscular layer of the posterior wall of the uterus.

In the **middle layer** the fibres have no definite direction on account of the numerous bloodvessels traversing them. They

Fig. 28.

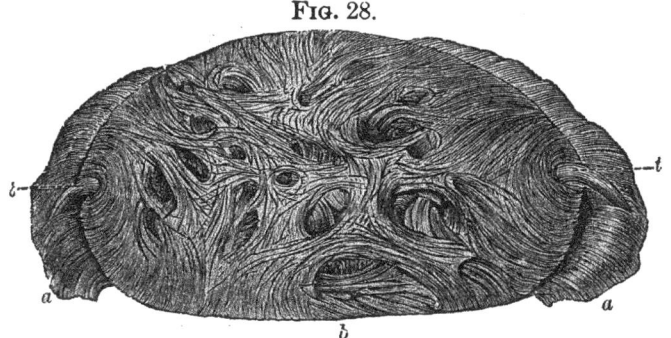

Middle muscular layer at the fundus : *a, a,* superficial layer dissected back ; *b,* branches belonging to the inner layer ; *t, t,* tubes.

pass in every direction—longitudinal, transverse, and oblique— twisting and curving about the vessels. Frequently they are arranged in the form of a figure-of-eight, forming rings about the vessels, thus constituting living ligatures (Fig. 28). This layer is probably the thickest, and is most marked in the upper segment of the uterus.

In the **inner layer** some fibres are arranged in a series of concentric rings about the orifices of the tubes (Fig. 29). Other fibres pass directly across from one cornu to the other transversely; while others pass downward longitudinally to the cervix, in the middle line of the anterior and posterior walls.

FIG. 29.

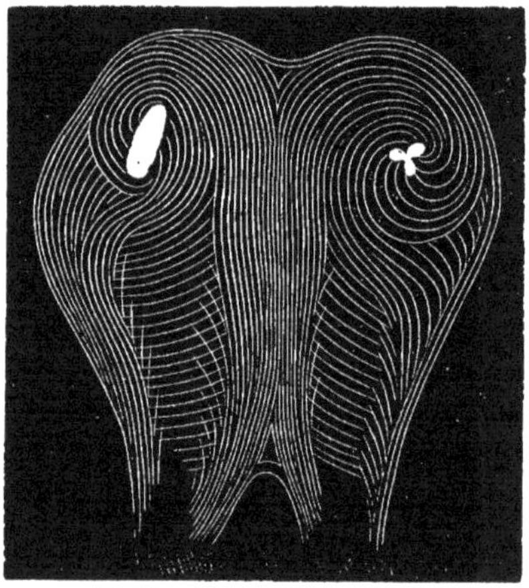

Internal surface of the uterus as shown after incision in t e median line of the anterior wall. (Parvin.)

These layers are not all distinct, but shade imperceptibly into one another. In the *upper* part of the uterus the arrangement of layers is fairly distinct; but in the *lower* part the fibres are more loosely arranged, passing chiefly in a longitudinal direction.

Uterine segments: Hence the uterus may be divided into two portions, the upper of which has a firmer muscular arrangement than the lower.

These portions are termed respectively the *upper* and the *lower uterine segments.*

The line of separation between the segments lies nearly at the level of the uterovesical fold of the peritoneum, and is termed the *retraction-ring,* or *Bandl's ring.*

The upper segment plays an active *rôle* in labor, while the lower has but a passive *rôle.* The lower segment along with the cervix must undergo dilatation preparatory to the expulsion of the fœtus.

The upper segment includes roughly the upper two-thirds of the entire body of the uterus; while the lower segment and the cervix, which are nearly of equal lengths, form the remaining one-third.

The **round** and the **broad ligaments,** which have become hypertrophied during pregnancy, serve as guys to steady the uterus during its contractions, so that its long axis corresponds to that of the pelvic inlet.

The **peritoneum** covering the uterus is firmly attached to this organ as far down as the retraction-ring; below this its attachment is loose and it may easily be stripped off. Thus the site of the retraction-ring, or Bandl's ring, is at the lower border of firm peritoneal attachment.

The peritoneum at term has in front of and behind the uterus the same relations as in the non-pregnant condition; but at the *sides* it has been so lifted up by the enlarged uterus that it does not descend into the pelvis. The broad ligaments have become so elevated that their bases are only at the pelvic brim, extending on either side from the iliopectineal eminence to the sacro-iliac joint. Thus there exists on either side of the uterus at term a large triangular area uncovered by peritoneum. Owing to the drawing up of the uterosacral ligaments the *pouch of Douglas* becomes much deeper than in the non-pregnant condition.

The Relation of the Full-term Uterus to Contiguous Structures.

The **intestines** do not descend behind the uterus at all, and in front only as low as the umbilicus. A portion of the rectum lies behind the uterus, and occasionally a loop of the sigmoid flexure of the colon.

The **urinary bladder** lies wholly within the pelvis before the onset of labor, its highest point being below the symphysis pubis, except when distended.

The **cellular tissue** about the uterus exists as a thin layer behind; but in front there is a broad band between the cervix and the bladder. At the sides of the uterus it is enormously increased as compared with the non-pregnant condition. At the bases of the broad ligaments (defined above) there exists only cellular tissue (no peritoneum) between the uterus and the pelvic wall; this deposit extends upward and backward between the layers of the broad ligament into the iliac fossæ.

The **ureters** enter the pelvis just in front of each sacro-iliac joint and pass downward, forward, and inward to the neck of the bladder in such a way that they are not in the least liable to pressure between the uterus and the bony pelvis.

5—Obst.

The shape and position of the uterus as well as the direction of the axis of its cavity change as the organ passes from its relaxed state to one of active contraction. These will therefore be discussed later.

The Pelvi-genital Canal.

Bony Pelvis.

Definition: The pelvis is the bony basin, or canal, which forms the most important part of the birth-canal (Fig. 30).

FIG. 30.

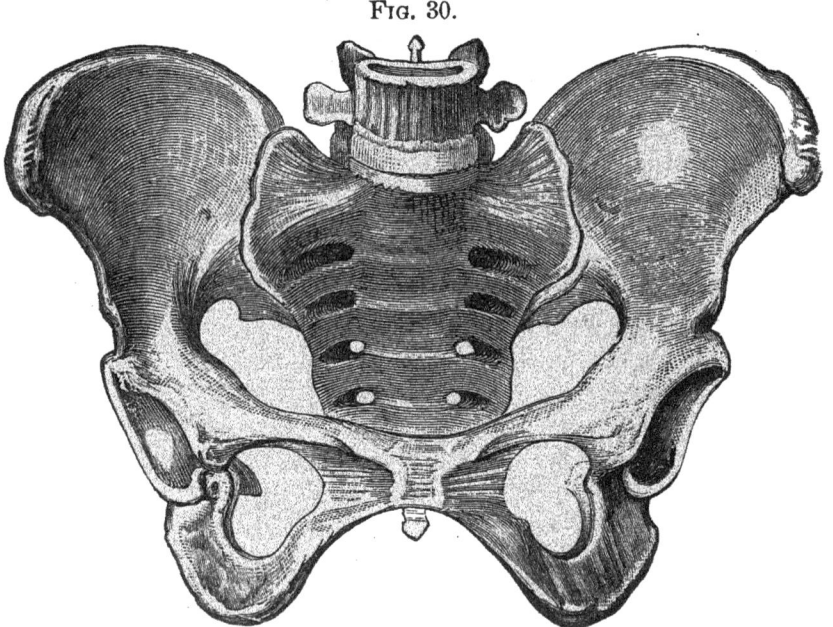

The female pelvis. (Jewett.)

The term is derived from the Latin *pelvis,* a bowl. The pelvic canal is irregularly funnel-shaped, flattened from before backward, the larger end looking upward and forward, the smaller downward and backward, when the woman is in the erect position. It contains in the non-pregnant state the essential organs of generation, and in labor the child is expelled through it.

An intimate knowledge of the pelvis as related to ·the mechanism of labor is essential to complete understanding of the problems of the art of obstetrics.

General description: The pelvis is composed of the sacrum, the coccyx, and the two ossa innominata. Each of these bones is made up of separate parts which become united by the twentieth year of life. The *articulations* of the pelvis, which are of considerable obstetrical importance, are the sacro-iliac joints, the sacrococcygeal joint, and the symphysis pubis.

The sacro-iliac joints: The opposed surfaces of each bone forming these joints are covered with thin plates of cartilage. These become separated by spaces containing a small quantity of glairy fluid, but no synovial membrane can be demonstrated. Each of these joints has anterior and posterior ligaments and intercartilaginous bands; of these, the posterior are by far the most important. Each of these posterior ligaments is formed of three fasciculi; the two superior run nearly horizontally from bone to bone; while the inferior passes obliquely downward and inward from the posterior superior spine of the ilium to the third and fourth sacral vertebræ.

The **sacrococcygeal joint** has an interosseous fibrocartilage which permits recession of the coccyx. Its ligaments are of no importance.

The symphysis pubis: The slightly convex surface of each pubic bone is covered with a thin plate of cartilage sufficient only to fill out any irregularities in the bones forming the joint. The opposed surfaces are held together by an intervening mass of fibrocartilage, which constitutes the *interpubic disk.* A small cavity is frequently present in the centre of this disk, the result of absorption of the fibrocartilage; it is non-synovial in character.

The *ligaments* of this joint are four in number—anterior, posterior, superior, and inferior; of these, the most powerful is the inferior, often termed the *ligamentum arcuatum.* It is a strong fibrous bundle passing across from one descending pubic ramus to the other, blending at the median line with the interpubic disk.

Besides the ligaments which are associated with the pelvic joints, we have the **sacrosciatic ligaments**, which play a very important part in the mechanism of labor.

The **greater sacrosciatic ligament** arises from the posterior inferior spine of the ilium and from the side of the sacrum and coccyx. It narrows and thickens in its middle part, becoming broad again at its anterior attachment to the inner surface of the ischial tuberosity.

The **lesser sacrosciatic ligament** takes its origin from the side of the sacrum and coccyx, and, passing in front of the greater, is inserted into the spine of the ischium.

Mobility of the pelvic joints: Toward the end of gestation there obtains a certain degree of swelling or œdema of all the interarticular structures of the pelvic articulations, which permits of some slight expansion of the pelvis during labor, under the wedge-like advance of the fœtal head. The sacrum permits of a slight rotation on its transverse axis. There is also a hinge-like motion of the coccyx on the sacrum which permits an enlargement of the anteroposterior diameter of the pelvic outlet.

The pelvis presents two **divisions**, the *false* and the *true* pelvis, the dividing-line being at the plane of the brim—*i. e.*, the plane cutting the upper end of the sacrum, the top of the symphysis pubis, and the iliopectineal line on either side.

The **false pelvis** has but little obstetric interest; it simply forms with the vertebral column and the abdominal walls a funnel-shaped approach to the true pelvis, and is included in the abdominal cavity.

The **true pelvis** constitutes that portion of the pelvis lying below the iliopectineal lines. It is a deep basin-shaped cavity, the *posterior wall*, formed by the sacrum and coccyx, being sharply curved with an anterior concavity. The *anterior wall* is formed by the symphysis pubis and is short and straight. The *lateral walls*, which are formed by the lower portions of the ilia, the rami and tuberosities of the ischia, the sacro-iliac ligaments, and parts of the descending rami of the pubes, are irregular in outline, sloping inward, so that the transverse diameter of the pelvis is less at their lower than at their upper extremities.

The true pelvis may be divided into **three portions**: 1, the inlet, or superior strait; 2, the outlet, or inferior strait; 3, the excavation, or cavity.

(1) The **inlet**, or superior strait, of the pelvis, sometimes termed the *brim*, is usually described as being heart-shaped, though in

the fresh state it is more nearly circular. Its boundaries are defined by the top of the sacrum behind, the iliopectineal lines on either side and the top of the symphysis pubis in front.

(2) The **outlet, or inferior strait** (Fig. 31), is bounded by the subpubic ligament, the descending rami of the pubes, the rami, tuberosities, and spines of the ischia, the sacrosciatic ligaments, and the coccyx. Its outline is roughly triangular in shape, but when distended by the advancing head in labor, it becomes ovate, owing to the distensibility of the sacrosciatic ligaments and the yielding character of the coccyx and sacro-iliac joints.

Fig. 31.

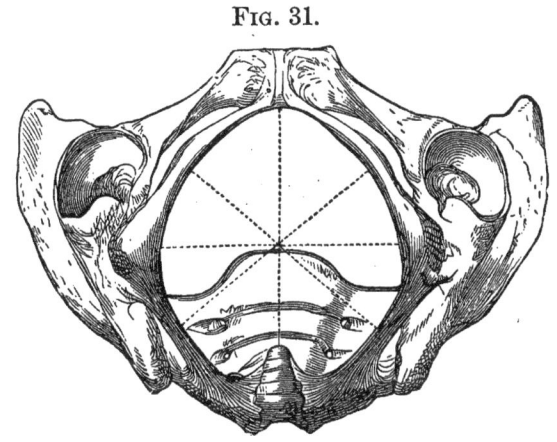

Outlet of pelvis. (Leischman.)

(3) The **excavation, or cavity of the pelvis,** is bounded by the superior and inferior straits, and comprises all that portion of the pelvis between them.

Posteriorly, the cavity is bounded by the sacrum and coccyx ; *anteriorly,* by the pubic bones and their rami ; *laterally,* by the lower portions of the ilia, the bodies, tuberosities, spines, and rami of the ischia, and by the sacrosciatic ligaments.

The *posterior wall* is concave from above downward ; its depth, following the sacral curve, is 11.5 to 12.5 cm. (4½ to 5 inches).

The *anterior wall* is concave from side to side ; its depth at the symphysis is 4 cm. (1⅝ inches).

The *lateral wall* is about 9 cm. (3½ inches) in depth.

For description each must be divided into three portions, which may be mapped out in Fig. 32.

The *first portion* is triangular in shape, its base being a line drawn from the iliopectineal eminence to the top of the sacro-iliac joint, its lateral boundaries meeting at the iliac spines. This portion is bony throughout, and is smooth and curved.

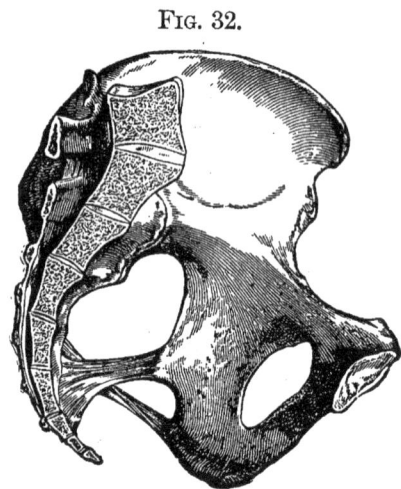

FIG. 32.

Side view of pelvis.

The *second portion* lies forward and somewhat below the first, and has but little bone in its composition, being chiefly made up of the membranous tissues of the foramen ovale covered by the obturator muscle.

The *third portion* is made up mainly of the pyriformis muscle and the elastic sacrosciatic ligaments; its borders are bony, being composed posteriorly of the lateral borders of the sacrum and coccyx, and anteriorly by the posterior edge of the ilium. During descent of the head these ligaments and muscles are put on the stretch, and this portion is thus converted into a long, spiral groove, which deepens as it descends and turns forward.

Obstetric planes of the pelvis : The pelvic canal varies in size and shape at different parts of its course ; these variations are best understood by means of a series of transverse planes through the pelvic cavity at different levels. Three of these are of special importance obstetrically : the plane of the brim, the plane of the outlet, and middle plane of the cavity.

Plane of the brim : The anatomical brim of the pelvis is at the level of the true pelvis, while the *obstetrical plane of the brim* is situated at the level of least expansion of the upper part of the pelvic canal. This lies at the level of the summit of the sacral promontory, the iliopectineal line, and *the posterior surface* of the symphysis pubis, at a point 1 cm. ($\frac{2}{5}$ of an inch) *below* its upper margin (Fig. 33).

Plane of the outlet : At the outlet also the anatomical and obstetrical planes differ. The obstetrical plane of the outlet

Fig. 33.

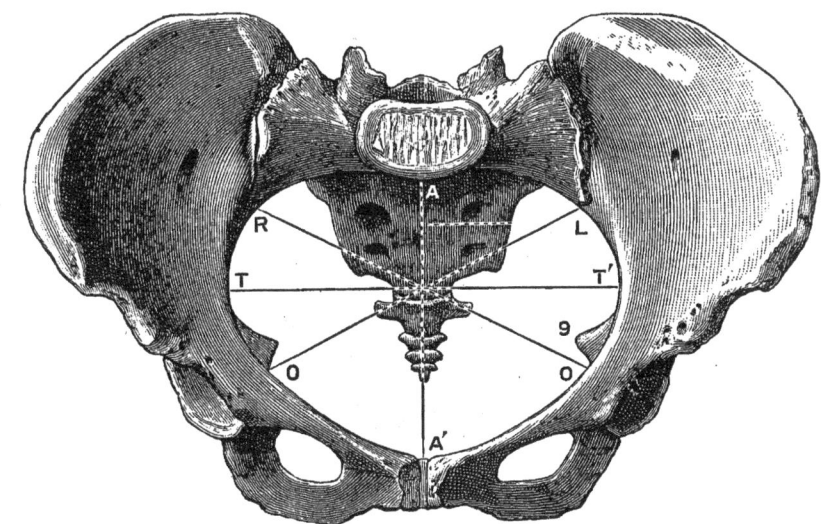

Obstetric diameters of the pelvic brim: A A', conjugate diameter; T T', transverse
diameter; L O, left oblique diameter; R O, right oblique diameter.   (Jewett.)

Fig. 34.

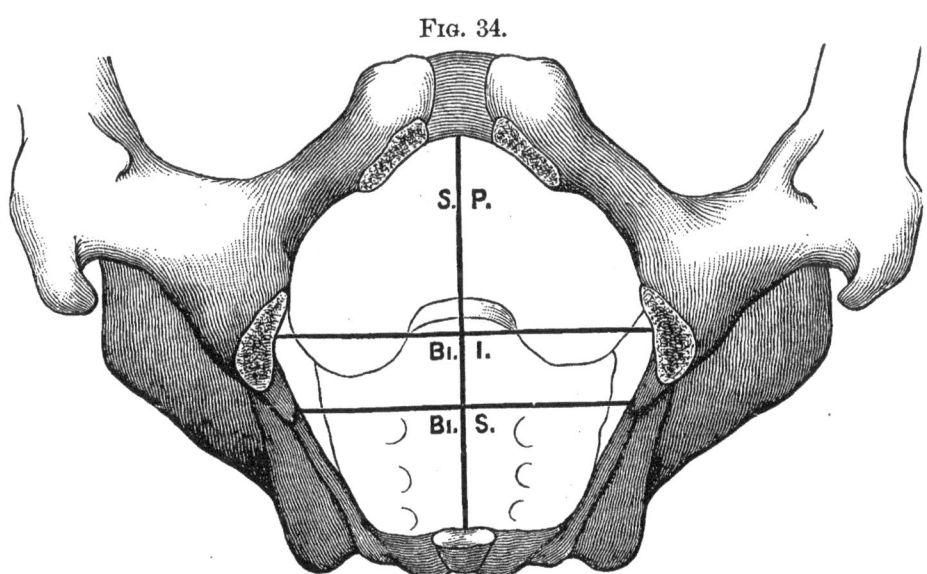

Obstetric diameters of the pelvic outlet: S. P., sacropubic diameter; Bi. I., bisischial diameter; Bi. S., bisischiatic diameter.   (Jewett.)

is defined by the tip of the sacrum, the lower border of the ischial spines, and the lower border of the symphysis pubis at a point just above the lower margin (Fig. 34).

Plane of the cavity : The middle plane of the pelvic cavity lies at the level of the upper end of the third piece of the sacrum, the middle of the symphysis pubis, and the centre of the acetabular cavities (Fig. 35).

Internal pelvic diameters : The dimensions of *each plane* are measured in four directions : the anteroposterior, the transverse, and the two oblique.

At the plane of the brim : The *anteroposterior diameter* of the brim is the least distance between the sacral promontory and the symphysis pubis. It is measured from the middle of the sacral promontory to the posterior surface of the symphysis, at a point 1 cm. ($\frac{2}{5}$ inch) below its upper margin. It is termed the *conjugate,* or *true conjugate,* and measures 11 cm. ($4\frac{3}{8}$ inches) (Fig. 33).

The *transverse diameter* (Fig. 37) is the greatest distance between the iliopectineal lines, and measures 13.5 cm. ($5\frac{1}{4}$ inches).

The *oblique diameters* (Fig. 37) are measured one from the right and the other from the left sacro-iliac joint where it intersects the iliopectineal line, to the opposite iliopectineal eminence. The right oblique springs from the right, and the left oblique from the left, sacro-iliac joint. They each measure about 12.5 cm. (5 inches).

At the plane of the cavity : The *anteroposterior diameter* is the distance from the upper margin of the third piece of the sacrum to a point midway on the posterior surface of the symphysis (Fig. 36), and is 12.5 cm. (5 inches).

The *transverse diameter* is the greatest diameter of the pelvis at this plane, and measures 12 cm. ($4\frac{3}{4}$ inches).

The *oblique diameters* of this plane are valueless from an obstetrical point of view.

At the plane of the outlet : The *anteroposterior diameter* is a line drawn from the tip of the sacrum to a point just above the lower border of the symphysis pubis (Figs. 34 and 35). It measures 11 cm. ($4\frac{1}{2}$ inches).

The *transverse diameter* at this plane may be measured in two places (Fig. 34). The greatest transverse diameter is the bisischial line, which is measured from a point on the inner surface of one ischial tuberosity at the middle of its posterior border, to the same point on the opposite side. This measures 11.5 cm. ($4\frac{1}{2}$ inches).

FIG. 35.

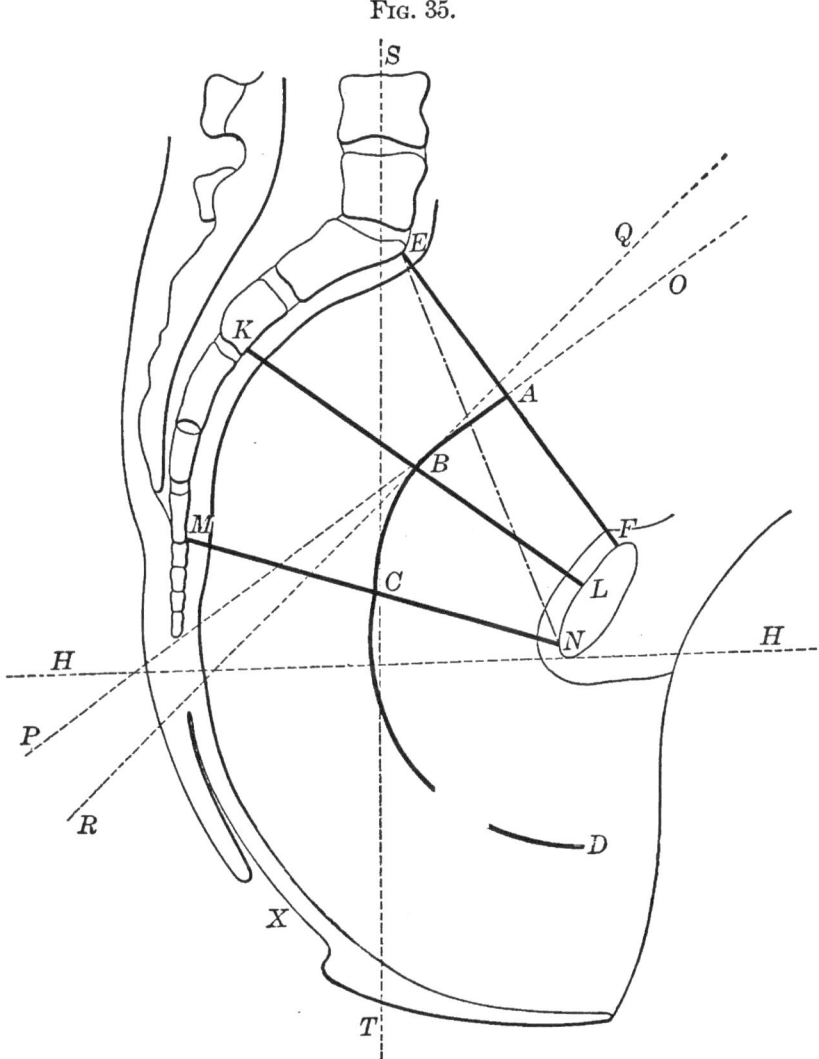

Diagram showing axes and planes of pelvis : *A B C D*, axis of entire parturient canal ; *X*, anus as distended at acme of expulsion ; *E F*, plane of brim ; *K L*, mid-plane of cavity ; *M N*, plane of outlet ; *O P*, axis of brim ; *Q R*, axis of mid-plane : *S T*, axis of outlet ; *H H*, horizon ; *E N*, diagonal conjugate diameter.

The least transverse diameter is the distance between the ischial spines, the bisischiatic diameter, which measures 10.5 cm. ($4\frac{1}{8}$ inches).

Fig. 36.

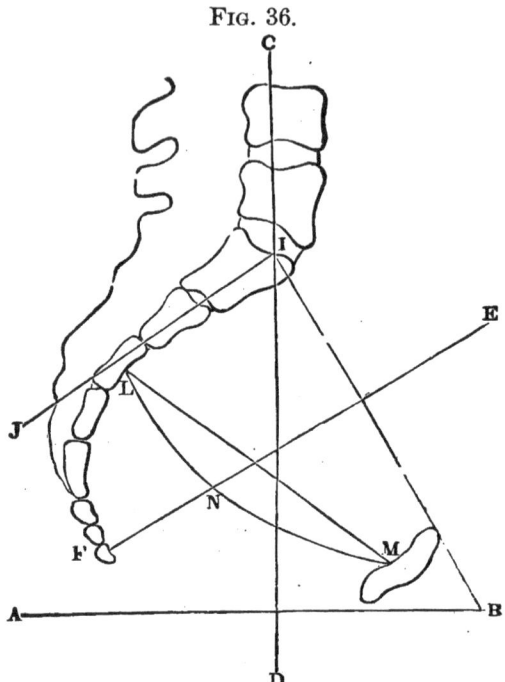

Planes of the pelvis with horizon: A B, horizon; C D, vertical line; A B I, angle of inclination of pelvis to horizon, equal to 60°; B I C, angle of inclination of pelvis to spinal column, equal to 150°; C I J, angle of inclination of sacrum to spinal column, equal to 130°; E F, axis of pelvic inlet; L M, mid-plane in the middle line; N, lowest point of mid-plane of ischium. (Playfair.)

Fig. 37.

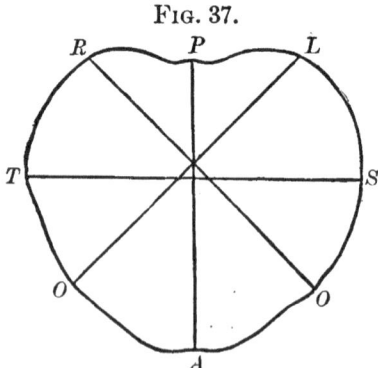

The inlet, or superior strait.

A P, anteroposterior diameter,   4 3 to 4 5 inches, or 11–11½ centimetres.
T S, transverse,   5.3   "   ,or   13½   "
R O, right oblique,   4.7 to 4 9   "   or 12–12½   "
L O, left oblique,   4 7 to 4 9   "   or 12–12½   "
The circumference of the inlet is 15 8 inches, or 40 centimetres.

The *oblique diameters* at this plane are of no importance.

It will be **noted** by comparing the dimensions at the different planes, that the transverse diameter of the pelvic canal grows progressively smaller from the brim to the outlet; the difference between these being 2.5 cm. (1 inch); and also that the anteroposterior diameter of the pelvic canal is 0.5 longer at the outlet than at the brim.

Measurements: The *internal diameters* of the bony pelvis as stated in the following table are sufficiently accurate for all practical purposes, and should be memorized:

	Anteroposterior.	Oblique.	Transverse.
Brim,	10 cm. (4 inches).	11.5 cm. (4½ inches).	12.5 cm. (5 inches).
Cavity,	11.5 " (4½ ")	11.5 " (4½ ")	11.5 " (4½ ")
Outlet,	12.5 " (5 ")	11.5 " (4½ ")	10.0 " (4 ")

Inclination of the pelvis: The inclination (Fig. 36) of the plane of the pelvic brim to the horizon, with the woman in the erect position, may be stated as fifty-five degrees. The inclination of the pelvis, of course, differs with changes of posture. In the erect position the symphysis pubis is nearly 9 cm. (3½ inches) below the level of the promontory; and the coccyx is 2 cm. (¾ inch) above the level of the lower border of the symphysis pubis, the pubococcygeal line making an angle of ten degrees with the horizon.

The Soft Parts of the Pelvic Canal.

The lower segment of the uterus and the cervix form a part of the birth-canal; while the upper segment is the chief source of the propelling power. This portion of the soft parts has already been described.

The *soft parts which line the bony pelvis* and those which contribute to the formation of the *pelvic floor* are of great obstetric importance. The former diminish somewhat the diameters of the bony cavity; the latter form the lower portion of the birth-canal.

The **psoas** and **iliacus muscles**, which lie at the brim, diminish the transverse diameter of this portion of the pelvis a quarter of an inch on either side, thus bringing this diameter down to about the size of the oblique diameter.

The external iliac vessels run along the inner borders of

these muscles, and the main trunk of the lumbar plexus follows the course of the psoas, the crural nerve running between the psoas and iliacus muscles.

The **obturator internus,** which is but a thin muscle-sheet, covers portions of the anterior and lateral walls and a part of the small sciatic notch.

The **pyriformis,** which is a thin fan-shaped muscle, lies a little over the edge of the sacrum and completely fills the great sciatic notch.

The anterior wall of the pelvis is not covered by muscle, but during pregnancy the **bladder** lies in relation with it. During labor the greater part of this viscus is drawn up above the inlet; but its base may, in tedious labors, be subjected to prolonged pressure between the head and the pubes, thus damaging it to such an extent that sloughing may occur and vesicovaginal fistula result.

The **rectum** lies in front of the left sacro-iliac joint. It runs forward and inward, descending in the median line down the anterior surface of the sacrum and coccyx. When distended it may encroach on the pelvic space to a very considerable extent. Its presence in this portion of the pelvis is supposed to account for the greater frequency with which the long diameter of the fœtal head occupies the right oblique diameter at the onset of labor.

The **pelvic floor** comprises the soft structures which close the outlet of the bony pelvis. Its function is to support the pelvic viscera. Its upper limit is the peritoneum, its lower, the skin; it is perforated by the rectum, vagina, and urethra.

Hart has divided the pelvic floor into **two segments,** as follows: the posterior vaginal wall and the soft structures behind it constitute the *sacral segment;* the anterior vaginal wall and the soft structures in front of it compose the *pubic segment.*

In labor the pubic segment is drawn upward and the sacral segment is pushed downward and distended as the fœtus descends. The resiliency of the sacral segment holds the fœtal mass in close relation with the ischiopubic rami during the latter part of labor, and assists in its final expulsion.

The pelvic floor when stretched by the fœtus **measures,** from the tip of the sacrum to the anterior border of the pubic segment, about 5 inches (12.75 cm.). It is mainly composed of muscles and fasciæ.

The muscles forming the pelvic floor are the levator ani, the sphincter ani, the transverse muscles of the perineum, and the sphincter vaginæ.

Fig. 38.

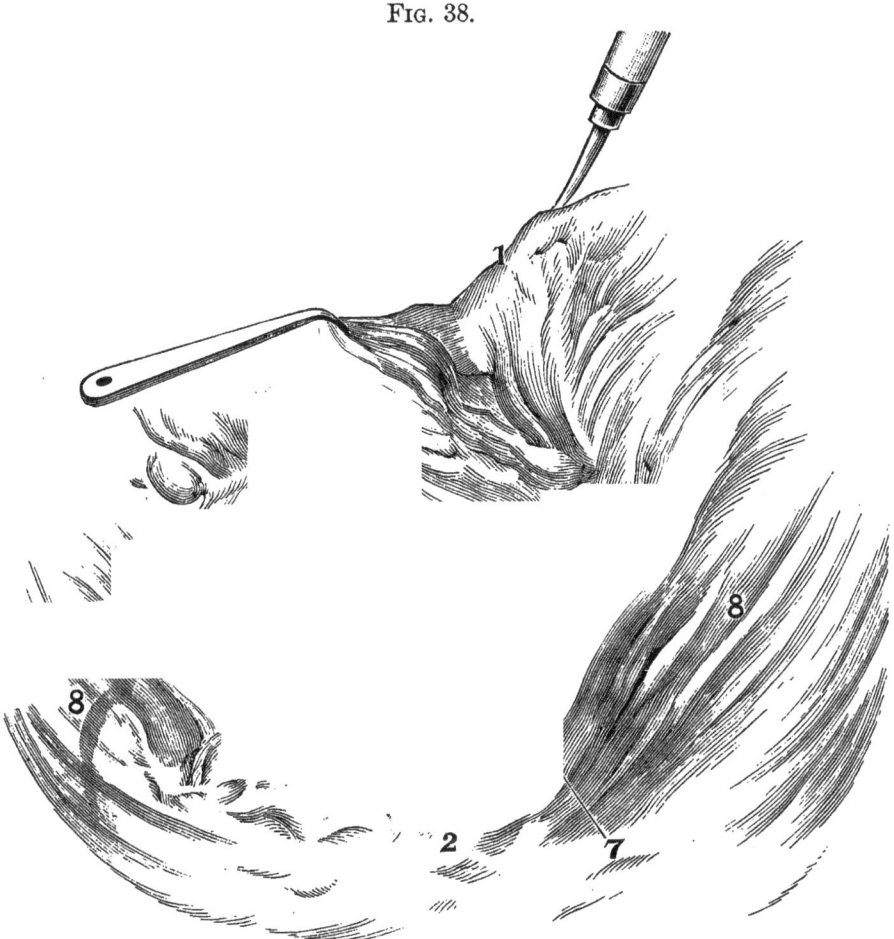

Drawing from a photograph of a dissection made at the Long Island College Hospital: 1, symphysis; 2, coccyx; 3, anus; 4, superficial fibres from the pubic origin of the levator ani; 5, deeper fibres from the pubic origin; 6, fibres from the "white line"; 7, fibres from the spine of the ischium; 8, gluteus maximus muscle. (Browning.)

The levator ani muscle, which is the most important, takes its origin from the posterior layer of the triangular ligament, from the spine of the ischium, and from the whole length of the "white line" (Fig. 38).

Those fibres which arise from the pubes pass backward to be inserted into the last two pieces of the coccyx, and on their way send fibres to the urethra, vagina, and the internal sphincter ani, and a few to unite with those of the opposite side behind the anus. That part arising from the " white

FIG. 39.

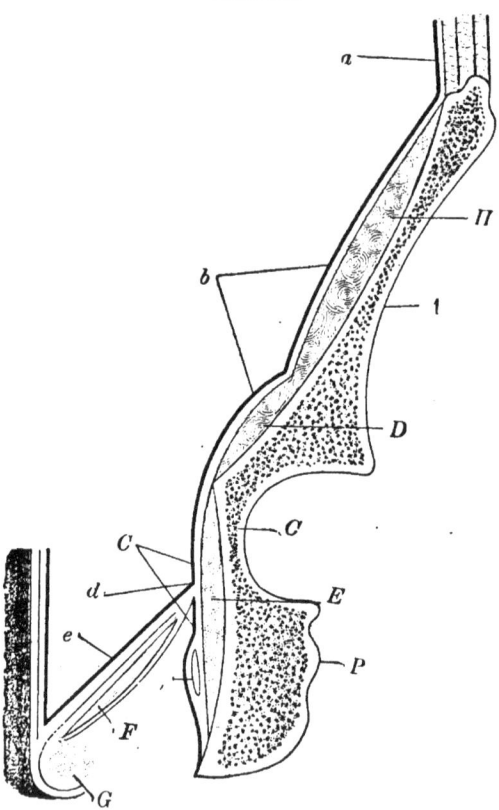

Coronal section of the pelvis: *A*, ilium; *P*, ischium; *C*, acetabulum; *D*, psoas magnus muscle : *E*, obturator internus; *F*, levator ani; *G*, sphincter ani externus; *a*, transversalis fascia ; *b*, iliac fascia ; *c*, obturator fascia ; *d*, " white line " ; *e*, recto-vesical fascia ; *f*, Alcock's canal. (Browning.)

line " and the rest of the line of origin which forms the greater bulk of the muscle, runs backward, downward, and inward to the side of the coccyx and lower end of the sacrum. The muscle thus forms a diaphragm with the concavity upward.

The other muscles entering into the formation of the pelvic floor form a second layer thinner than that formed by the levator ani. They all meet at the central point of the perineum.

The **fascia** forming the pelvic floor is probably a more important element obstetrically than the muscle layer. It may be described in two portions, a parietal and a visceral layer (Fig. 39).

The **parietal layer**, which is the less important, covers the muscles, padding the sides of the pelvis; in front it forms the posterior layer of the triangular ligament, and is perforated by the urethra and vagina; at the back it helps to cover the sciatic notches.

The **visceral layer** is continuous with the fascia covering the sides of the pelvis. From its line of origin at the " white line" the visceral layer passes downward and inward to the middle line, where its fibres fuse with the connective tissue at the base of the bladder, the vagina, and the rectum, thus slinging these structures in the pelvis. On its lower surface is the levator ani muscle.

The **perineum** may be defined as that portion of the body lying between the anus and the orifice of the vagina. It is formed by the *perineal body* (Fig. 40), which is the aggrega-

Fig. 40.

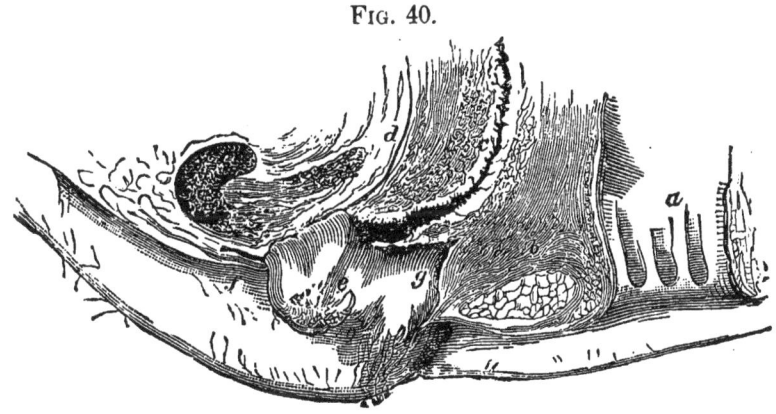

The external genitals, as seen in mesial section: *a*, anus; *b*, perineal body; *c*, vagina; *d*, urethra; *e*, labium minus; *f*, clitoris; *g*, fossa navicularis, in front of which is the hymen. (Henle.)

tion of the tissues lying between the rectum and vagina below their point of contact. On section the perineal body is triangular in outline and pyramidal in form. Its skin surface (base) from the anterior part of the anus to the posterior part of the vaginal orifice measures about 2.5 cm. (1 inch).

The parturient axis: The mathematical axis of the pelvic canal is a line which pierces each pelvic plane perpendicularly at its central point. This axis is a curved line with its concavity forward, and represents very closely the course the fœtal head follows in its descent through the pelvis in normal labor (Fig. 41).

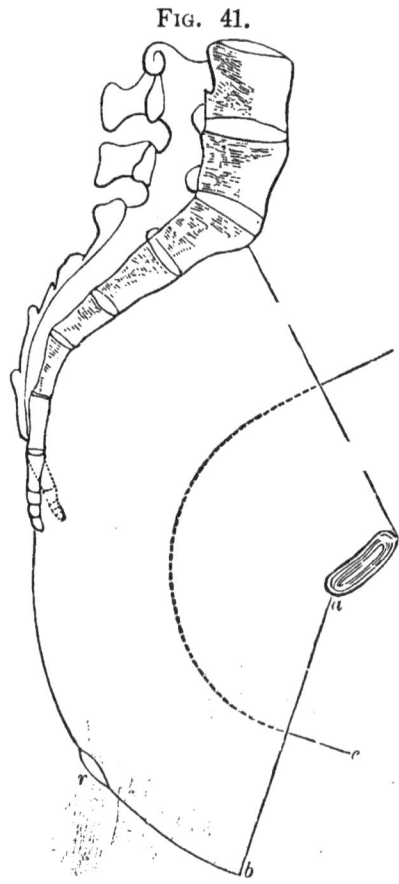

FIG. 41.

Axis of the birth-canal : *r,* anus; *a b,* plane of outlet of completed canal; *e,* perpendicular to plane or axis of expulsion.

The **axis of the brim** if prolonged would strike the tip of the coccyx below, above it would touch a point on the abdomen near the umbilicus.

The **axis of the bony outlet,** if prolonged upward, would pass immediately in front of the sacral promontory. The *axis of the plane of the vulvo-vaginal ring* at the moment when the head is expelled, is a line directed upward almost parallel with the lower part of the abdominal wall of the mother (Fig. 35).

Hirst points out that the direction of the pelvic canal depends entirely on the curve of the sacrum, and that this differs in every pelvis.

The Fœtus.

The **third anatomical element** concerned in labor is the body to be expelled. This consists of the whole ovum, viz., placenta, membranes, and fœtus. The anatomy of the placenta and membranes has already been described, therefore this section will be concerned with the fœtus only.

The **mature fœtus**: At term the fœtus *measures* usually between 46 and 51 cm. (18–20 inches) in length. Its *weight* averages from 3150 to 3290 grammes (7–7¼ pounds), males being somewhat heavier than females. Not rarely the weight may reach as high as 5400 grammes (12 pounds), the phenomenal weight of 9000 grammes (20 pounds) has been recorded.

The *head* bears a much larger proportion to the trunk than in the adult. Its diameters are greater than those of any part of the trunk, and are more incompressible. It therefore offers the principal resistance to the passage of the child through the pelvis. In the mechanism of labor it is with the head that obstetric problems are mainly concerned.

The *whole body* of the fœtus before and during labor forms a roughly ovoid mass. So long as the long diameter of the fœtal ovoid coincides as nearly as possible with the axis of the parturient canal the mechanism is a normal one. This is the case whichever extremity, head or breech, the fœtus presents.

The head: Obstetrically, the fœtal head presents two divisions: (1) *the cranial vault*; (2) *the cranial base and face.*

The **vault**, which is compressible, is composed of thin, membrano-cartilaginous plates, which are in themselves flexible and are, with the exception of the frontal bone, united to the base and to each other by membrane only.

The **base** is formed of bones which are solid and firmly ankylosed. It is, therefore, incompressible, thus affording protection during birth to the ganglia at the base of the brain.

The **attachment between the base and the vault** of the cranium is along a line drawn through the junction of the orbital and "squamous" parts of the frontal bone, continued backward by the squamous suture and downward by the hinge-like junction of the tabular part of the occipital bone to the basilar and condylar portion.

The **bones forming the cranial vault** are the two parietal, the frontal, and the "squamous" portions of the occipital and of the two temporal bones. These are united only by the unossified external periosteum and by the dura mater.

6—Obst.

The plasticity of the vault is due to the cartilaginous character of the bones and to the existence of the membranous interspaces.

The **sutures of the vault** are the membranous intervals between two adjacent bones. The most important are the *sagittal,* running between the two parietals; the *frontal,* between the two portions of the frontal bone; the *coronal,* between the frontal and parietals; and the *lambdoidal,* between the parietals and the occipital bone (Figs. 42 and 43)

FIG. 42.   FIG. 43.

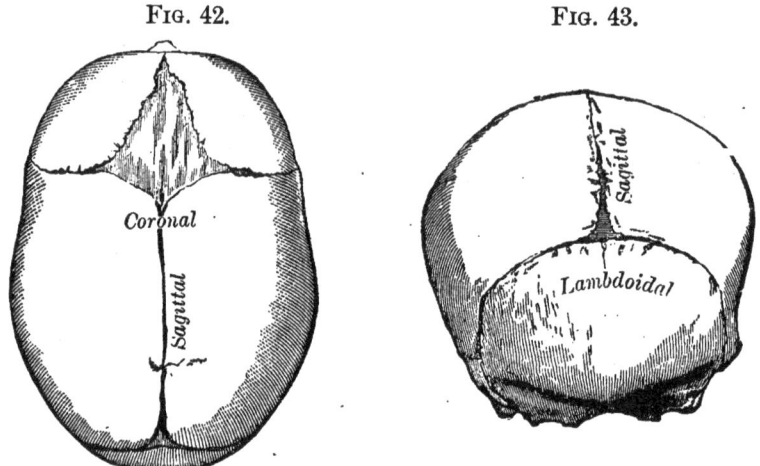

Anterior and posterior fontanelles, sagittal, lambdoidal, coronal, and frontal
sutures.

The **fontanelles** are the larger spaces formed by the widening out of the sutures between the angles of three or four adjacent bones.

The largest is the *anterior fontanelle,* or *bregma,* situated at the junction of the sagittal, the coronal, and the frontal sutures. It is kite-shaped, or quadrangular, with its most acute angle forward. Its average diameter is about one inch, but its size varies in different heads. Four lines of sutures run into it.

The *posterior, or small, fontanelle* is formed at the junction of the sagittal and lambdoidal sutures, and is merely felt as a small triangular depression. There are three lines of sutures running into it.

Temporal fontanelles : At the junction of the temporal with

FIG. 44.

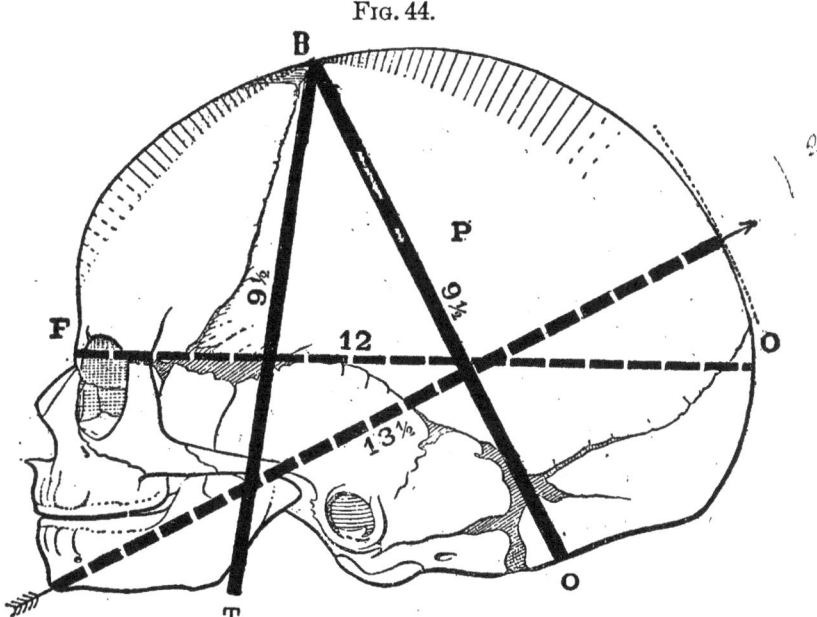

The diameters of the fœtal head: O F, occipitofrontal; O B, suboccipito-bregmatic; B T, cervicobregmatic. The maximum diameter, occipitomental, is indicated by the long dotted arrow. Measurements are centimetres. (Farabeuf and Varnier.)

FIG. 45.

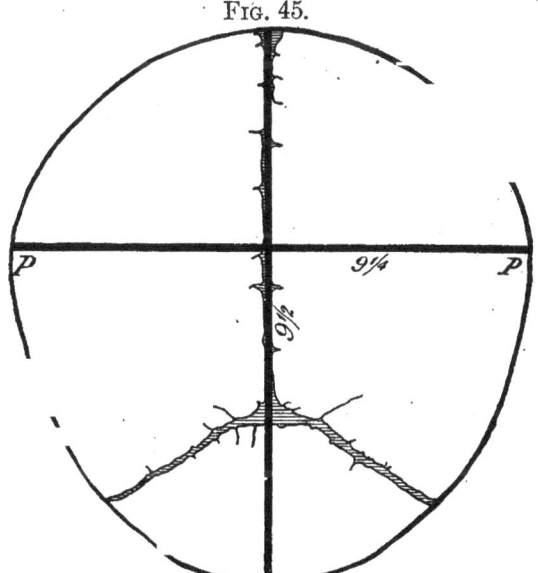

Engaging diameters of the flexed head: *P P*, Biparietal diameter, 9¼ cm (After Farabeuf and Varnier.)

the parietal and occipital bones, on either side of the head, there exists a small quadrilateral fontanelle.

False fontanelles are occasionally observed either in the body of the bone or in the course of a suture. These are due to some defect in ossification. A quadrilateral false fon-

FIG. 46.

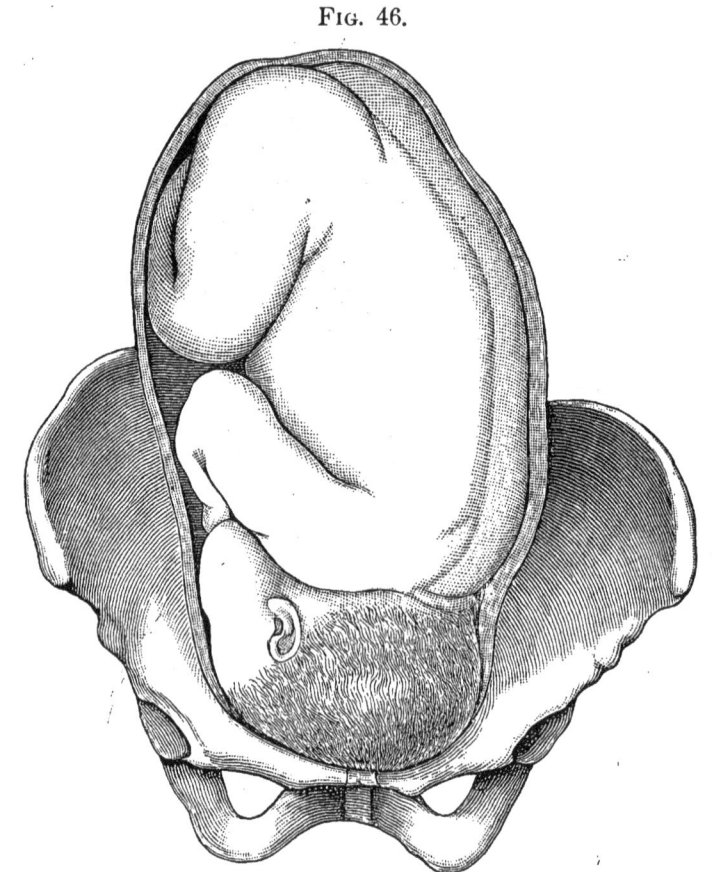

Vertex.　Left occipito-anterior position.　(Ribemont-Dessaignes and Lepage.)

tanelle is not infrequently to be felt in the line of the sagittal suture a short distance from the usual small fontanelle.

Obstetric landmarks: Certain landmarks about the *fœtal head* are of considerable obstetrical importance.

The *vertex* is that portion of the head between the anterior and posterior fontanelles, and extending laterally to the parietal eminences.

The *occiput* is that portion of the head behind the posterior fontanelle.

The *sinciput* is that portion of the head in front of the bregma.

·FIG. 47.

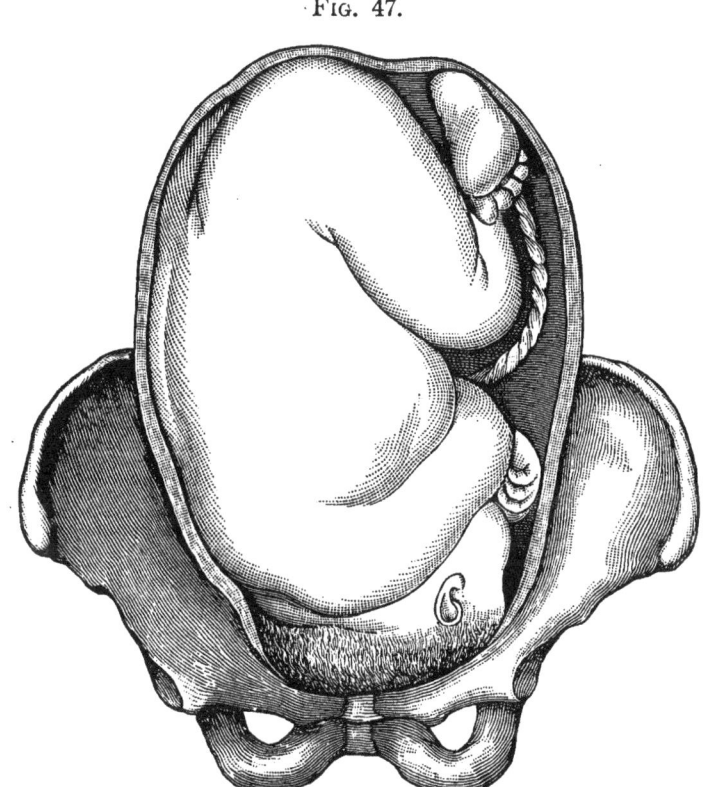

Vertex.   Right occipito-anterior position.   (Ribemont-Dessaignes and Lepage.)

The *glabella* is the space over the root of the nose and between the supra-orbital ridges.

Five protuberances are presented by the cranial bones :

The *occipital protuberance* situated in the middle of the squamous portion of the occipital bone about 2.5 cm. (1 inch) behind the posterior fontanelle.   The *parietal protuberance* is the boss or eminence in the centre of each parietal bone.

The *frontal protuberance* is the eminence in the centre of each frontal bone.

Diameters of the fœtal head : *Occipitofrontal,* extending from the glabella to the most prominent portion of the occipital bone.　Measures 11.5 cm. (4½ inches).

FIG. 48.

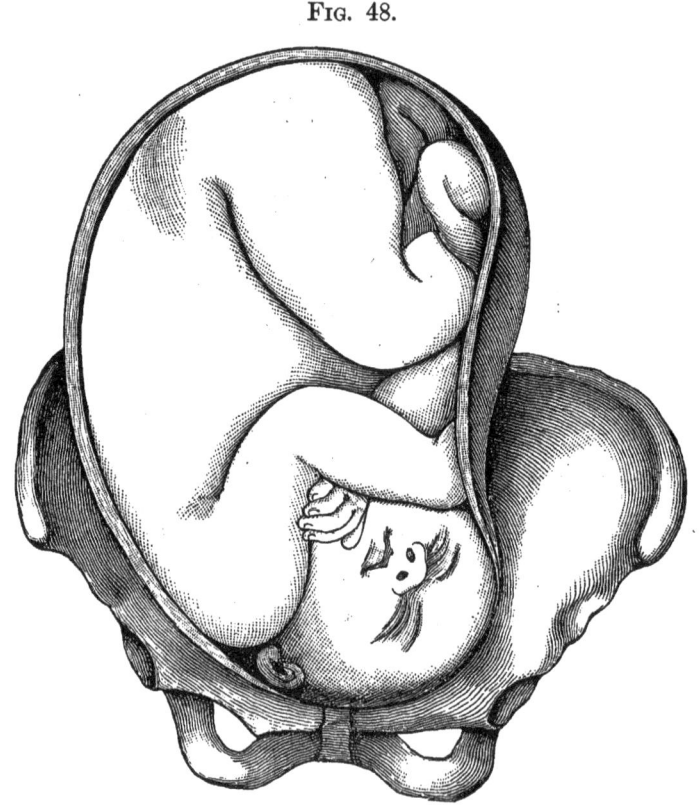

Vertex.　Right occipito-posterior position.　(Ribemont-Dessaignes and Lepage.)

Occipitomental, extending from the most prominent portion of the occipital bone to the tip of the chin.　Measures 14 cm. (5½ inches).

Suboccipitobregmatic, extending from the junction of the neck and occiput to the centre of the bregma.　Measures 9.5 cm. (3¾ inches).

Suboccipitofrontal, extending from the junction of the neck and occiput to the summit of the brow. Measures 11 cm. ($4\frac{3}{8}$ inches).

Biparietal, measures through the centre of the parietal eminences. Measures 9.5 cm. ($3\frac{3}{4}$ inches).

Frontomental, extending from the summit of the brow to the centre of the lower border of the chin. Measures 9 cm. ($3\frac{1}{2}$ inches).

FIG. 49.

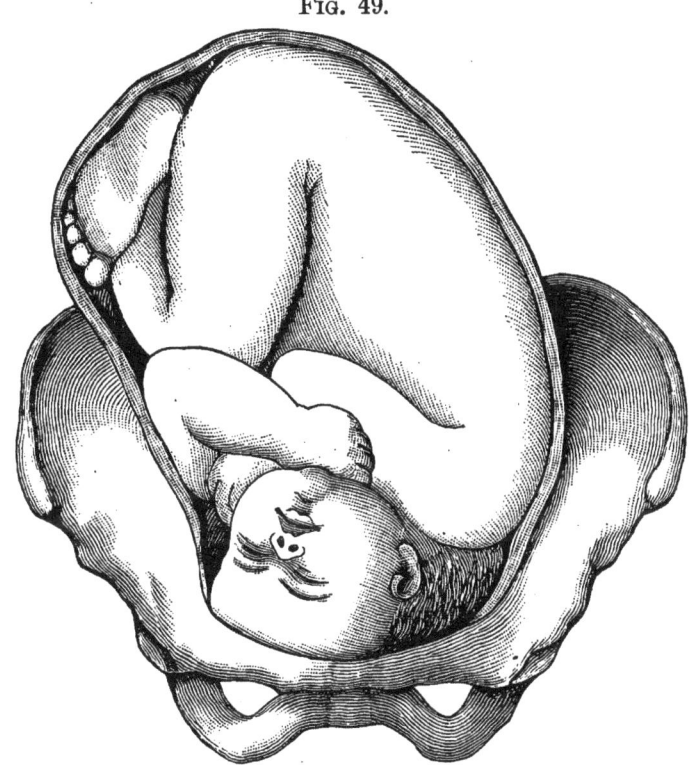

Vertex. Left occipito-posterior position. (Ribemont-Dessaignes and Lepage.)

Cervicobregmatic, extending from the junction of the neck and chin to the centre of the bregma. Measures 9.5 cm. ($3\frac{3}{4}$ inches).

The *above* diameters (Figs. 44 and 45) are all of them more or less *compressible.*

The *remainder* are *incompressible.*

Bimastoid, measured through the mastoid processes, 7 cm. ($2\frac{3}{4}$ inches).

Bimalar, measured through the malar eminences, 7 cm. (2¾ inches).

Bitemporal, measured through the lower extremities of the coronal suture, 8 cm. (3⅛ inches).

The *following table* is sufficiently accurate for all practical purposes and should be memorized :

FIG. 50.

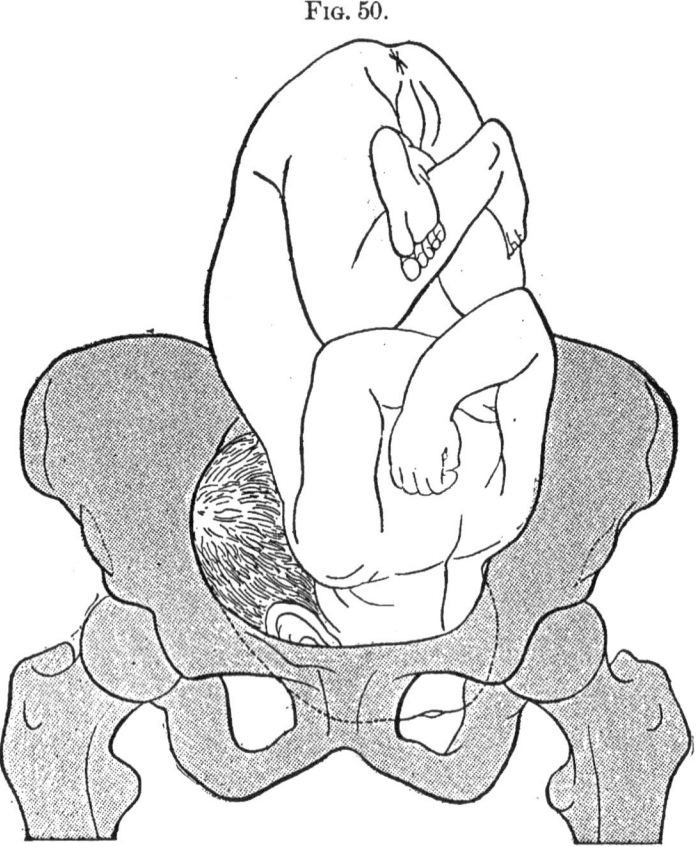

Face. Left mento-anterior position. (Farabeuf and Varnier.)

Diameters of the Fœtal Head (Jewett).

Biparietal,	9 cm. (3½ inches).
Suboccipitobregmatic,	9 cm. (3½ ").
Frontomental,	9 cm. (3½ ").
Occipitofrontal,	11.5 cm. (4½ ").
Occipitomental,	14 cm. (5½ ").

In the following table the **circumferences** of the most important planes of the fœtal head are given :

Circumferences of the Planes of the Fœtal Head.

Suboccipitobregmatic,   33 cm. (13 inches).
Suboccipitofrontal,   35 cm. (13¾ ").
Occipitofrontal,   34.5 cm. (13½ ").

Fig. 51.

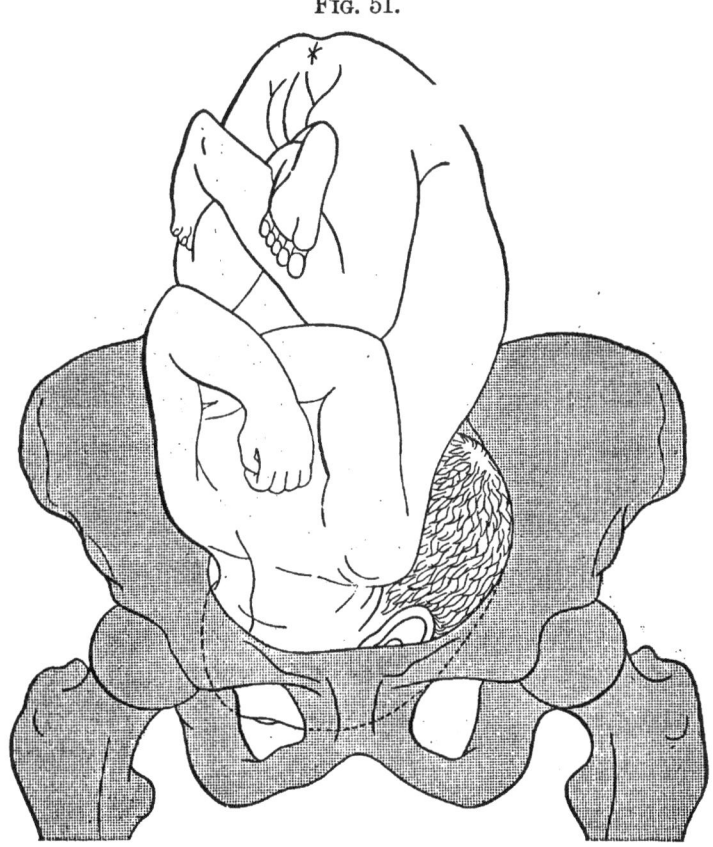

Face. Right mento-anterior position. (Farabeuf and Varnier.)

Importance of flexion of fœtal head : When the head is completely flexed, as it is in normal labor, its smallest plane (measured by its circumference) comes into relation with the different pelvic planes successively as the head descends. This smallest plane, as will be noticed in the above table, is the *sub-occipitobregmatic*. The importance of the maintenance of complete flexion of the fœtal head until almost the moment of its delivery will thus be easily comprehended.

FIG. 52.

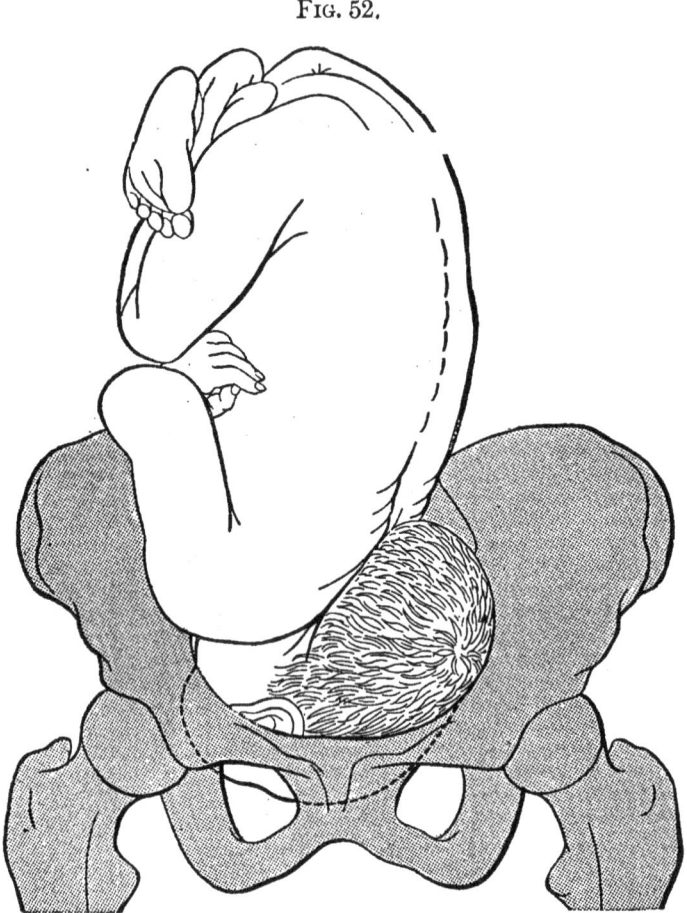

Face. Right mento-posterior position. (Farabeuf and Varnier.)

Moulding of the fœtal head: During labor the head undergoes more or less compression which results in its alteration in shape.

Moulding results from the overlapping of the cranial bones, which takes place in a definite way in all cases. The parietal bones override the occipital and frontal bones; and of the parietals the one most pressed upon, generally the one in relation to the promontory, always slips under the other. The

FIG. 53.

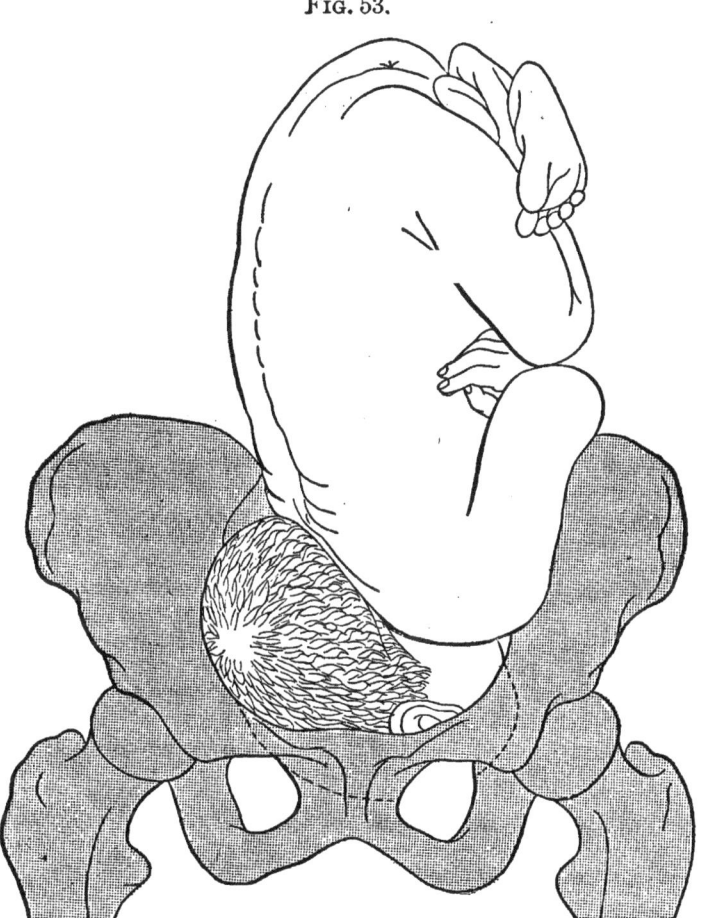

Face. Left mento-posterior position. (Farabeuf and Varnier.)

two halves of the frontal bone follow the same rule as the parietal bones.

The whole volume of the head is reduced by compression, the greater portion of the cerebrospinal fluid and of the contents of the cerebral bloodvessels being forced out of the cranial cavity during labor.

The fœtal trunk : The *diameters* of importance in the trunk are few, as the whole body is very incompressible.   The *bis-acromial* is the longest and measures 12 cm. (4¾ inches), and is reducible to the extent of 2 to 3 cm.

The *bitrochanteric* measures about 10 cm. (4 inches).

The *dorsosternal* measures 9 cm. (3½ inches).

Fig. 54.

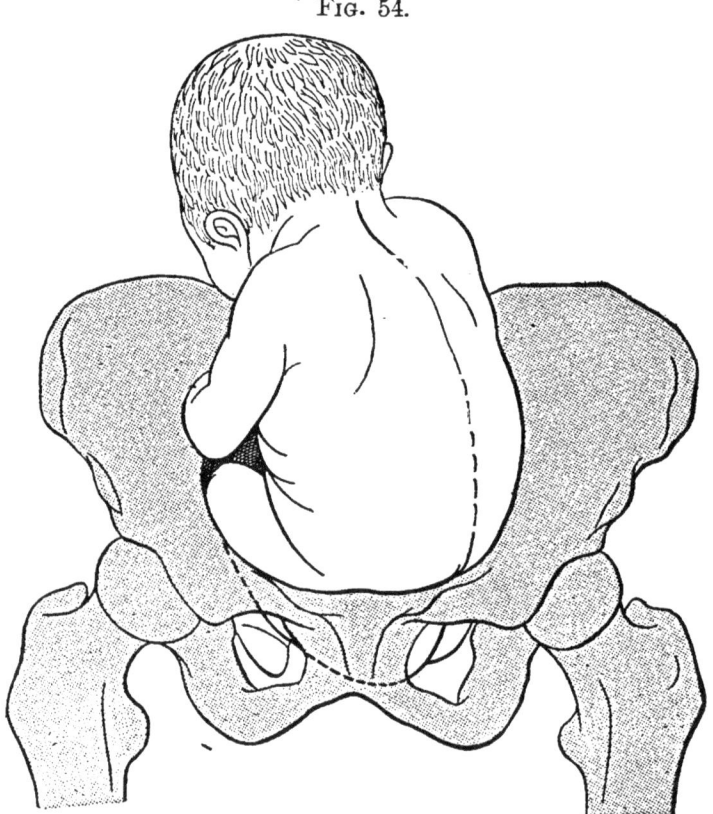

Breech   Left sacro-anterior position.   (Farabeuf and Varnier)

The *length of the fœtal ovoid*, that is, from the vertex to the breech, may be given as 24–24.5 cm. (9½ to 10 inches).

Mobility of the fœtal head and trunk : The movements of flexion, extension, and rotation of the *fœtal head* are of great importance in the mechanism of labor.   *Flexion* is limited by the pressure of the chin upon the chest.

Extension is limited by compression of the occiput against the back. *Rotation* is safe through an arc of 90 degrees on each side, till the chin points over the shoulder.

The *trunk* permits of a certain amount of rotation which is limited by the rotation of the vertebral bodies. A certain

Fig. 55.

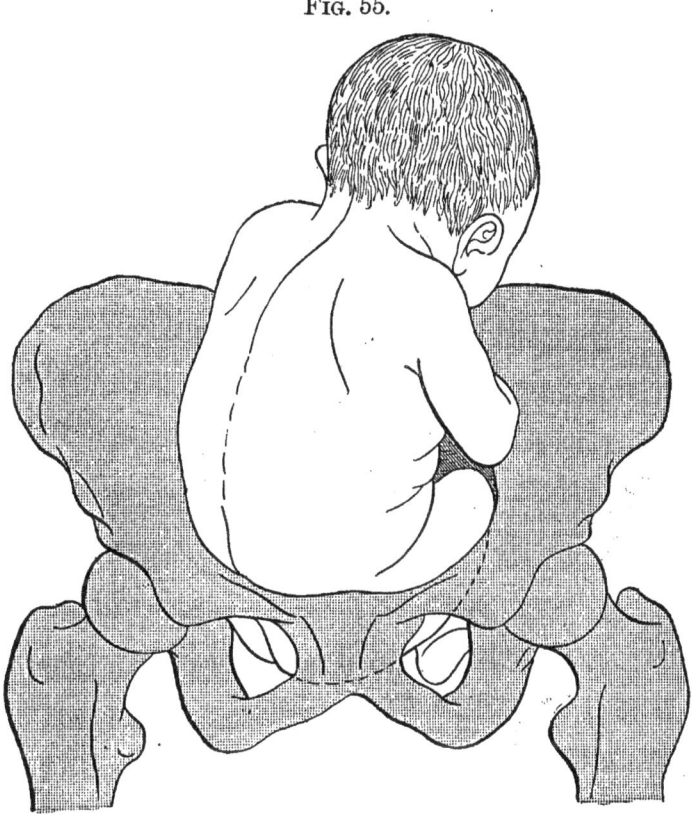

Breech. Right sacro-anterior position. (Farabeuf and Varnier.)

degree of lateral flexion is also possible as well as ordinary flexion and extension.

The **posture** of the fœtus is the relation which the trunk, head, and limbs of the child have to one another, independently of the relations of any part of the fœtus to any part of the mother.

The *normal posture* of the fœtus during pregnancy and

parturition is one of flexion, the head being flexed on the trunk, the thighs on the abdomen, and the legs on the thighs, the arms being folded on the chest.

The relation of the uterine and fœtal axes: During the latter part of pregnancy and in parturition the long axis of the fœtal ovoid may correspond to the long axis of the uterus (longitudinal); or may be at right angles to it (transverse).

Fig. 56.

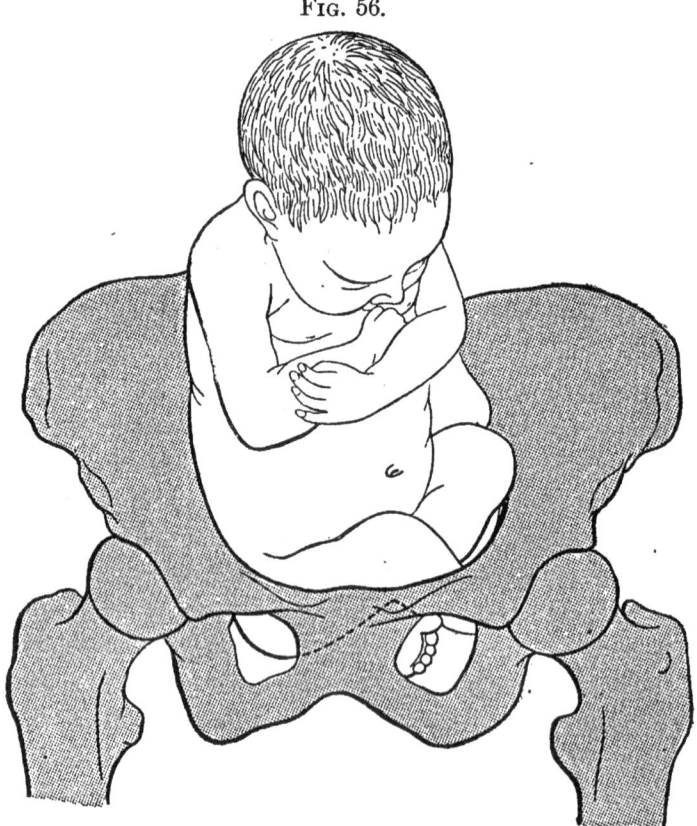

Breech. Right sacro-posterior position. (Farabeuf and Varnier.)

Normally the long axes correspond; any deviation from this relationship leads to serious complications in labor.

Commonly, obstetricians apply the term **presentation** to denote the relation of the long axis of the fœtal ovoid to the uterine axis. In our opinion the use of this term to denote this relationship is a misnomer. The term *presentation* should only be used to denote the part of the fœtus which presents at the pelvic brim and is accessible to the examining finger.

Presentations: Under the definition just given there are three *forms* of fœtal presentation : the *cephalic*, the *pelvic*, and

Fig. 57.

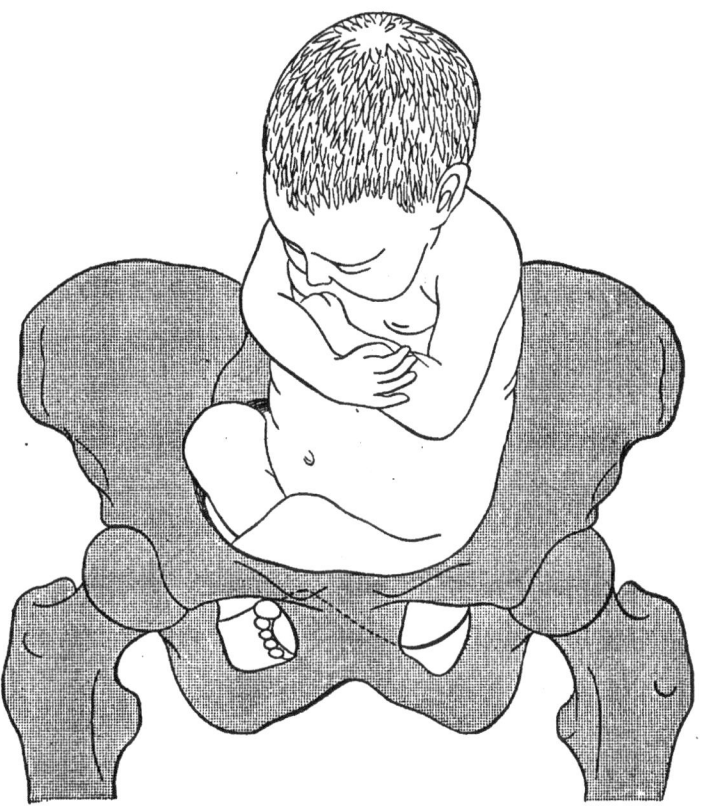

Breech. Left sacro-posterior position. (Farabeuf and Varnier.)

the *somatic*. There occur distinct varieties of each of these forms, as will be noted in the following table :

Table of Fœtal Presentations.

	Frequency.			
Cephalic,	97 per cent.—(*a*)	vertex,	(*b*) face,	(*c*) brow.
Pelvic,	1.6 per cent.—(*a*)	breech,	(*b*) leg,	(*c*) foot.
Somatic,	0.5 per cent.—(*a*)	shoulder,	(*b*) elbow,	(*c*) hand.

The *latter* form of presentation is often termed transverse or crossed birth.

Position : The pelvic brim is divided by the conjugate and transverse diameters into *four quadrants.* *Position* may be defined as the relationship of the presenting part of the fœtus to the quadrants of the pelvic brim. Thus for each presenta-

FIG. 58.

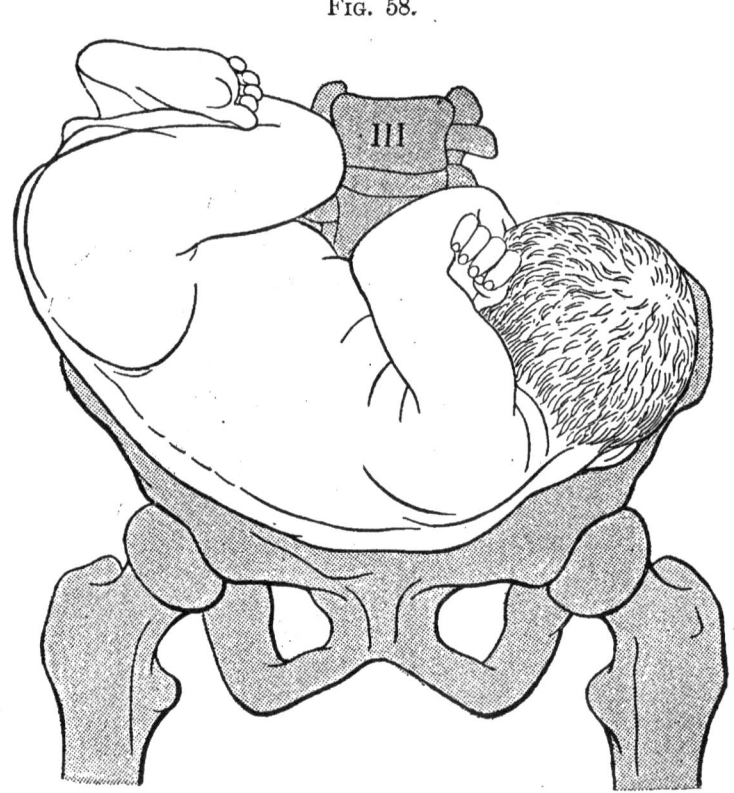

Shoulder.   Left scapulo-anterior position.   (Farabeuf and Varnier.)

tion there are four positions. They are named according to the particular quadrant confronted by the presenting part.

In **vertex, face, and breech presentations** the long diameter of the presenting part engages in one of the oblique diameters of the pelvic inlet.

In *vertex presentations* when the occiput confronts the left anterior quadrant of the pelvic brim, the *position* is left occipito-anterior, and so on.

Face presentations are named similarly according to the direction of the chin, left mento-anterior, etc.

Breech presentations are named according to the position of the sacrum, left sacro-anterior, etc.

Fɪɢ. 59.

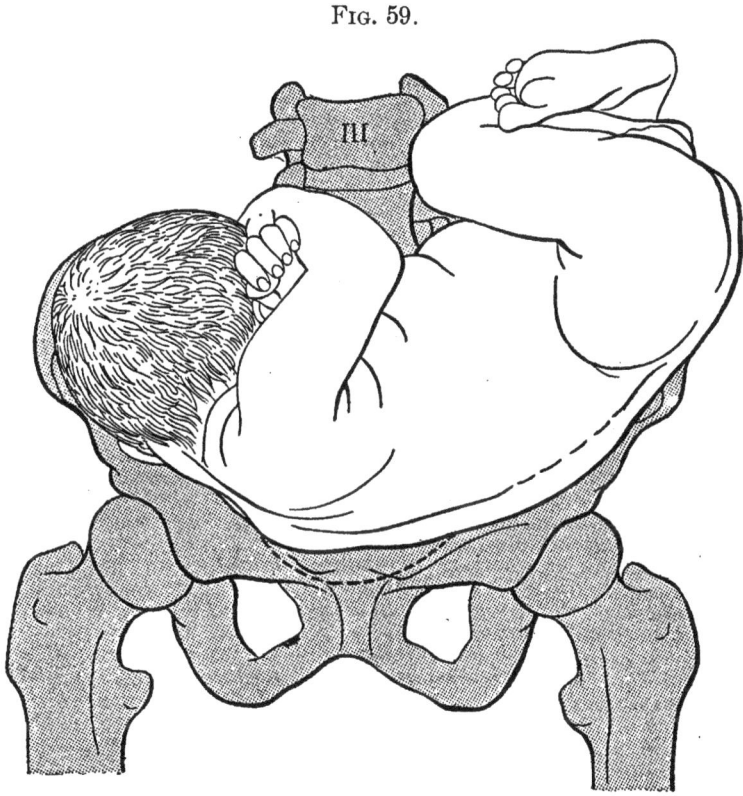

Shoulder. Right scapulo-anterior position. (Farabeuf and Varnier.)

Shoulder presentations are named according to the direction of the scapula, left scapulo-anterior, etc.

The **positions** are sometimes spoken of as first, second, third, or fourth, the left anterior being the first and the others following in order from left to right around the pelvic brim. This method is apt to mislead, as various authorities differ as to which is the first position in certain presentations, and con-

7—Obst.

fusion results.   It is better to designate each position in full or by the initial letters (Figs. 46–61).

FIG. 60.

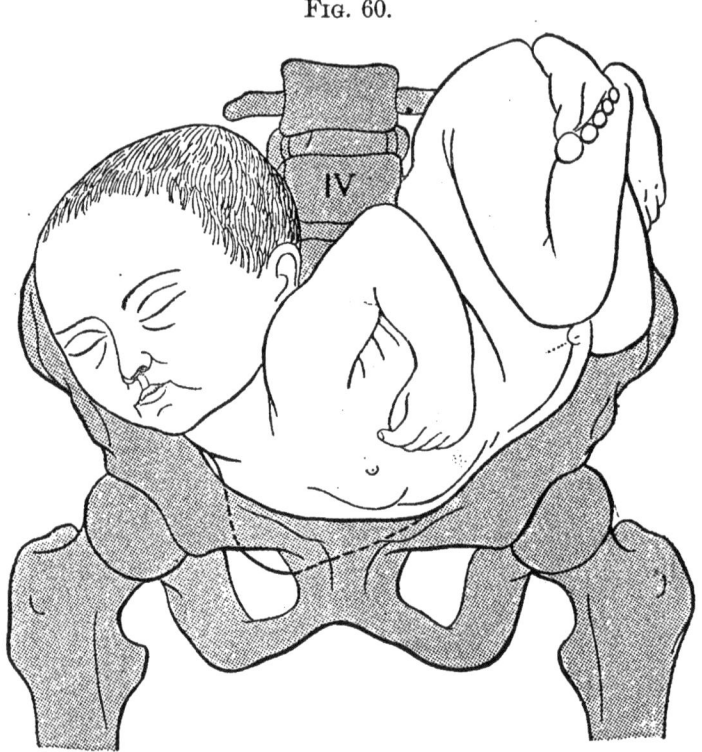

Shoulder.   Right scapulo-posterior position.   (Farabeuf and Varnier.)

Vertex positions :

> Left occipito-anterior, L. O. A.
> Right occipito-anterior, R. O. A.
> Right occipitoposterior, R. O. P.
> Left occipitoposterior, L. O. P.

Face positions :

> Left mento-anterior, L. M. A.
> Right mento-anterior, R. M. A.
> Right mentoposterior, R. M. P.
> Left mentoposterior, L. M. P.

Breech positions :

> Left sacro-anterior, L. S. A.
> Right sacro-anterior, R. S. A.
> Right sacroposterior, R. S. P.
> Left sacroposterior, L. S. P.

Somatic or shoulder presentations :

> Left scapulo-anterior, L. Sc. A.
> Right scapulo-anterior, R. Sc. A.
> Right scapuloposterior, R. Sc. P.
> Left scapuloposterior, L. Sc. P.

FIG. 61.

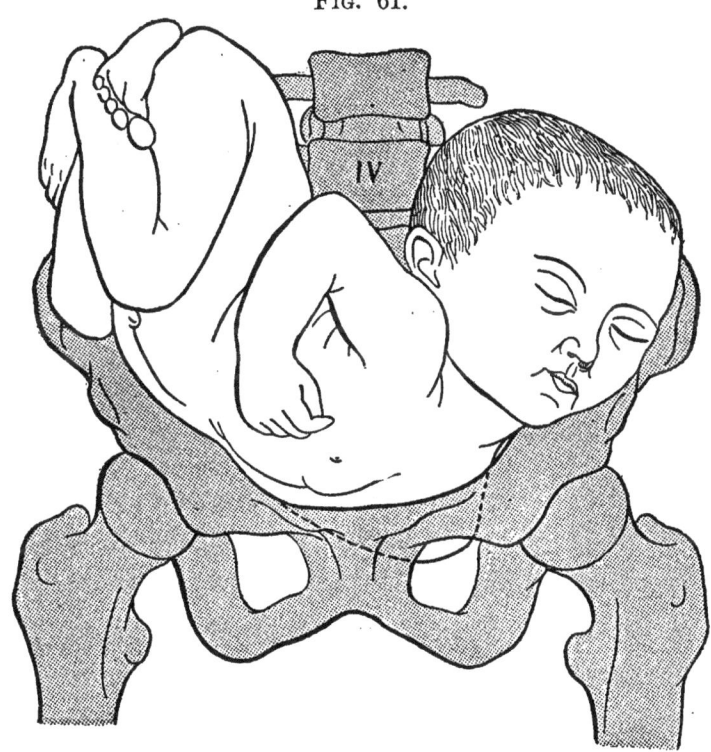

Shoulder. Left scapulo-posterior position. (Farabeuf and Varnier)

Face presentations are sometimes named according to the pelvic quadrant confronted by the brow, as left fronto-anterior, L. F. A., etc.

That some form of **cephalic presentation** occurs in 97 per cent. of all cases is not quite satisfactorily accounted for. There are three conditions each of which has some influence in bringing about this result. These are: 1, the position of the centre of gravity of the fœtus; 2, the relative shapes of the uterus and of the fœtus; 3, the movements of the fœtus:

1. Matthews Duncan long ago found that the **centre of gravity of the fœtus** lay somewhere about the shoulders, and nearer the right than the left, owing to the presence of the liver on the right side. Thus if a fœtus is immersed in a saline fluid of the same specific gravity as its own, it sinks into a position with the back of its right shoulder looking downward, this, therefore, becoming the lowest part of the body.

2. **The relative shapes of the uterus and of the fœtus:** The fundus is at term the most roomy part of the uterus; hence at term the more bulky breech finds greater accommodation in the upper segment, while the head readily adapts itself to the smaller lower segment.

The fœtal movements: The movements of the legs of the fœtus are probably more powerful than those of the arms. Hence if the child lie with the feet downward these will when in a state of motion come into contact with the resisting pelvic brim, which will result in lateral displacement of the child's body. The shape of the uterus will then tend to convert this attitude again into a longitudinal one. The action of the specific gravity of the fœtus will tend to bring the cephalic pole downward, and when once this position has been obtained its alteration is not likely to occur provided no abnormal conditions are present.

THE MECHANISM AND COURSE OF NORMAL LABOR.

Definition: The term *eutocia*, indicating normal labor, is applied to labors which terminate without artificial aid and without injury to the mother or child.

Under this definition, in this work, only *uncomplicated vertex presentations* will be classed as normal.

At this point it may be mentioned that a woman pregnant

for the first time is termed a *primigravida ;* one in labor or in the puerperium for the first time, a *primipara.*

If a woman has had several children or miscarriages previously she is termed a *multipara.* When it is desired to indicate the exact number of the labor she is spoken of as a i para, ii para, iii para, and so on.

Stages of labor: While there is frequently a premonitory stage before labor actually sets in, it is customary to divide labor itself into three distinct stages :

The *first stage,* or stage of dilatation, ends with the full dilatation of the os uteri, with which the rupture of the membranes is usually coincident.

The *second stage,* or stage of expulsion, ends with the complete birth of the child.

The *third stage,* or placental stage, ends with complete expulsion of the placenta and membranes and retraction of the uterus.

The **duration of normal labor**: The average duration of normal labor in primiparæ may be stated as eighteen hours ; while in multiparæ it is from eight to ten hours.

The average duration of the *first stage* in primiparæ is about twelve hours; in multiparæ from six to eight hours.

The *second stage* in primiparæ lasts about four to six hours; and in multiparæ from one to two hours.

The *third stage,* which is but rarely terminated spontaneously, lasts from a few minutes to two hours.

The Causes of the Onset of Labor.

No entirely satisfactory theory has been advanced to account for the onset of labor, which usually occurs on the two hundred and eightieth day after the beginning of the last menstrual period.

It is known that three motor centres exist which preside over uterine contractions ; a centre in the medulla ; the cervical ganglia ; and the ganglia in the anterior vaginal wall and the uterine walls.

Labor is not the result of the operation of one, but rather of a number of concurrent causes. These act by increasing the painless rhythmic contractions of the uterus present throughout the whole period of pregnancy.

Many causes have been suggested, among them :

1. Increasing distention of the lower uterine segment, leading to increased pressure on the nervous ganglia ;

2. Changes in decidua, senile and thrombotic in character ;

3. Senile changes in the placenta, formation of fibrous tissue ;

4. Excess of carbon dioxide in the maternal blood, acting on the centre in the medulla ;

5. Increase of fœtal metabolic products in the maternal blood, acting as above ;

6. Menstrual periodicity.

During pregnancy, at each menstrual epoch the irritability of the uterus is increased, hence the tendency to its interruption at such periods.

The senile changes in the placenta, and the changes in the maternal and the fœtal blood, metabolic in origin, associated with increased irritability of the uterus, are all at their maximum at term ; these combined probably tend to set in action the nervous mechanism concerned in the act of parturition.

The Forces of Labor.

The expellent forces of labor are :

1. Contractions of the uterus and of the vaginal and pelvic muscles ;

2. Contractions of the abdominal muscles and diaphragm ;

3. Gravity.

1. Contractions of the Uterus and of the Vaginal and Pelvic Muscles.

Uterine Contractions.

These are by far the most important factor in bringing about the expulsion of the ovum.

The contractions are **involuntary**, occurring independently of the woman's will ; though they undoubtedly are weakened or even inhibited by various agents. Emotion, such as the dread of pain, or nervousness caused by the entrance of the physician or a stranger, may inhibit them. A loaded rectum or a full bladder may reflexly inhibit uterine contractions.

They are **peristaltic**, the wave of the contraction being from the fundus to the cervix, and lasting from one-third to two-thirds the length of the labor pain.

They are **intermittent**. The contraction begins gradually, rapidly reaches an acme, and then slowly passes off. This may be demonstrated clinically by keeping the hand on the woman's abdominal wall throughout a contraction ; the uterus will be felt to harden gradually ; then, remaining in this condition for a short interval, to relax and become soft again.

Their **duration** averages about one minute. In the earliest stage of labor they occupy but a few seconds ; but in the expulsive stage they last longer and are stronger. The contractions are **rhythmical** in their intermissions. There is a certain regularity in their appearance and disappearance. The greater their frequency the longer their duration. At the beginning of labor the interval is long, say a quarter of an hour ; toward the end the interval between the pains may be but a few seconds, so that the contractions seem to be almost continuous.

The contractions are **painful**, hence the term "pains" usually applied to them. This pain is due to the forcible stretching of the cervix and its attachments, and of the vagina and vulva consecutively ; also in part to the fact that the uterus is contracting against resistance. A parallel to this latter occurs in the intestine when an obstruction exists. The pain is usually referred to the sacral region, especially in the earlier stages ; later, when the sacral nerves are pressed upon by the advance of the fœtus, the pain is felt down the limbs.

The individual *muscle-fibres* of the uterus during contraction become shorter and thicker than they are during relaxation.

Retraction is a process peculiar probably to all involuntary muscle-fibres ; but is most marked in those of the uterus. Retraction enables a muscle-fibre which has shortened during contraction to relax without returning to its original length. The fibres after contraction do not quite return to their original length, but remain persistently somewhat shorter and thicker.

Retraction is due in part also to a rearrangement of the fibres. These are assumed at the beginning of labor to be nearly end to end; in the course of retraction they come to lie almost side to side. Retraction is practically limited during labor to the muscle-fibres forming the *upper uterine segment.* This portion of the uterine wall as the ovum is pushed down becomes gradually thicker; thus its propulsive force during contraction augments, and it is enabled to remain constantly in contact with the upper end of the ovum until its expulsion from this segment.

The *lower uterine segment,* not possessing the power of retraction, becomes progressively thinner and dilates as the ovum is forced down through it. Retraction thus enables the uterus to preserve the expulsive results of contraction.

Polarity is a useful term to express the fact that throughout labor the expelling part of the uterus—the upper segment—is in a state of opposite function to the sphincter part—the lower segment and cervix.

During pregnancy the muscle forming the body of the uterus is practically at rest, while the cervix, especially the internal os, is in a state of tonic contraction, it is active. During labor this relation is inverted, the body contracts while the cervix is relaxed. This relation is taken advantage of when it is necessary to induce labor for any cause—that is, to set up active contractions in the muscle forming the body of the uterus. This is usually accomplished by dilating the cervix either manually or by instruments, which brings about the desired result.

Effect of uterine contractions: *In changing the shape and position of the uterus:* During a contraction the longitudinal and anteroposterior diameters of the uterus are increased, while its transverse diameter is decreased, the whole organ assuming a roughly cylindrical form (see also pp. 43 and 44). The fundus is held against the abdominal wall and becomes more prominent; this brings the long axis of the uterus into line with that of the inlet of the pelvis.

On the circulation in the uterus and placenta: During contraction the uterine sinuses are slowly obliterated and emptied, refilling as it passes off; but the fœtal portion of the placenta is not affected. Thus throughout the whole of pregnancy the . circulation of blood in the uterus is assisted by the regular rhythmical uterine contractions.

On the foetal heart: The foetal heart is slowed because the pressure on the placental site raises the general foetal blood-pressure.

On the maternal pulse: The maternal pulse-rate increases ten to twenty beats, thus contrasting with the foetal pulse-rate. The arterial blood-pressure is markedly raised.

Vaginal and Pelvic Muscles.

These muscles play but a very unimportant part in bringing about the expulsion of the ovum. They act only in the later stages.

2. Contraction of the Abdominal Muscles and Diaphragm.

The **muscles** entering into the formation of the abdominal walls, along with the diaphragm, when simultaneously in a state of contraction, increase the intra-abdominal pressure and thus render very important aid to the uterus. These muscles taken altogether form, as it were, a second layer of muscular tissue external to the uterus.

Their **mode of action** is as follows: A deep inspiration is taken, thus flattening out and depressing the diaphragm, which is then fixed by the closure of the glottis; then the muscles in the abdominal walls contract. The descent of the diaphragm pushes the fundus forward; this is resisted by the contraction of the muscles of the abdominal wall, so that the resultant of the combined pressure of these muscles is in the direction of the long axis of the uterus—that is, downward in the axis of the pelvic brim.

The action of these muscles is not exerted until the second or expulsive stage, and is at first entirely voluntary. In the later stages of the expulsive period their action is entirely involuntary.

At first they act only during the acme of a pain, when the woman voluntarily bears down; but later, when the pain lasts longer, the woman is compelled to open the glottis to

. respire, thus relaxing the pressure; but immediately another breath is taken, they act again, so that there are often several abdominal contractions to one pain.

3. Gravity.

The weight of the child and of the waters contained in the membranes exerts but a small influence in aiding expulsion, except perhaps during the first stage of labor, when the woman is more or less in the erect or semirecumbent position.

LABOR—FIRST STAGE.

Premonitory Signs and Symptoms of Labor.

The events which indicate the approach of labor are variable in their duration and may be so slight as quite to escape observation.

The **change of position** of the uterus which takes place during the last weeks of pregnancy has been referred to already.

Irregular pains, usually felt low down in the abdomen in front, are frequently complained of by patients for some days before the onset of true labor. They are sometimes severe, and may cause much suffering to sensitive women. These "false pains," as they are termed, may be distinguished from true pains by their irregularity and by their site; true labor-pains being felt chiefly in the sacral region. These false pains have absolutely no effect on the cervix, and no increase in the vaginal secretion accompanies them.

Frequency of micturition and, less often, **of defecation,** may be troublesome during the last few days, and are probably caused by increase in the nervous excitability of the pelvic structures usually present at this time.

Characteristic Signs and Symptoms of the Onset of Labor.

Regular uterine contractions: The interval between these is long at first, but shortens steadily as the labor progresses. The pains at this period are always referred to the sacral region.

Appearance of the "show": This is the term commonly applied to the mucus tinged with blood which escapes from the cervix and vagina at this time. The mucus comes chiefly from the cervix, and the blood from the separated surfaces of the membranes and the uterine walls just above the internal os.

Softening and shortening of the cervix: These changes can only be noticed by making a vaginal examination. The softening of the cervix is due to infiltration with serous exudate resulting from the interference with the return circulation caused by the uterine contractions. The shortening of the cervix results from the yielding of the internal os, which is undoubtedly a physiological relaxation analogous to that which takes place in sphincter muscles.

Mechanism of the First Stage.

The uterine contractions during this stage are occupied entirely with **dilating the cervix,** there being little or no expulsion of the ovum, this being limited to the slight advance of the bag of membranes through the internal os.

Dilatation of the cervix results from: (1) the yielding of the internal os, which is a physiological relaxation; (2) the hydrostatic pressure of the bag of waters; and (3) the action of the long muscular fibres in the outer muscle-layer of the uterus.

1. **The first** of these has already been discussed.

2. **The hydrostatic pressure of the bag of waters:** The first result of uterine contraction is an *increase in the general intrauterine fluid pressure.* When the waters are abundant and the membranes intact the effect of this pressure is *nil* so far as the fœtus is concerned; as the law of fluid pressure is that it is equal and opposite in all directions.

The *direction* of the force of the uterine contraction is centripetal; this is opposed centrifugally by the bag of waters. The force of the contraction is centripetal, while the force exerted by the bag of waters in opposition is centrifugal.

These two forces would then *equalize one another* if: (1) the uterine wall were of equal thickness throughout, and therefore of equal strength throughout; and if (2) the uterine wall were in a state of equal contraction throughout at the same moment of time.

Both these conditions fail in that : *first,* the uterine wall is not of equal thickness throughout, the lower segment being thinner ; and having a solution in its continuity (the yielding internal os), it is weaker and therefore must expand ; *secondly,* the uterine wall is not in a state of equal contraction throughout at the same moment of time, in that the contraction is vermicular, beginning at the fundus and spreading downward to the cervix, so that when the fundus is in a state of contraction the cervix is relaxed. This may be demonstrated clinically by keeping the finger-tip on the lowest point of the bag of waters, when at the onset of a pain this will be felt to become tense some seconds before the woman complains of the pain which causes the increase of pressure.

For these reasons the force of the centrifugal pressure of the waters is exerted most markedly on the lower uterine segment and cervix ; hence *dilatation of these parts* takes place as a result of the increase in the general intra-uterine fluid pressure.

As dilatation proceeds the membranes, having become loosened from their attachment to the uterine walls, insinuate themselves into the opening. Since the fluid within the membranes transmits the force of the uterine contraction equally in all directions, the bag of waters is distended laterally as well as downward, thus exerting an expansive action directly on the walls of the cervix, and finally on the margins of the external os. As the cervix and external os dilate this lateral pressure of the bag of waters increases proportionately.

3. **The action of the longitudinal muscle-fibres of the uterus:** The contents of the uterus being practically incompressible, the pull of the longitudinal fibres will result in drawing the lower uterine segment and cervix, whose structure is thinner than that of the upper segment, up over the contained body. In this action the oblique fibres assist to a considerable extent.

The wave of contraction probably passes through the longitudinal fibres more rapidly than through the circular fibres, hence the former will tend to draw the cervix up over the presenting part while the lower segment is relaxed.

When the cervix and external os have become well dilated the **membranes usually rupture.** This, as a rule, occurs during a pain, and is announced by a gush of waters from the vagina. The quantity escaping will depend on how rapidly the presenting part of the fœtus descends and occludes the lower uterine segment.

The rupture of the membranes may **occur at** or before the onset of labor; or may not take place till the end of the expulsive stage; but it is very rare that a full-term child is born with the membranes unruptured; though it has happened that in precipitate labors the whole ovum has come away entire.

On the rupture of the bag of waters, the **presenting part of the fœtus takes its place as a dilator.** The fluid still retained in utero then transmits the effective intra-uterine pressure to that portion of the fœtus in contact with the margins of the os.

In **dry labors**—*i. e.*, in cases where the membranes rupture prematurely, thus permitting the escape of the waters before dilatation has progressed to any extent—the first stage of labor becomes tedious, for the reason that no part of the fœtus can act as a dilator so satisfactorily as the hydrostatic pressure exerted by the bag of waters. In these cases the long fibres of the uterus practically draw the cervix up over the wedge-like presenting part of the fœtus, whatever that part may be.

These longitudinal fibres when in a state of contraction produce a **downward traction of the fundus** upon the fœtus tending to force it downward; this force is transmitted to the presenting part, in vertex or in breech cases, by the vertebral column of the child.

This downward traction of the fundus exerted by the longitudinal fibres when in a state of contraction, does not cause a drawing down, or descent, of the fundus uteri, because the circular fibres by their more powerful action tend, as it were, to straighten out the somewhat bowed fœtus; with the result that the position of the fundus in relation to the abdominal wall throughout labor does not vary; but the whole resultant of the forces exerted by the contractions of these two sets of fibres is transmitted down the vertebral column of the fœtus to the presenting part, which is thus forced to advance, while at the same time the cervix is dilated and drawn up over it.

Os uteri during first stage of labor: On making a vaginal examination very early in labor, in a *primipara*, that portion of the cervix not yet taken up may be felt as a soft appendage to the spherical surface of the distended lower pole of the uterus. Possibly the external os may be sufficiently soft and dilated to permit the insertion of the finger-tip. Under the same circumstances in a *multipara* the os may be quite patent long before the cervix is taken up, so that the finger may easily be inserted into the uterus. Under these circumstances the only way to be certain of the extent of cervix still remaining to be taken up is to insert the finger till the membranes can be felt, then, while withdrawing it making firm pressure on the posterior wall, note the length of cervix before the margin of the external os is reached.

Later, when the cervix is completely taken up, during a pain the sharp edges of the external os can be distinguished, and the smooth surface of the membranes can be felt stretching across the aperture.

In primipara the edge of the external os is at first thin and sharp; later it becomes more œdematous. In multipara it may be thick, and as a result of laceration in a previous labor the external os may have a very irregular shape.·

The degree of dilatation may be described by stating that the os will admit one, two, or three fingers; or it may be compared with the size of a ten-cent piece, quarter, etc.

Clinical Phenomena of the First Stage.

The initial labor-pains come on, as a rule, in the earlier part of the night; and they differ but little from the false pains, except that they occur more regularly and gradually increase in strength and frequency.

The pains are sharp and nagging, many patients finding them more difficult to bear than those of the expulsive stage. Many prefer to walk restlessly about, bending over a chair or the foot of the bed during the acme of the pain. Usually a plaintive cry or moan is uttered with each pain, and the patient's face becomes congested owing to involuntary fixation of the respiratory muscles.

Reflex vomiting is of frequent occurrence as dilatation progresses.

The patient is compelled frequently to **evacuate the bladder and rectum** on account of the increased nervous irritability of the organs.

The **pulse** and **respiration** are not markedly affected, as a rule, in this stage, though in cases where it is prolonged the rate of both may be considerably accelerated; and the **temperature** may rise to 100° F., or even higher.

Anatomy of the Soft Parts at the End of the First Stage.

The **external os** is, as a rule, dilated so as to admit three fingers. The **cervix** is completely taken up. The whole **lower segment** of the uterus is thinned out somewhat from stretching; while the **upper segment** is slightly thicker than before the onset of labor.

The **bladder**, as a rule, is drawn upward with the cervix, the upper end being displaced forward over the pubes. The upper end of the **vagina** is somewhat distended.

LABOR—SECOND STAGE.

Mechanism of the Second Stage.

During this stage the **fœtus is expelled from the maternal passages.**

Vertex presentations being considered in this work as normal, and the left occipito-anterior position being by far the most common, the corresponding mechanism will be fully described at this point; while the mechanism of the other positions will be described only in so far as they differ from it.

The mechanism of this stage is concerned chiefly with the **movements** which the **fœtal head** and **trunk** undergo in their passage through the birth-canal.

The most important part of the mechanism is that relating

to the *head,* on account of its size and the incompressibility of its diameters as compared with the trunk.

The Head Movements.

These are : descent ; flexion ; internal rotation ; extension ; and finally, after expulsion, restitution or external rotation.

Descent: Descent of the head begins, as already mentioned, with the rupture of the membranes, or as soon as it comes into complete contact with the lower uterine segment, or os. It is *caused* by the uterine contractions reinforced by the action of the abdominal muscles and diaphragm, and persists throughout this stage, resulting in the other movements about to be described.

Flexion: The position of the head is naturally one of partial flexion, as it lies in the lower uterine segment at the onset of the second stage. As the head descends this flexion increases as the result of various *causes:*

(*a*) At the beginning of this stage the intra-uterine fluid pressure acts on the whole base of the skull, and flexion results from the different angles at which the anterior and posterior slopes of the vertex meet the resistance of the lower uterine walls. The friction offered by the wall to the anterior end of the head is greater and this end is more impeded in its descent, hence flexion is assisted. This is reinforced by the action of the circular fibres of the cervix compressing the head. The force exerted by these fibres not being equal and opposite, flexion of the head is favored.

(*b*) When the waters drain away sufficiently to permit the fundus to come into direct contact with the fœtus, then a more powerful force is exerted to produce flexion of the head. The propulsive force of the uterine action transmitted down the vertebral column of the fœtus acts on the head along a line running nearer the occipital than the sincipital pole.

The head is so attached to the trunk that its sincipital is longer than its occipital pole; it corresponds to a lever with unequal arms, the occipito-atlantoid articulation being the pivotal point, and the sincipital the long arm of the lever. Hence the sincipital pole is more acted on by the resistance offered to descent, while the occipital pole receives the maxmum pressure from above (Fig. 62).

Thus is flexion produced and maintained.

The **advantage** of flexion is that it brings the smallest, or suboccipito-bregmatic, circumference of the head into relation with the girdle of resistance offered by the pelvis and soft parts. It also results in the occiput reaching the pelvic floor in advance of any other part of the head, a point of very considerable importance, as will be seen later.

When **flexion is complete** the posterior fontanelle is brought within easy reach of the examining finger. At this time if the sagittal suture be felt, it seems to lie nearer to the posterior than to the anterior wall of the pelvis, and the head seems to occupy a somewhat oblique position in the pelvis as regards the plane of the brim, the anterior or right parietal bone seeming to be at a lower level than is the left parietal bone. This led Naegele to infer that the head usually

Fig. 62.

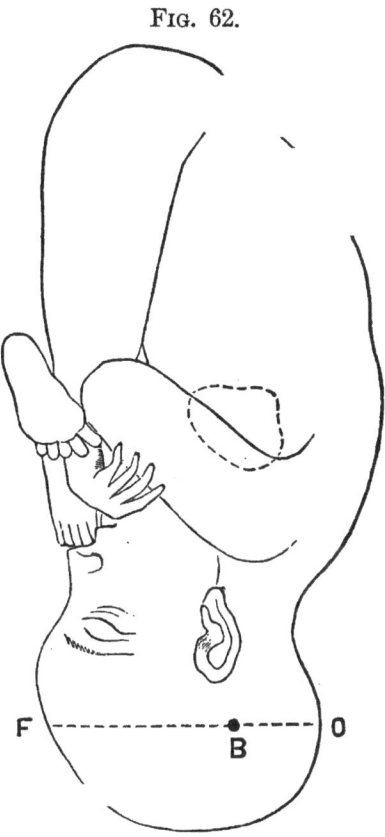

Illustrating the different lengths of the frontal arm, F B, and the occipital arm, B O, of the lever presented by the fœtal head. (Jewett.)

entered the pelvis with the sagittal suture nearer to the promontory than to the pubes. This is not a real but an apparent obliquity, and is due to the pelvic inclination. The head normally enters the pelvis with its horizontal plane in complete coincidence with the plane of the brim. This condi-

8—Obst.

tion is known as *synclitism*. The absence of the proper relation of these planes is known as *asynclitism*, a condition which usually occurs when any deformity of the pelvis is present.

Internal rotation: The long diameter of the fœtal head occupies the right oblique diameter of the brim when the position is L. O. A., but it must emerge at the outlet with its long diameter directed anteroposteriorly, because this diameter of the outlet is the greater. The movement by which the

FIG. 63.

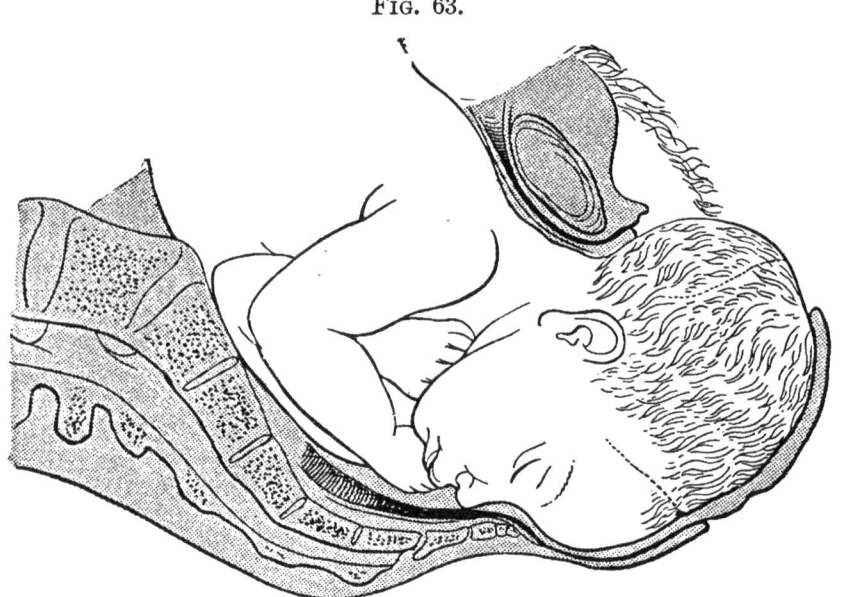

Beginning extension of head. (Farabeuf and Varnier)

oblique position at the brim is converted into an anteroposterior position at the outlet is termed *rotation*.

To secure internal rotation there must be good flexion of the head, strong uterine contractions, and a fairly resistant pelvic floor. When all these factors are present, the occiput, reaching the pelvic floor first, follows the line of least resistance, which is downward, inward toward the middle line, and forward in the direction of the symphysis pubis. The pressure of the head causes the pelvic floor to bulge, thus forming a trough with its outlet under the pubic arch.

The resistance of the pelvic floor drives the occiput toward the symphysis pubis, thus causing its rotation forward.

In anterior positions of the occiput its rotation is through one-eighth of a circle; while in posterior positions, as in R. O. P., it is through three-eighths of a circle, thus requiring a

Fig. 64.

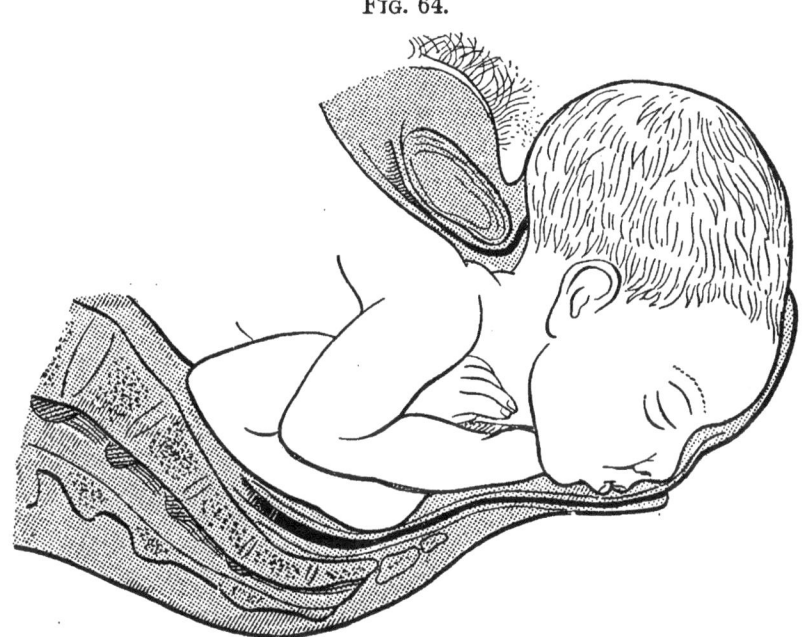

Maximum distention of pelvic floor. Equator of head about to pass. (Farabeuf and Varnier.)

greater driving force and a longer time for its accomplishment.

The head then descends into its new position, still retaining its flexion, further distending the perineum, until the occiput clears the lower border of the pubic arch.

At this time the rima of the vulva has been pressed apart, and the child's head can be seen forcing the lips apart during each pain.

Extension: The occurrence of the next movement depends

on the width of the pubic arch and the size of the child's head. If the arch is wide and the head well molded, the occiput soon pivots on the subpubic ligament and the extension takes place.

With extension the occiput comes out under the pubic arch, the chin leaves the sternum, and the face of the child emerges from the border of the distended perineum, which retracts from it, and the head is born (Figs. 62–65).

FIG. 65.

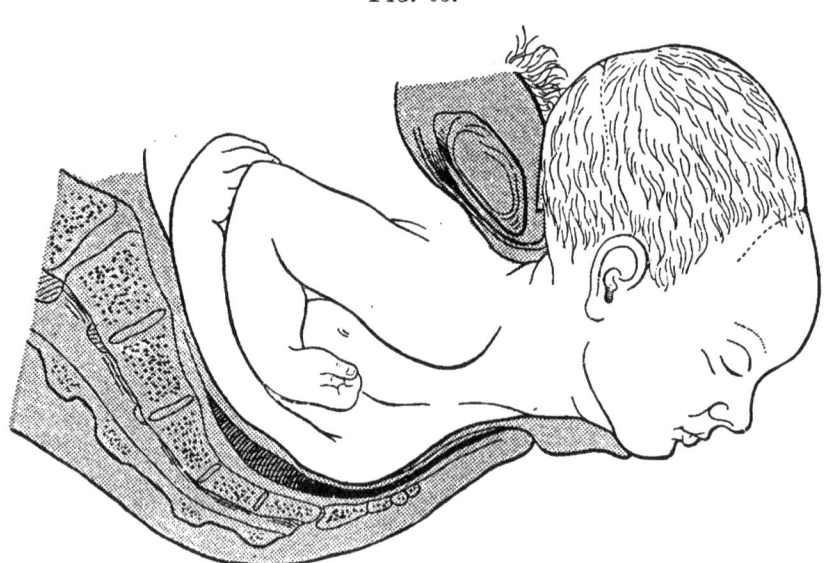

Occiput rides up in front of symphysis Pelvic floor retracts. (Farabeuf and Varnier.)

Restitution or external rotation : Directly after the head is born, it resumes its usual relation to the shoulders, namely, with its occipitomental diameter at a right angle to the bisacromial.

The shoulders enter the brim in the opposite oblique to the head ; thus in L. O. A. position they enter in the left oblique diameter, and as they descend the right shoulder comes to the front. Hence the head, when it escapes from the vulva, turns so that the occiput points to the left side of the mother, which is the same position it occupied at the brim. This movement of the head is termed *restitution,* and is of interest, as it indicates usually its primary position (Fig. 66).

Fig. 66.

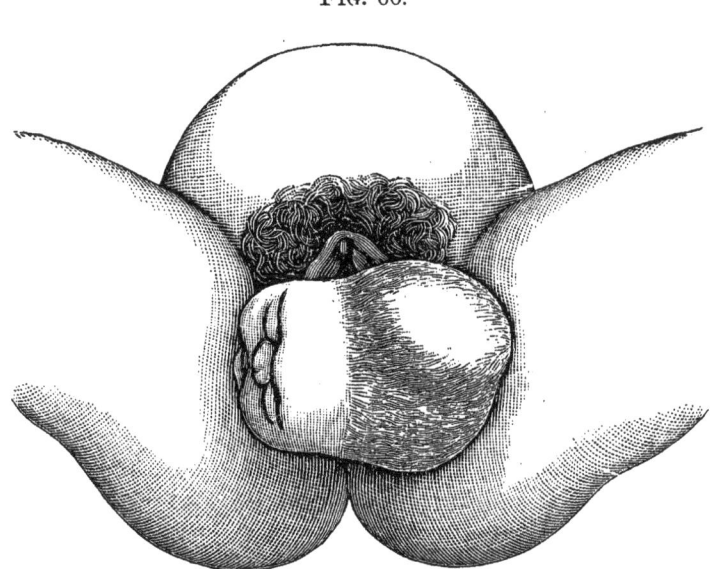

Fœtal head after restitution. Shows also caput succedaneum. (Ribemont-Dessaignes and Lepage.)

Delivery of the Trunk.

The anterior shoulder is, as a rule, arrested at the lower border of the symphysis, so that the posterior passes over the perineum and appears at the vulva first. After the posterior shoulder escapes the anterior descends and is delivered. The hips emerge with the bisiliac diameter in the anteroposterior position.

Clinical Phenomena of the Second Stage.

At the conclusion of the first stage the **pains** not infrequently cease for a time, and the more or less exhausted woman has a few moments of rest and possibly of sleep. Especially is this the case if chloral has been administered.

The pains are more severe during the second stage and last longer; but the patient becomes more hopeful as a rule, for she realizes that with each pain definite progress is being made. When the pelvic floor is reached the perineum begins to distend from the pressure of the head, and the sphincter ani relaxes, so that not infrequently a quantity of fæcal matter or mucus escapes from the anus.

At this time the contractions of the abdominal muscles are involuntary, and the patient is forced to **strain down** with each pain, holding her breath as she does so. As a rule, the woman grasps any support near by firmly with her hands and braces her feet, to assist her expulsive efforts.

In the **intervals between the pains** she rests quietly and may fall asleep.

When **the vulvar ring is being distended** the sufferings of the woman may become so intense as to result in a condition bordering on delirium. At this period the head advances rapidly with each pain, coming plainly into view as it does so. In the intervals it recedes, thus permitting the circulation of blood in the perineum to be resumed.

If this recession does not take place, œdema of the parts rapidly comes on, and may be very marked in some cases.

Usually there is a **pause** when the head is born.

Accompanying the delivery of the body there is a **gush** of waters and blood.

After the birth of the child the woman soon quiets down, no matter how noisy she may have been; the freedom from pain affording her great satisfaction and a keen sense of rest. Her temperature at this time may be slightly elevated; especially if the labor has been difficult. The pulse-rate rapidly subsides and in a few moments resumes its normal frequency.

Moulding of the Fœtal Head.

The child's head, even in normal labor, undergoes considerable alteration in shape as it is forced through the maternal passages.

The **manner** in which the bones overlap has been already referred to.

The **degree** of moulding depends on the relative size of the head and the pelvis, and also upon the extent of ossification present.

The moulding of the head is **essential** to the mechanism of the expulsive stage in that it leads to adaptation of the head to the pelvis; and also because its *elongation* favors rotation by increasing the dip of the leading pole, so that it is more easily directed forward.

Elongation: In L. O. A. and L. O. P. positions the elongation of the head is along a line joining the chin to the posterior upper angle of the right parietal bone.

In R. O. A. and R. O. P. positions the elongation of the head is along a line joining the chin to the posterior upper angle of the left parietal bone.

This deformity is accentuated by the *caput succedaneum.*

Caput Succedaneum.

Definition: The caput succedaneum is an œdematous swelling which is developed on the presenting part in the course of birth, usually after rupture of the membranes. The vessels of the presenting part become engorged during the pains, and serous exudation takes place into that portion of the fœtal surface which escapes the pressure of the girdle of resistance.

Its **size** varies with the degree of force producing it; hence it is large in difficult and prolonged labors. Its size is an indication of the degree of obstruction encountered by the fœtus in its passage through the pelvis.

Its **location** indicates the position in which the head has descended. In anterior positions it is situated on the posterior, and in the posterior positions on the anterior aspect of the summit of the head. In left positions it is on the right; and in right positions it is on the left of the median line.

The exact position of the caput may be modified if the head has been subjected to prolonged pressure at the outlet or at the vulva.

Anatomy of the Second Stage.

When the head is in the distended perineum the shoulders lie just within the dilated cervix.

The **uterus** has retracted on that part of the fœtus remaining inside it. The differentiation between its upper and lower segments has become marked; and if the labor is a difficult one, the retraction-ring may be felt running obliquely across the uterus a short distance above the pubes. The higher this ring is felt the more serious is the obstruction which has been encountered by the fœtus.

The **bladder** is now wholly above the pubes and the urethra is greatly elongated; hence catheterization is difficult and urination impossible, the pressure of the head increasing the difficulty.

The **structures in the sacral segment** of the pelvic floor have been pushed downward and backward; the contents of the rectum are forced out by the pressure of the head; and the anus has become widely distended, permitting the anterior wall of the rectum to come into view. The edges of the vulva are forced apart and they may be œdematous.

LABOR—THIRD STAGE.

This stage of labor is occupied with the detachment and expulsion of the placenta and the membranes.

Mechanism of the Third Stage.

Separation of the Placenta.

The placenta is separated by **retraction** and **contraction** of the uterus.

Many theories have been advanced to explain the **method** of placental separation; and the following description is but a summary of those most generally accepted.

As a result of retraction of the uterus after expulsion of the child the placenta is compressed to about one-half its original size before detachment occurs.

The method of its detachment depends on its *site*.

If the **site** be confined to the wall and does not encroach on the fundus, the separation probably begins at the margins and advances toward the centre. If the placental attachment is to any extent fundal, the placenta, as the result of uterine retraction, becomes bent over at an angle, and detachment will begin at its lower margin and detrusion will occur. That is, the placenta will slip down sideways as detachment goes on, being detached by the expulsive force of the uterine contractions.

As **separation advances** uterine vessels are torn across and some hemorrhage takes place.

In some cases this **retroplacental hemorrhage** plays an important *rôle* in placental detachment; and in all cases it renders easier the shrinkage of the placental site away from the placenta.

Separation of the Membranes.

As a result of the **protrusion** of the "bag of membranes" through the os, in the first stage of labor, some separation of the membranes from the walls of the lower uterine segment takes place.

After rupture of the membranes and escape of the waters the non-elastic membranes become thrown into folds and wrinkles, and as a result become partially detached in some places. The placenta, in the process of expulsion, strips the membranes completely off the uterine walls as it descends.

It is important that the amnion and the chorion remain **firmly united**: failure of these structures to adhere to one another results in portions of the chorion being left behind in the uterus, a condition it is desirable to avoid.

In cases where too early rupture of the membranes occurs, there is no "bag of waters," hence the membranes adhere to the uterine wall too closely, and no detachment of these can occur until the placenta in its expulsion strips them off.

Expulsion of the Placenta and Membranes.

As the result of uterine contractions, the placenta is **expelled.**

It usually **presents** at the vulva by some spot on its fœtal aspect about two inches from its lower margin. The presentation of the fœtal aspect is *caused* by the retroplacental hemorrhage leading to an inversion of the placenta, which has to strip from the uterine wall a portion of the membranes between its lower margin and the os ; hence this part is delayed to a certain extent (Fig. 67). The higher in the uterus the placenta is situated the more membrane has to be stripped off between its lower margin and the os, and the greater is the degree of inversion, or folding over of the placenta. The placenta never presents by its margin at the vulva unless its lower edge was originally situated close to the internal os.

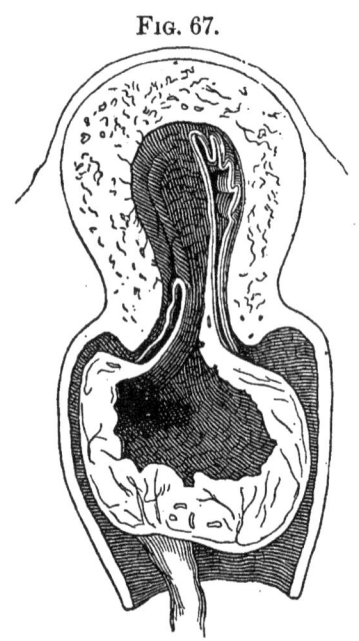

FIG. 67.

Inversion of the ovum and expulsion of the placenta as an inverted umbrella. (Schultze.)

The **membranes are dragged** out by the descent of the placenta ; hence they are usually inverted and the amnion appears outermost.

The whole mass of placenta and membranes is **accompanied** by a variable amount of clots and fluid blood, these coming from the placental site.

After expulsion of the afterbirth the uterus is found retracted and contracted to about the size of the fœtal head. Its *size* varies with the amount of retraction and with the size of the child.

The **position of the fundus** immediately after labor is about half-way between the pubes and umbilicus. Later, when the paralyzed lower segment has regained its tone by retraction, the fundus rises to a position about the level of the umbilicus.

Labor is now completed, and the puerperal period begins.

Blood lost in labor: The average amount of blood lost in labor is about six to ten ounces. The total quantity varies considerably. Women who menstruate profusely habitually lose more than those whose menstruation is usually scanty.

THE MANAGEMENT OF NORMAL LABOR.

In the management of a case of labor it is the duty of the physician to assist the woman in the processes of labor when required, in order that she may be spared unnecessary suffering and discomfort; and also to protect her from any infection which might be imported from without.

It has already been mentioned that it is desirable in every case to make a preliminary examination of the patient about four weeks before the expected confinement. Besides the ordinary obstetric examination, the *general condition* of the patient should be noted at this time. Any irregularities should be corrected, and everything should be arranged so that at the date of the expected labor the patient's strength and vitality shall be the best possible.

OBSTETRIC ANTISEPSIS.

In 1847 Ignatius P. Semmelweis, having been deeply impressed by the heavy mortality in the Vienna Maternity, first applied the antiseptic method to the management of labor. By simply compelling students attending all cases of labor to cleanse the hands thoroughly in chlorine-water, he reduced the mortality in the maternity clinic from 12 per cent. to under 2 per cent. in less than a year.

Since that date the mortality from puerperal sepsis in all maternity hospitals has been reduced to considerably under 1 per cent.

That the application of the antiseptic method to the management of *private labor cases* has not been as widespread is evidenced by the fact that the mortality-returns, both in Britain and America, show there has been but little decrease in the number of deaths due to puerperal sepsis in recent years.

The great numbers of women who throng the gynecologic clinics in all parts of the country, suffering from disease dating from a previous confinement, are witnesses to the fact that the application of the antiseptic method to the conduct of labor is still far from being as general as it should be.

Antiseptic Agents.

Soap and hot water are probably the most valuable agents. Many who practise obstetrics neglect these, while making use of some *antiseptic drug* in solution, which blinds them to the fact that asepsis is more important than antisepsis.

The plentiful use of soap and hot water accompanied by muscle and common sense would greatly reduce not only mortality, but also morbidity in obstetric work, even if antiseptics had never been heard of.

The use of these agents should always precede the employment of antiseptics.

Heat, either dry or moist, is the most general and available germicide.

All **utensils** employed about a puerperal woman should be at least scalded thoroughly with hot water, and where possible should be boiled.

All **dressings** or material which it is intended to use as vulvar pads should be boiled or steamed before labor, and kept carefully wrapped up until used.

All **instruments** should be boiled for at least five minutes in a 1 per cent. soda solution, after which they may be placed in sterilized water.

All **water** used in the labor-room should be boiled, and then kept covered until wanted.

In fact, **cleanliness** in all that pertains to the woman, not only during labor, but for two weeks subsequently, is absolutely necessary if it is desired to have fever-free obstetric cases.

In all **details** the method followed should be as simple as possible.

Chemical Antiseptics.

The most useful chemical germicides are *mercuric chloride; lysol;* and *formalin.*

Creolin and permanganate of potassium are also very commonly employed in obstetric practice.

It should be **remembered** that soap decomposes mercuric chloride and permanganate of potassium, rendering them inert;

that carbolic acid and permanganate of potassium are incompatible ; that mercuric chloride is decomposed in the presence of albumin, forming therewith an inert albuminate of mercury.

Convenience and accuracy are secured by using **tablets** containing *mercuric chloride.* Sublimate solutions are used in strengths of from 1 : 5000 to 1 : 500.

Formalin solutions are now replacing sublimate solutions for douching purposes, as they are free from the objections connected with the use of the latter. Formalin solutions vary in strength from 1 : 2000 to 1 : 500 as ordinarily used. The strength of the usual commercial *formalin* is 40 per cent. of the gaseous compound formaldehyde in water.

In the **application** of the antiseptic method to the conduct of labor not only are the *obstetrician* and the *nurse* concerned, but also the *patient.*

The Obstetrician.

The obstetrician should always be careful to keep **his hands** not only clean, but also in good condition. He should avoid as far as possible any work which will render his hands rough and hard. Care should be taken to keep the skin intact, for cuts, scratches, and chapping all render the making of the hands surgically clean an impossibility. Should there be any of these conditions present, it is the duty of the obstetrician to wear aseptic **rubber gloves** when conducting a case of labor. Care should be taken not to *handle septic material ;* if compelled to do so, the hands should be sterilized repeatedly subsequently.

The **nails** should receive particular attention. They should be cut short and well filed, so that ragged edges may not be left to scratch or injure in the slightest degree the maternal soft parts.

There are **two methods of sterilizing the hands**, both of which are probably equally efficacious. These may be designated respectively (1) the *sublimate method ;* (2) the *permanganate method.*

The Sublimate Method.

(*a*) The hands and forearms are **scrubbed** thoroughly for five minutes with a nail-brush, using water as hot as can be borne and a good soap; either an ethereal or alcoholic solution of green soap being the best for this purpose. Special attention must be paid to the nails and subungual spaces.

(*b*) After thorough rinsing in plain sterilized water, the **nails** should be cleansed with a nail-cleaner or sterilized manicure-stick.

(*c*) Then the hands and forearms are laved with **pure alcohol**, to dehydrate the skin, for at least one minute.

(*d*) The next step is to immerse the hands in a *hot* 1 : 2000 solution of **mercuric chloride** for from three to five minutes.

The Permanganate Method.

The hands and forearms are **scrubbed** and cleaned as in steps *a* and *b* of the preceding method.

(*c*) They are then immersed for five minutes in a hot saturated solution of **potassium permanganate**, vigorous friction being applied by means of a sterilized swab, till the skin is stained a rich mahogany-brown.

(*d*) Then they are bathed in a hot saturated solution of **oxalic acid** till the brown stain has been completely removed. This may be followed by rinsing in plain sterilized warm water or a 1 : 1000 sublimate solution.

It is much to be desired that the obstetrician should follow the operating surgeon's example not only in the preparation of his hands, but in wearing a freshly laundried, or, better, **sterilized, long coat-gown** of linen or duck, when attending a case of labor.

The Nurse.

The nurse should be no less particular in her attention to detail, in the application of the antiseptic method to the conduct of labor.

The nurse should make an entire **change of clothing**, after taking a bath, before assuming charge of a patient in labor.

Her clothing should be absolutely clean, and she should wear wash-dresses.

If she has recently been **exposed to sepsis**, it is her duty to inform the physician of the fact before taking charge of a case of labor.

Before attending to the vulva of the patient the nurse should sterilize her **hands** thoroughly, and the process should be repeated each time she has occasion to cleanse the parts.

The Patient.

The aseptic preparation of the patient **should begin** weeks before the expected date of labor. She should be informed of the importance of strict *personal cleanliness*. Any *diseased conditions* of the rectum, vulva, or bladder should receive treatment.

At the onset of labor the patient should take a warm bath and then put on clean linen. The lower bowel should be emptied by an enema.

The nurse should then thoroughly **scrub** the lower part of the abdomen and thighs with green soap and hot water, making use of a soft hand-brush, or a jute swab, for this purpose.

The *vulvar hair* should be clipped if it be too long.

Then these parts should be washed with a warm solution (1:500) of **formalin** or of (1:2000) **mercuric chloride**.

After the parts have been dried with an aseptic towel a **sterile vulvar pad** should be applied. The pad should be worn during the first and second stages of labor.

The **normal vaginal secretion** of a pregnant woman has been proved to be germicidal; therefore in normal cases no antepartum vaginal injections should be permitted. Not only is vaginal irrigation useless, but it may cause actual harm in impairing the secretive activity of the vaginal walls, thus interfering with nature's protection against sepsis.

PREPARATIONS FOR LABOR.

On the Part of the Physician.

The physician should give the patient a list of those things he wishes her to provide and have ready for the labor.

The patient, if a primipara, should be **warned** of certain conditions which may arise at the onset of labor, such as premature rupture of membranes, hemorrhage, etc., and instructed to send for the physician early.

The **call** to a case of labor should always receive the physician's immediate attention, such a summons taking precedence over everything.

He should go *provided with* such instruments and drugs as are likely to be needed in the conduct of ordinary labor and in the more important obstetric emergencies. These can all be carried in a hand-bag.

The **obstetric bag** should contain the following :

A pair of obstetric forceps.

Two pair of hæmostatic forceps.

One needle-forceps for suturing.

Needles, curved and straight, of various sizes.

A pair of scissors.

A Sims speculum.

A pair of long uterine dressing-forceps.

A double tenaculum.

A pelvimeter, and a measuring-tape.

A hypodermic case, well equipped.

A gravity syringe for douching, etc.

A long uterine douche nozzle, either of glass or metal.

Two soft-rubber catheters, Nos. 8 to 12.

Catgut, silk, and silkworm-gut for suturing.

Two nail-brushes.

A small package of sterile iodoform gauze.

A two-ounce bottle of chloroform.

A quarter-pound tin of ether.

A two-ounce bottle of syrup of chloral.

Antiseptic tablets or solutions.

An **apparatus** for the **subcutaneous injection of sterile salt solution** should also be carried. This may consist of a fair-sized exploring-needle, attached to a piece of soft-rubber tubing one yard in length, and a four-ounce glass or aluminum funnel.

Many physicians carry also a freshly laundried linen coat and duck apron, as well as a pair of rubber gloves. These latter may be sterilized and wrapped up in a package, not to be opened till required.

On the Part of the Patient.

The labor-room: Where practicable, a large, high, well-ventilated room should be selected for the lying-in chamber. It should not be exposed to contamination from defective plumbing.

The room selected should be thoroughly cleaned a few days before the expected labor if possible, and all unnecessary hangings and furniture removed, especially those likely to collect dust. It is well to have two or three **small tables** available for holding basins, instruments, etc.

All **linen** and other things provided for the labor should be kept under cover in this room, so as to be immediately available as required.

One dozen towels and a half-dozen freshly laundried sheets should be ready.

Two **rubber sheets**, or sheets of some impervious material, to reach across the bed, about four feet wide, should be provided.

The patient should also make or obtain a **labor-pad**, about three feet square and about three inches thick, made of cheese-cloth and filled with surgical cotton or other absorbent material.

Also two dozen **vulvar pads** made of the same material should be provided. These should be two inches thick, four inches wide, and ten inches long, and have tail-pieces attached to either end to fasten them to the binder. Two or three linen or cotton **binders** should be ready; each should be a yard and a half long and half a yard wide.

The labor-pad, vulvar dressings, and binders, as well as half a dozen towels, should be wrapped in four separate parcels, **steamed** for half an hour, and then put away and not opened till required for use.

9—Obst.

The following should also be provided : a bed-pan, a bottle of antiseptic tablets for solution, a fountain-syringe, four ounces of tincture of green soap, a half-pound package of absorbent cotton, and a one-ounce bottle of vaseline, as well as a skein of bobbin.

On the Part of the Nurse.

The nurse's **first duty** is to prepare the patient for labor, as has already been described.

The **labor-bed** should then be made ready. This should by preference be a single bed, with a stiff spring and a fairly hard hair-mattress. Over this a rubber sheet should be spread and then covered by an ordinary sheet, which should be securely pinned at each corner under the mattress. In the middle third of the bed another rubber sheet is then laid, covered over by a folded draw-sheet, both being securely pinned under the mattress at each side of the bed. On this the labor-pad is placed when it is required. The bed should be accessible from both sides.

The nurse should see that **everything likely** to he needed in the course of labor has been provided and is at hand for immediate use.

The nurse should see that plenty of **hot water** is at hand, and make ready two jugs of sterile water, covering the tops and placing them where the water will rapidly cool.

A pair of scissors and the necessary ligatures **for the cord** are to be sterilized and placed within reach.

A small bowl containing a solution of boric acid, and a few small cotton swabs, should be ready for **washing out the child's eyes and mouth.**

Wrappings to receive the child should also be prepared, and in winter kept warm till wanted for use.

Use of Anæsthetics in Labor.

Obstetric anæsthesia differs from surgical anæsthesia in that in the former the object is to blunt and not wholly to abolish the sensibilities.

The **prolonged** and **too free use** of anæsthetics during labor is capable of harm ; but at the same time it is the duty of the physician to relieve the patient of needless suffering and to spare her unnecessary exhaustion.

The **rule** should be to use an anæsthetic when the pains are not well borne without it. The degree of pain which some women can endure is wonderful, while in other cases the limit of endurance is soon reached.

Anæsthetics are usually **indicated** toward the end of the second stage of labor. At the acme of expulsion surgical anæsthesia should be induced, as a rule.

Chloroform or **ether** may be employed. Chloroform is generally preferred, as the necessary quantity is less bulky, and it is pleasanter to take. When partial anæsthesia is all that is desired chloroform is the more satisfactory ; but in cases requiring surgical anæsthesia for any length of time ether is undoubtedly the safer and the better.

Chloroform is said to weaken, and ether rather to stimulate, uterine contractions. Ether should not be employed when bronchitis is present, or when the patient is the subject of atheroma.

Administration : In cases requiring only *partial anœsthesia* the administration can be entrusted to the nurse, acting under the physician's direction. A mask or folded towel is held over the patient's face, and at the approach of each pain the nurse is instructed to sprinkle a few drops upon it. It is well in all cases to smear the patient's face with a light coating of vaseline, as the anæsthetic may occasionally fall on skin and cause considerable irritation subsequently should this precaution be overlooked.

Care should also be taken to remove any false teeth before commencing the administration of the anæsthetic.

When *surgical anœsthesia* is required for any length of time its administration should never be left to the nurse, but a physician should be called for this purpose.

MANAGEMENT OF THE FIRST STAGE OF LABOR.

Preliminary Conduct of the Physician.

The **physician** is usually the one person to whom the woman in labor looks for help and encouragement in her hour of trial.

His **duty** is to win the absolute confidence of the patient, and to inspire her with hopefulness and courage throughout the labor.

His **bearing** should be quiet and confident, and his manner, while firm, should be sympathetic and gentle.

The **effectiveness of a woman's labor** depends very considerably on the preservation of her self-control and the absence of strongly inhibiting emotions. The physician cannot afford to lose the intelligent assistance of his patient. Nor is he justified in adding fear or despair to her sufferings. Thus, whatever he may tell her relatives, he should, after his examination, give his patient the impression that all is satisfactory.

The physician is sent for at this time because the patient believes herself to be in labor. In this she may be mistaken.

On **entering the lying-in-room** the physician should not proceed at once to examine the patient ; but should try to set his patient at ease and permit her to become accustomed to his presence.

In a quiet, conversational manner, information as to the time of onset, the frequency, and the duration of the pains should be obtained.

The condition of the patient's general health since the last visit of the physician should be learned, etc.

While thus engaged the physician may watch for himself any symptoms of labor which may be manifest, and at the same time he should observe his patient carefully for any obvious sign of disease as shown in her face or bearing, and seek to estimate for himself the character and type of woman with whom he has to deal.

Should it be evident that **labor has commenced** the nurse may then be instructed to prepare the patient, if this has not been done already.

In any case the patient should have the **bladder and bowel evacuated** before any physical examination is made.

Obstetric Examination.

External Examination.

Preparation: The patient should be placed in the dorsal position close to the edge of the bed with her limbs extended and her head on a low pillow. The clothing should be arranged so as to expose the abdomen from the ensiform cartilage to the pubes. The physician, having washed his hands in hot water, may then take a position alongside the patient, either sitting or standing as may be more convenient.

Inspection: The prominence and contour of the abdomen should first be observed. The condition of the umbilicus, whether depressed or prominent, the presence or absence of striæ, pigmentation, or scars, and the condition of the flanks should all be noted. Evidence of uterine contraction and of fœtal movements should be looked for.

Percussion: The abdomen should then be percussed. In normal cases the dulness should be limited to central regions of the abdomen extending from a short distance above the navel to the pubes, while the flanks and epigastric regions should give a clear note.

Palpation.

Before proceeding to the actual palpation the character and temperature of the skin should receive attention. Then the degree of panniculus adiposus, and the presence or absence of œdema in the hypogastric region, should be noted. The shape of the uterus and the height of the fundus should then be made out.

The **upper borders of the pelvis** should then be examined by placing the tips of the fingers of each hand on either iliac crest, with the thumb-points resting on the anterior superior iliac spines. The relationship of the spines as regards the crests should be observed, and a rough estimate of the width of this part of the pelvis made.

The upper border of the pubes should then be located, for beginners are very apt to mistake the pubes for the head when endeavoring to explore the pelvic excavation from above.

The next point is to **explore the excavation** of the pelvis in order to ascertain whether it is full or empty, and, if full, the characteristics of that part of the fœtus occupying it. In order to do this the hands should be placed over the lateral aspects of the lower abdomen with their palmar surfaces almost facing each other, the finger-tips being directed toward

FIG. 68.

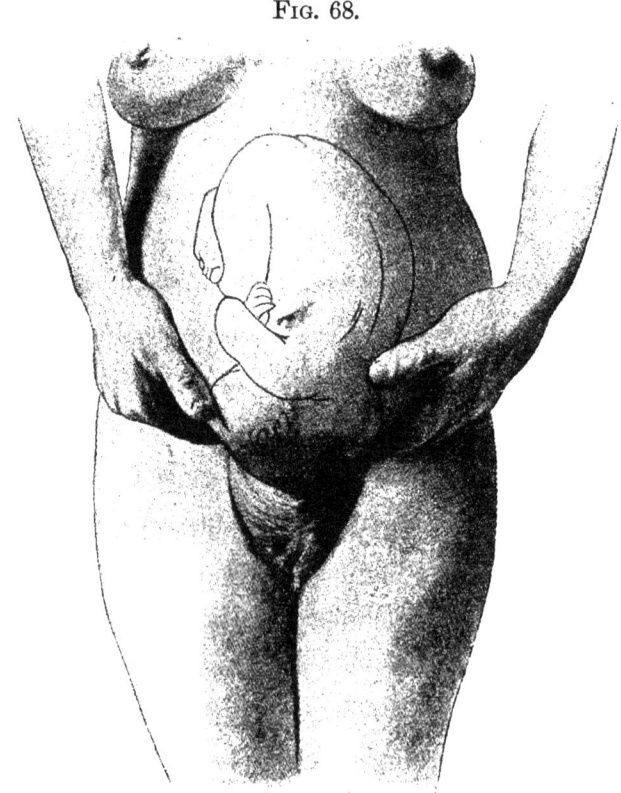

Palpation of lower fœtal pole.

the patient's feet and resting about an inch and a half above Poupart's ligaments.

The patient is then directed to breathe deeply, and with each expiration the finger-tips are pressed downward and backward into the pelvis, care being taken to avoid the pubes. In sensitive patients the pressure exerted may cause pain; in such cases this manœuvre can be carried out by a series of ballottement-like movements, and the information desired thus obtained with the minimum of discomfort to the patient.

If the excavation be occupied, the finger-tips are quickly arrested in their descent. The only part of the fœtus which

FIG. 69.

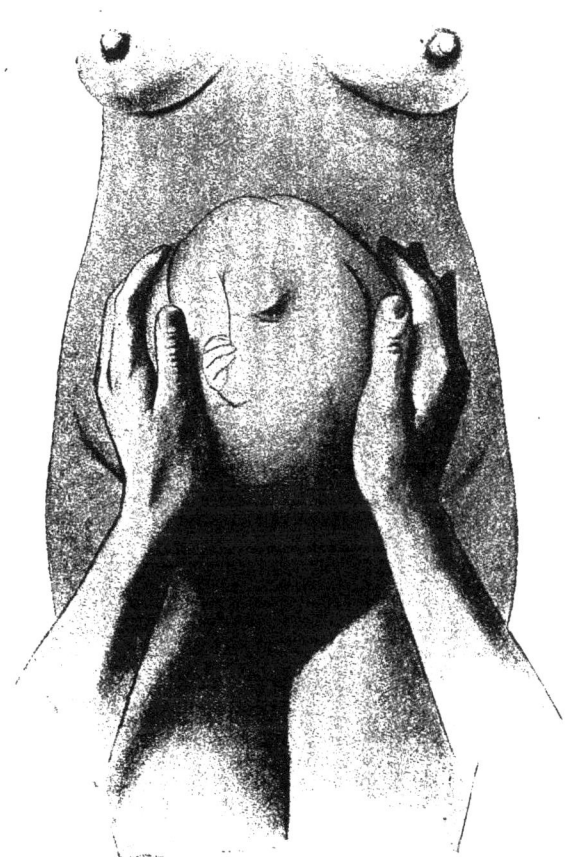

Palpation of fœtal back and limbs.

sinks into the pelvis before or very early in labor is the head. This may be recognized by its hardness and by its globular outline, which can be readily defined. The breech, on the other hand, is soft and bulky, and its outline very difficult to define.

Should the **head** of the fœtus **occupy the pelvis in the normal condition of flexion** (Fig. 68), it will be noted that one hand is arrested above the brim, while the other sinks to a lower level before meeting with resistance.

The part of the head which is thus most accessible is the brow. This condition is most marked in occipitoposterior

FIG. 70.

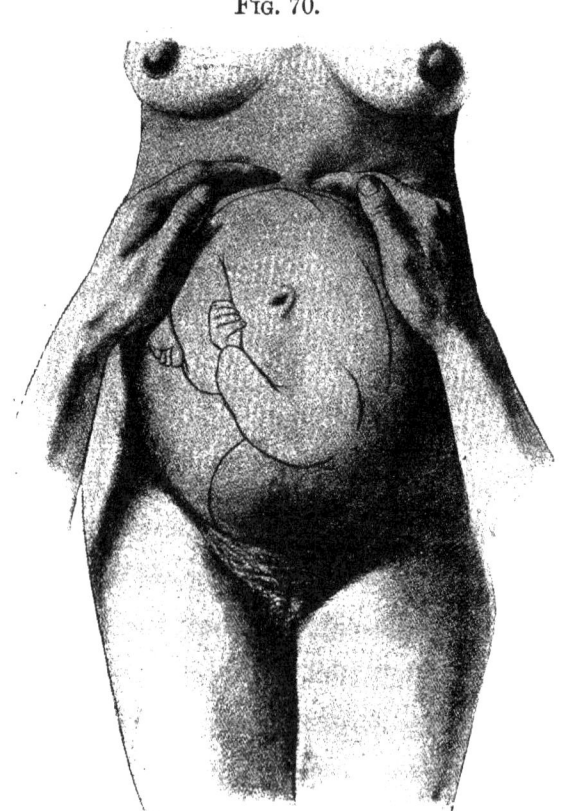

Palpation of upper fœtal pole.

positions of the head. Hence, if this fact be noted the position of the fœtus is pretty well indicated.

If the **head be located at the brim** and the excavation of the pelvis not be accessible, it should be noted whether it is engaged—that is, fast in the brim—or whether it is movable. If the head be found to be freely movable, an attempt should be made to engage it by pressing it downward and backward in the axis of the pelvic inlet, and thus to estimate the relative proportions of these parts.

The **upper pole** of the uterus is palpated by grasping the fundus firmly between both hands, having the finger-tips directed toward the head of the mother. By thus steadying the fundus between the hands, by flexing the fingers the upper *fœtal pole* can be palpated for the distinguishing marks of the head or the breech. When the *head is at the fundus* it can be readily felt and is very susceptible to ballottement. The *breech* is not so movable, is much more bulky, and is more difficult than the head to define.

The fœtal back and limbs must then be located.

The **back** offers a broad resisting surface, which is somewhat convex from end to end. In certain positions it is not possible to feel the back, but in this case the lateral plane of the fœtus can be felt; it is narrower than the back, not convex, and the shoulder can generally be located without difficulty by making firm pressure downward on the fundus with one hand; the back, if directed to the front, can be more readily palpated with the other. This pressure in the long axis of the fœtus increases the convexity of the dorsal plane and renders it more accessible.

The **limbs** are felt as small nodules, knees, heels, elbows, etc., which slip about freely under the touch.

If the **small parts** are numerous and found near the middle line of the abdomen, a posterior position of the fœtus is indicated. Finding of the small parts in one section of the abdomen confirms the location of the dorsum in the opposite region; thus, small parts to the right indicate a left, and small parts to the left indicate a right, position of the fœtus.

Auscultation.

Auscultation is **best practised** with the binaural stethoscope. It is a mistake to press the bell of the instrument firmly on the abdominal wall; it should be allowed to rest lightly upon the skin, being steadied by the slightest touch of one finger on the cross-bar.

The *first object* is to locate the point at which the fœtal heart is heard with maximum intensity.

The **fœtal heart-sounds** are transmitted most loudly through the back, generally about the lower angle of the left fœtal scapula.

In *anterior vertex presentations* the heart-sounds are heard best at a point midway between the umbilicus and the anterior

FIG. 71.   FIG. 72.

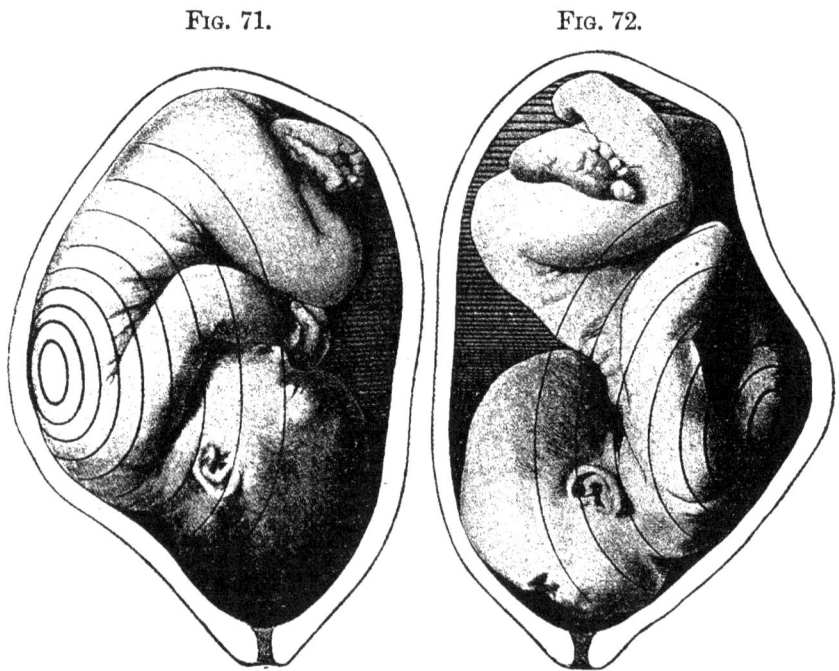

Auscultation for fœtal heart-sounds.

superior spine of the side to which the fœtal back is directed ; while in *posterior vertex presentations* their point of maximum intensity is in the corresponding flank.

Fig. 73 illustrates the points of maximum intensity of the fœtal heart-sounds in the various positions and presentations.

The sounds produced by the fœtal heart have been compared to the muffled ticking of a watch under a pillow, the rate being about 120–160 per minute.

It should be remembered that in dorsoposterior positions, in hydramnios, and in certain other conditions the heart-sounds may not be audible.

The loud rhythmic swishing-sound occurring synchronously with the maternal heart-beat, occasionally heard low down on one or other side of the uterus, is termed the **uterine bruit**. This sound is caused by the rushing of blood through the

Fig. 73.

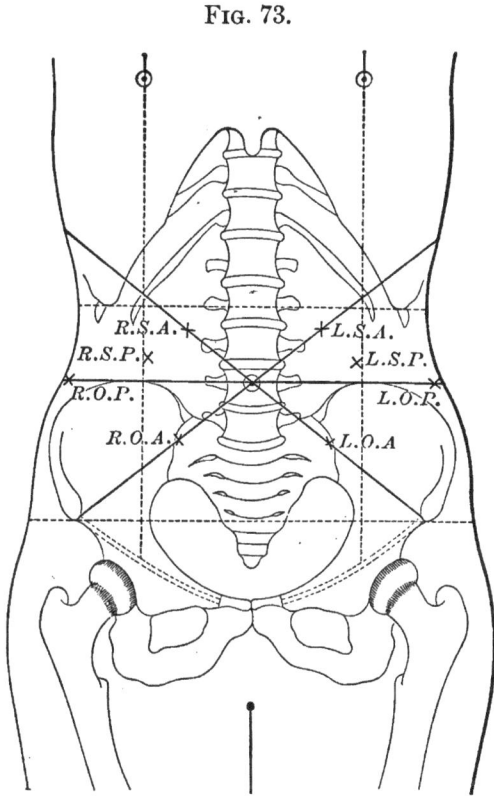

Illustrating the points of maximum intensity of fœtal heart-sounds in vertex and breech presentations.

enlarged uterine vessels, and is generally to be heard loudest in the neighborhood of the placenta.

Rarely a high-pitched hissing or blowing sound, which is synchronous with the pulsations of the fœtal heart, may be heard. This is termed the **funic souffle**, and is caused by the blood rushing through the vessels of the cord. It is, as a rule, only heard when the cord is twined around the body of the fœtus.

Vaginal Examination.

In cases in which the pelvis is normal and the vertex is presenting firmly engaged in the brim, and the fœtal heart-sounds are normal, vaginal examination is not necessary and may be avoided.

Should delay or any other complication occur in the course of labor, a vaginal examination may then be undertaken.

Preparations: The patient is placed on her left side, with her hips brought well to the edge of the bed and her lower limbs flexed. The clothing should be so arranged as not to interfere with the access of the examining hand, and a sheet is then draped over the patient. While this is being attended to, the physician should cleanse and sterilize his hands, according to the directions already given.

The Examination.

Everything being in readiness, the physician seats himself facing the patient's genitalia. The nurse is then directed to lift the sheet covering the patient, so as to expose the buttocks.

With his left hand the physician then gently cleanses the vulva with a pledget of absorbent cotton wet with an antiseptic solution.

Having moistened his right hand in the same solution, he then separates the lips of the vulva by means of the thumb and middle finger of this hand, holding the examining forefinger well flexed into the palm so that it will not come into accidental contact with any part of the patient.

Having thus exposed the orifice of the vagina, he then extends his forefinger, passing it gently in in the direction of the hollow of the sacrum.

Having already noted the condition of the vulva and vaginal discharge, he now examines the perineum and the posterior vaginal wall. The finger is then passed upward following the curve of the sacrum, which should be noted, until it reaches the posterior vaginal fornix.

The posterior lip of the cervix will now be felt, and is to be traced down till the margin of the external os is reached.

The finger is then swept round the external os, note being taken of its condition and of the degree of dilatation present.

The **bag of waters** is then felt if present; if not, the finger is inserted within the os until the presenting part of the fœtus is reached. This is then explored for **landmarks** and its position in the pelvis ascertained.

On withdrawing the finger ·the **anterior lip** of the cervix should be followed; and the anterior vaginal wall as well as the posterior surface of the pubes should be explored.

FIG. 74.

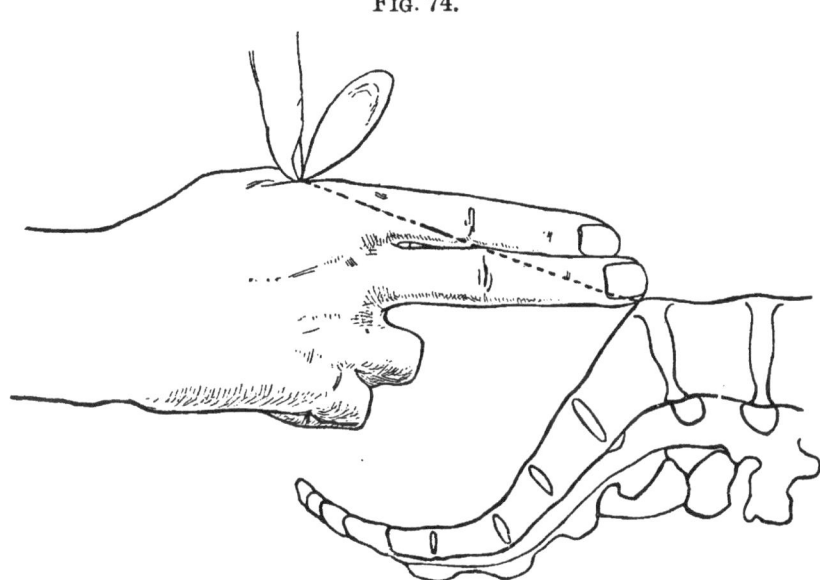

Manual method of measuring the diagonal conjugate.

The **capacity of the pelvis** should then be ascertained by sweeping the finger about in various directions. If possible, an attempt may be made to reach the promontory of the sacrum; if this can ʼreadily be touched, there is some degree of pelvic contraction present.

The **diagonal conjugate** should therefore be measured.

For this purpose the finger should be withdrawn and the whole hand again immersed in an antiseptic solution. The first and second fingers are then inserted into the vagina, and the tip of the second finger placed in contact with the most prominent point of the promontory; the radial edge of the hand is then raised until it rests against the subpubic ligament (Fig. 74). This point of contact is then marked by a finger-nail of the other hand. On withdrawing the hands the distance between the two points of contact is then measured and the true conjugate estimated (see Pelvimetry).

Succeeding the Examination.

Having now gathered all his facts the physician is enabled to make a **diagnosis**. It is unwise to venture a diagnosis till all the facts are in hand.

Predictions as to the probable duration of the labor should be avoided; but at the same time the patient should be given all the encouragement and assurance possible.

If the presentation be favorable and the part well engaged in the pelvic brim, the patient may be **allowed the liberty of her room**, and indeed should be encouraged to move about.

The **attendance of the physician** during the first stage of labor is not required, in the absence of any complication.

The **nurse should be instructed** to give the patient small quantities of *liquid nourishment* at short intervals. It is well to leave a couple of 15-grain doses of chloral to be administered to the patient, with an interval of twenty minutes between each, should her suffering become acute. The nurse should also be instructed to *keep the patient in bed*, and *to summon the physician* when the membranes rupture or on the occurrence of bearing-down pains.

Should the membranes not rupture after six to eight hours of moderately strong pains, a vaginal examination may be made, and then, should it be found that the tenseness of the bag of waters remains the same during the pains as in the intervals, or should the os be dilated so as easily to admit three fingers, then **the membranes may be ruptured**.

This is accomplished by a scratching movement of the forefinger, accompanied by pressure. Should this fail, a sterilized probe or straightened-out hairpin may be employed for this purpose, the greatest care being exercised not to injure the maternal tissues nor the skin of the presenting part of the fœtus.

MANAGEMENT OF THE SECOND STAGE OF LABOR.

During the second stage of labor the patient should be kept in bed. Her ordinary night-clothing should be turned up and pinned at the shoulder, so as to prevent its being soiled.

Position: The patient may assume any posture during this stage in which she can secure the greatest amount of comfort, provided there is no reason why she should be constantly kept in one position.

She should be encouraged to bring all her expulsive efforts into operation, and to this end her feet may be braced against some object, and she may be allowed to assist herself by either pulling upon the hands of a bystander or on a sheet-sling fastcued to the foot of the bed.

In **rapid cases** these measures should be avoided, and the patient instructed not to bear down, but to relax her muscles by short, panting breathing or by crying out aloud during the acme of the uterine contractions. In this way too rapid distention and rupture of the perineum may be avoided. The physician should be in constant attendance during this stage.

There is but little occasion to make a **vaginal examination** when the second stage of labor is established. Should it be found that advance does not occur in spite of apparently good uterine action, then a vaginal examination should be made to establish if possible the cause of delay ; but frequent examinations should be avoided.

During the second stage an **anæsthetic** may be employed to control and limit the expulsive efforts of the patient should this be desired, as well as to relieve her suffering. Not infrequently it is necessary to employ it in the first stage for the latter object. It should only be administered during the pains, according to the directions already given.

When the **anus begins to distend** with each pain, the head has reached the pelvic floor and rotation is under way.

Perineal stage: It is now the duty of the physician to watch the effect of each contraction of the uterus in advancing the head.

As the perineum begins to distend with each pain, not infrequently a small quantity of fæcal matter is expelled from the anus. This must be washed away, from before backward, so as to prevent infection, with pledgets of absorbent cotton soaked in an antiseptic solution.

Laceration of the perineum occurs in about 35 per cent. of primiparæ, and in about half that number of multiparæ. Prevention of this accident depends on the distensibility of the pelvic floor and the smallness of the engaging circumference of the fœtal head. Slow delivery of the fœtal head, by gradual stretching of the perineum, minimizes the possibility of rupture. Half the injuries occurring to the pelvic floor in general obstetric practice are preventable by skilful management of the perineal stage of labor.

The patient should at this time be **placed** on her left side, with her hips close to the edge of the bed. Her legs should be flexed and a folded pillow placed between her knees.

The **physician** should sit close to the edge of the bed, facing its foot. Near at hand on a chair or low table should be a basin containing an antiseptic solution, in which he may dip his hands from time to time, as well as ligatures for the cord, scissors, swabs, etc., which he will require as the case proceeds.

The rate of the descent of the head is **moderated** by controlling the expulsive efforts of the patient and by direct pressure upon the perineum. Should there be evidence of *œdema* of this region, hot fomentations may be applied, care being taken first to anoint the parts with sterile vaseline, so as to prevent burning.

As the **moment of delivery** of the head approaches the physician should slip his left hand over the patient's abdomen and between her thighs, so as to place his fingers on the occiput as it emerges below the pubic arch (Fig. 75). By exerting pressure with this hand too early extension of the head can be prevented, and any of the soft structures of the pubic segment of the pelvic floor, which may be caught in front of the occiput, can be pushed back in the intervals between the pains and held out of the road, so as to permit its early escape under the arch of the pubes.

The fingers of the right hand are held on the lower side of the vulva, and the thumb on the upper, while the palm covers the perineum.

As the **occiput escapes** under the pubic arch pressure is

made with the fingers and thumb of the right hand, so as to push the head forward, and at the same moment the left hand firmly grasps it in order to moderate the rapidity of its escape ; then the right hand is free to prevent the perineum slipping too rapidly over the face.

As the **head escapes from the vulva** it is well to have the nurse extend the limbs of the patient somewhat, which movement results in a certain degree of relaxation of the perineum.

Fig. 75.

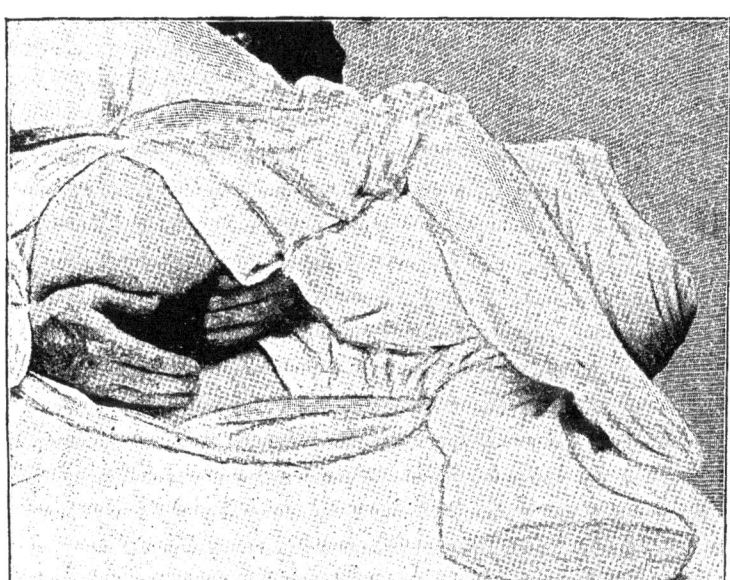

Protection of pelvic floor and delay of fœtal head. (Davis.)

With the hands placed as directed above to control the delivery of the head, this extension of the limbs interferes in no way with the physician's work.

During the **moment of delivery** the anæsthetic should be pushed so as to induce surgical anæsthesia, in order to prevent any unexpected movement of the mother and also to spare her agonizing pain.

Having **delivered the head,** the physician removes the mucus,

10—Obst.

etc., from the child's face before proceeding to examine the neck to see if it be **encircled by the cord.**

Should this be the case, he may draw down the cord and loosen the loop sufficiently either to pass it over the child's head or to deliver the shoulders through it; if this be impossible, it must be tied, cut, and the child rapidly delivered.

No effort for a couple of minutes should be made to **deliver the shoulders** after the head has been born, except when the labor has been long and difficult. Should they not advance, then the anterior shoulder should be reached if possible by passing two fingers over the dorsal surface till the arm is reached, when it is delivered by flexing the fingers, so that it moves over the chest.

The physician should then place his left hand over the fundus of the uterus, making firm pressure upon it, while at the same time with his right he pushes the head and body of the child forward toward the pubes as it escapes from the vulva.

Immediate care of the child: The nurse should then take charge of the fundus, while the physician attends to *clearing the mucus* from the child's mouth and to *cleansing its eyes.* Efforts should then be made to *establish respiration*, should the child not cry, by slapping it briskly or by sprinkling it with cold water. When once it cries lustily it should be laid on its side. The mother is then placed in the dorsal position.

The **cord may now be tied** an inch from the navel. A short distance beyond this a second ligature is placed, and the cord slipped between the middle and third fingers of the left hand, which is placed with its dorsum resting on the child's abdomen. The ligatured part of the cord thus lies in the palm of the hand, so that in cutting it there is not the slightest danger of the child's being injured by the points of the scissors.

The *fœtal end* of the cord should then be washed and examined to see that it has been firmly tied, when it may be wrapped in a dry piece of sterile gauze.

The **child** is then wrapped up warmly and put in a safe place till it can be washed.

MANAGEMENT OF THE THIRD STAGE OF LABOR.

In order to insure firm and continuous uterine contraction, either the nurse or physician should take charge of the

FIG. 76.

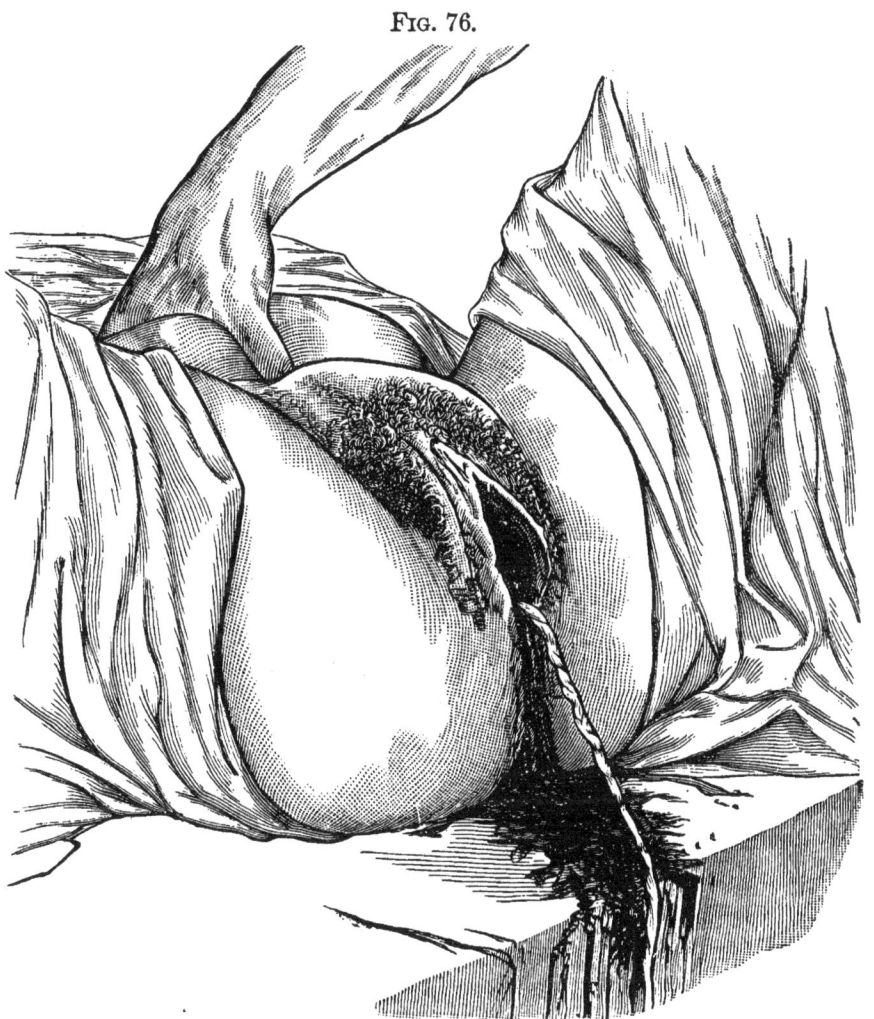

Credé's expression of the placenta   (Beers, from a photograph by H. F. J. After Jewett)

fundus from the moment the head is delivered till the uterus remains firmly contracted.   Should the uterus become relaxed, a few circular movements of the hand over the fundus will stimulate contraction and prevent hemorrhage.

A **sterilized bed-pan** or soup plate may now be placed under the buttocks so as to catch any blood that may escape from the vagina and also to receive the after-birth.

Lacerations: While waiting for the placenta to be delivered many physicians place the nurse in charge of the fundus while they utilize this time to examine the vulva and perineum for the presence of lacerations.

Should the lacerations not be extensive, they may be immediately sutured according to the directions given in the *Treatment of Lacerations.* The sutures should not be tied until the placenta has been expelled; but their ends may be caught in a pair of artery-forceps meanwhile. The advantage of passing the sutures at this time is that the patient is still partially under the influence of the anæsthetic, and the operation causes no pain.

Should the *placenta not have been expelled* in half an hour after the birth of the child, preparations should be made to deliver it by **Credé's method of expression.**

The patient's limbs are drawn up till her feet rest on the bed as close as possible to the buttocks, her knees being widely separated. The sheet covering her is then arranged so as to expose only the vulva. The physician should then sterilize his hands, for in cases where the placenta is found firmly attached to the uterine wall, in whole or in part, it is desirable that the hand be ready for immediate entrance into the uterus.

With his left hand placed upon the fundus so that the fingers are behind and the thumb in front of it, and the thumb and forefinger of the right hand grasping the cord just within the vulva, the physician, after kneading the uterus to secure good, firm contraction, makes strong, steady pressure downward in the axis of the pelvic inlet, at the same time squeezing the organ firmly. When the placenta is felt to detach itself, gentle traction may be made upon the cord so as to guide it out of the vagina.

Should the first attempt fail, it is repeated with each successive contraction until the after-birth is expelled.

Should the membranes be caught, they may be grasped by the fingers of the right hand and gentle traction made upward toward the pubes and parallel with the vulva, in order to separate them.

The nurse is now given charge of the fundus while the physician carefully **examines the placenta and membranes** in a good light in order to assure himself that no fragment has been left behind. Having satisfied himself on this point, he may now take charge of the fundus while the nurse proceeds to wash the vulva and remove all soiled linen from the bed.

Retraction of the uterus: Should the fundus not retract firmly after delivery of the placenta, a drachm dose of the fluid extract of ergot should be administered to the patient. In all cases the fundus should be gently kneaded for half an hour after the delivery of the placenta. When retraction is complete the binder or bandage may be put on, a fresh pad applied to the vulva, and the patient made comfortable.

The physician, before proceeding to wash up and collect his instruments, etc., should carefully **examine the infant** for the possible existence of developmental anomalies, and to ascertain that no injuries have been received in the course of delivery.

For *further directions* as to the care of the newborn the reader is referred to the compend of this Series on *Children's Diseases.*

Final measures: Before leaving the patient the physician should assure himself as to the condition of the fundus, the lochia, and the pulse. The nurse should be given full instructions with reference to the care of the mother and the child. It is well to leave the nurse one or two half-drachm doses of ergot to be administered should the fundus show any tendency to relax; she may also be left a prescription for relieving the after-pains should they prevent the patient resting.

THE PUERPERAL STATE.

The **puerperal period,** or **puerperium,** begins at the termination of labor; and concludes when involution and regeneration of the genital organs are completed.

This period varies in individual cases, but averages about six weeks.

The **physiological phenomena** of the puerperium are: the involution of the uterus and vagina; disintegration of the decidua and the regeneration of the endometrium; retrograde changes in the uterine ligaments, pelvic peritoneum, cellular tissue, lymphatics, bloodvessels, and nerves; alterations in the blood and circulatory system; changes in body-weight, temperature, and skin, as well as in the urinary and alimentary systems; and finally the establishment of lactation.

The two opposed processes of decay and regeneration occur simultaneously with great rapidity in the puerperium. These processes, which involve whole systems and organs, take place in the natural healthy woman without affecting her subjective condition.

The puerperal state, though it is physiological, borders so closely on the pathological that conditions of disease may very readily arise.

Hence during this period the woman is so beset with difficulties and dangers that accidents and complications are likely to occur unless she is guarded and cared for with knowledge and skill.

Anatomy of the Parts Immediately After Labor.

The Uterus.

Position: This organ lies in an anteverted and anteflexed state with its fundus in contact with the anterior abdominal wall. Its *shape* is usually an irregular ovoid.

The **upper uterine segment** is thick-walled ($1\frac{1}{2}$ inches, 3 to 4 cm.), and is pale pink in color on section.

The **lower uterine segment** is separated from the upper by a well-marked line. Its walls being much thinner, are thrown into folds by the weight of the upper segment.

The **cervix** can roughly be made out, its walls being rather thicker than the lower segment. The lips are usually everted, resting on the posterior vaginal wall, and are flattened by the weight of the uterus.

The lower segment and cervix are much congested, and thus contrast with the bloodless body of the uterus.

The **placental site,** which measures roughly 4 by 3 inches, has a ragged surface, and is somewhat elevated. It shows the openings of the sinuses filled with clots. The **area of the attachment of the membranes** is paler in color and smoother than the placental site. Shreds of decidua are scattered over the surface.

The **cavity of the uterus** measures 6 to $6\frac{1}{2}$ inches (15 to 16 cm.) in length.

The Vagina.

It retains its usual shape, but is much distended. Its walls are thickened and their surface smooth and œdematous; they also present more or less evidence of contusion or abrasion.

The Vulva.

The **vaginal orifice** is stretched and torn to a variable degree. All the external parts are frequently somewhat bruised and lacerated, and may also present more or less œdema.

The **pelvic floor** is greatly relaxed and not infrequently torn, the edges of the wound in this case gaping somewhat.

The Bladder.

This lies in its usual position, and is once more a pelvic organ.

The Peritoneum and Broad Ligaments.

The peritoneum over the *body* of the uterus is smooth; but at the *sides* and at Douglas's pouch it is thrown into folds. The *broad ligaments* lie folded and to a certain extent compressed between the body of the uterus and the pelvic walls. This compression of the broad ligaments must retard the circulation in the vessels contained in them, and so lessen the engorgement of the uterus.

The **abdominal walls** are relaxed and the skin usually thrown into folds and wrinkles.

Physiology of the Puerperal Period.

Involution.

The uterus : Immediately after the expulsion of the placenta the fundus of the uterus may be felt about half-way between the umbilicus and the pubes ; but in a short time, from one to six hours, it will be found to occupy a position at or slightly above the umbilicus. The dilatation of the lower uterine segment and cervix necessary to permit the passage of the child results in more or less complete loss of tone, so that the weight of the upper segment compresses them ; but as tone is regained they become capable of supporting the superimposed weight and the fundus becomes elevated slightly.

From this time the uterus diminishes rapidly in size, so that the fundus gradually sinks, and at the tenth day may be found at the level of the pelvic brim.

Involution of the uterus proceeds most rapidly between the third and the twelfth day of the puerperal period. The uterus never quite returns to its virginal condition, its cavity in the parous woman being about half an inch longer than in the virgin.

Changes in the muscle-cells : The firm contraction and retraction of the uterus, after labor, cut off its blood-supply to a very considerable extent, and thus being deprived of nourishment the muscle-cells rapidly undergo fatty degeneration. At the same time a portion of the cell-contents is converted into a peptone, which is absorbed into the blood and discharged through the kidneys.

It is doubtful if any cells are destroyed *in toto ;* for Sänger's observations prove that reduction of the uterus after labor is effected by a diminution in size of the individual cells and not by their destruction.

Changes in the uterine vessels and nerves : The bloodvessels, lymphatics, and nerves have all participated in the general growth during pregnancy. These all take on retrograde changes. The bloodvessels, which are closed by thrombi, are compressed, thus bringing their walls in apposition. Partly by organization of the clots and partly by excessive growth of connective tissue in the walls, the vessels become obliterated.

Uterine mucosa: The ovum when it is cast off carries with it chiefly the upper layer of the decidua, which remains attached to the chorion, and leaves behind on the uterine wall the lower cellular layer and the glandular portion.

Diminished blood-supply from uterine retraction soon results in loss of vitality in the lower portion of the decidua, fatty degeneration and disintegration of the cells rapidly ensue, and they are cast off in the *lochial discharge*. This process soon lays bare the glandular layer from which the new mucous membrane originates. The epithelial cells of the glandular layer as well as the interglandular connective tissue rapidly proliferate and form the new mucous membrane. This process takes about eight weeks to complete.

Lochia: The term *lochia* is applied to the discharge which comes from the vagina of the puerperal woman.

It is **composed** of blood, degenerated epithelial cells, débris of clots, mucus, and quantities of harmless micro-organisms. It **begins** after the placenta has been delivered, and lasts from ten to fourteen days.

Its **character** changes as the puerperium advances. At first it mainly consists of pure blood mixed with cervical mucus and small clots—*the lochia rubra*. In two or three days it becomes paler and consists of serum and mucus—*the lochia serosa*. About the sixth day it becomes thicker and is chocolate colored; but as the blood disappears and leucocytes become more abundant, it is white, having the appearance of thin pus, which it practically is—*the lochia alba*.

Frequently when the patient first assumes the erect posture the lochia again becomes tinged more or less with blood.

Its **quantity** was formerly greatly overestimated by Gassner, who gave it as about fifty ounces. Recently Giles, from careful measurement in a large number of cases, estimated the total quantity as being only ten and a half ounces.

Its **odor** is peculiar. The lochia rubra has the odor of fresh blood; but later the mucus from the vulvar glands gives it a peculiar and somewhat penetrating odor. Practically the odor may be defined as an acid odor when the discharge is normal. Ammoniacal or alkaline odor always suggests that putrefactive germs have gained access to the vagina.

Vulva and vagina: In primiparæ the hymen and fourchette

are invariably torn ; the remains of the former persist around the vaginal orifice in the form of small irregularly shaped elevations which are termed *carunculæ myrtiformes.*

More extensive tears of the vulva and perineum, if not sutured, heal by granulation and cicatrization, occasionally leaving extensive scars.

The vagina rapidly becomes smaller and narrower ; its walls from being smooth, gradually become rugated though the rugæ are never so marked as in the nullipara. As the hyperæmia of the parts passes off, the vulva and vagina assume more their previous color and proportions.

Involution also takes place in the **uterine ligaments, ovaries** and **tubes, abdominal walls,** and **pelvic joints,** all gradually returning more or less to their condition as before the occurrence of pregnancy.

Changes in the Circulatory System.

Pulse : The pulse-rate shortly after labor falls to about 60, or even lower. The cause of this lies in the reduction of the general blood-pressure due to changes in the constitution of the blood and also to the decreased intra-abdominal pressure.

The **blood,** probably as the result of hemorrhage during and after the third stage of labor, becomes deficient in red blood-corpuscles and hæmoglobin.

The **heart,** which has become slightly hypertrophied during pregnancy, quickly resumes its former condition.

Changes in the Urinary System.

The **urine** is not markedly increased in quantity. Peptone and acetone are said to be normally present in the urine of puerperal women. The occurrence of sugar is not unusual, especially when there is distention of the breasts. Albumin may be present for a few days, but its persistence is always of grave import.

The **bladder** not infrequently becomes overdistended in puerperal women and micturition impossible. The *causes* of this condition are twofold : First, the bladder is now subjected to less pressure than it was, because the greatly distended uterus has been emptied, in consequence of which the intra-abdominal pressure is greatly decreased and the abdominal walls flaccid ; hence the bladder has more room to distend and less resistance is offered to it. Second, small fissures about the vulva smart severely when the urine trickles over them, hence the woman is led almost unconsciously to retain her urine as long as possible.

The Skin.

During the puerperium the *sweat-glands* become unusually active. The skin is more moist and not infrequently during sleep profuse perspiration takes place.

The Digestive Apparatus.

The power of digestion of solid food is for a time enfeebled.

Thirst is usually present, and is easily accounted for by the great drain of water from the body by perspiration, the lochia, the milk, and the urinary secretion.

The **bowels** are apt to be sluggish, constipation being usually present, probably caused by the decrease in intra-abdominal pressure, the lax condition of the abdominal wall, and the great drain of water from the system referred to above.

Loss in weight takes place rapidly, as elimination exceeds ingestion during the puerperium. This loss is very marked in most cases, and has been estimated at from one-twelfth to one-eighth the body-weight in the first seven days. This diminution should cease by the tenth day.

Lactation.

By **lactation** is meant the suckling of the infant. It usually commences on the third day and lasts for about a year ; though after the seventh or eighth month there is a falling off in the quality of milk secreted.

The **mammary glands** are two large racemose glandular organs situated on the upper portion of the chest, anterior to the muscular structures of the thoracic walls. They occupy the space bounded above by the third rib, and below by the sixth rib; on the inner side by the edge of the sternum, and on the outer by the anterior axillary line.

They are epiblastic in origin and belong essentially to the skin; as do the sweat and sebaceous glands.

They are globular, and vary in size in different women.

At the summit of each breast is a small conical elevation known as the **nipple**, which is surrounded by an area of pigmented skin, termed the *areola*, in which there is a number of large sebaceous glands—the *glands of Montgomery*.

Internally each mammary gland is composed of from fifteen to twenty-four *lobes*, united by a certain amount of connective tissue and fat. Each lobe is divided into *lobules*, and these are further subdivided into a large number of acini or vesicles, in which the milk is secreted.

The *vesicles* empty their contents into small ducts; these excretory ducts from contiguous lobules unite to form a single large *lactiferous canal*.

Of these latter there are fifteen or more in each breast, each conveying the milk from a separate lobe to the nipple. The epithelium lining these canals is continuous with that of the integument.

Colostrum: Until the establishment of lactation the breasts contain only "colostrum," which is a yellowish fluid resembling milk, but differing from it chemically, in that it contains more sugar, fat, and salts. It has a laxative effect on the child, due to the excess of fats and salts it contains. *Microscopically* it can be recognized by the large, so-called colostrum-cells, which are simply large epithelial cells studded with fat-globules.

Milk is the secretion of the mammary glands. It is a yellowish-white fluid of an alkaline reaction having a specific gravity of 1024 to 1034.

Good human milk has approximately the following chemical composition:

	Per cent.
Fat,	4.00
Sugar,	7.00
Proteid (casein),	1.50
Salts,	0.20
Water,	87.30

The fats, sugar, and proteids are produced from the cells lining the acini of the glands; the plasma and salts are derived from the blood.

The **quality** of the milk is altered by varied conditions of the mother; mental and physical disturbances may so change the milk as to render it unwholesome.

The **quantity** of milk secreted varies in different women and at different times. At first about 200 c.c. is secreted daily, but after the tenth day the amount increases to from one-half to two litres.

The **secretion of milk** usually begins about forty-eight hours after labor. The breasts distend, become engorged with blood, and are painful or tender when touched.

When the breast is full it is hard and nodular to the feel, and milk may be expressed from the nipple on the slightest pressure.

The **establishment of lactation** may be painful, and may give rise to considerable emotional disturbance on the part of the patient, causing a slight elevation of temperature; this is, however, rare except in primiparæ. There is no such thing as the so-called "milk fever"; if fever occur at this time, it is a traumatic fever, and the result of infection only.

The Management of the Puerperium.

The **lying-in-room** should be in the quietest part of the house if possible. It should be well ventilated, and the light should be so arranged as to cause no inconvenience to the patient. It should be kept thoroughly clean and well dusted. The temperature of the room should be maintained at between 65° and 70° F. Soiled linen should be taken from the room as soon as possible after being removed from the patient. The patient's linen and draw-sheet should be changed daily.

Friends and relatives should not be permitted to use the room as a general meeting-place.

The care of the genitalia: The vulvar dressings should be changed at least every three hours during the first twenty-four; after this as often as soiled, or three or four times daily.

When the pad is removed the external genitals should be cleansed of lochia by means of swabs dipped in a 1 : 2000 bichloride solution and squeezed dry, before a fresh dressing is applied.

All manipulations should be carried out with the strictest aseptic precautions.

Care of Breasts, Nursing, Etc.

The child should be **put to the breast** for a few moments every six hours until the secretion of milk is established. This may be supplemented by an occasional ounce of sweetened water should the infant prove restless.

When **lactation is established** the child should be suckled every two hours from 6 A. M. to 10 P. M. Usually it is necessary to give one nursing during the night for the first six weeks. The importance of regularity in nursing should be impressed upon the mother, for without regularity it is scarcely possible for mother or child to do well. Overfrequent and irregular nursing deranges the infant's digestion and impairs the quality of the milk.

The **nipples** should be cleansed with a saturated boric-acid solution, both before and after suckling.

In drying the nipples only absorbent cotton or soft gauze should be employed, and care should be taken not to rub them.

Should they become tender or abraded, they may be painted with compound tincture of benzoin or with a 2 per cent. solution of silver nitrate, and a moist boracic acid pad applied to each.

It may be necessary to use a well-fitting *glass nipple-shield* for a short time, should the act of suckling give rise to irritation of the nipples.

Not infrequently, usually in women with large, pendulous breasts, considerable discomfort, even amounting to pain, is suffered when the glands **become distended with milk.** In these cases a snugly fitting *breast-binder* will afford great ease and comfort. Either the Murphy or the Y binder may be employed.

Contraindications to suckling : While suckling benefits the mother by promoting involution through reflex nervous action, and while there is certainly no food so suitable for the infant as mother's milk, there are still certain conditions which may render it unwise for the patient to nurse her child.

A feeble state of health, tuberculosis, and persistent albuminuria all contraindicate suckling. The same applies to cases in which syphilis has been contracted late in pregnancy, for it is possible the child may have escaped infection.

Inversion of the nipples, or severe and painful fissures, mastitis, or defective secretion, all act as contraindications of suckling.

Nourishment: As the process of digestion is usually impaired during the first days of the puerperium, the diet at this period should consist chiefly of fluids. Milk, clear soup, gruel, cocoa, week tea, toast, stale bread, and soft-boiled eggs may be permitted. After the third day a gradual return to the usual diet may be made. Malt liquors and wines may be permitted in small quantities if patients are accustomed to their use.

Rest: Everything about the patient should be so disposed that she may obtain absolute mental and physical rest. It is not necessary, *provided uterine retraction be firm*, for the patient to remain constantly on her back ; she may gently turn over to one or other side should she so desire. After the first day she may be allowed to rise almost to the sitting posture for a short time, should there be occasion, the use of the catheter thus being rendered unnecessary. All movements should be slow and deliberate, sudden changes of position being always avoided.

After-pains: In primiparæ after-pains due to uterine contractions are seldom severe enough to demand relief. In multiparæ, on the other hand, they may be so troublesome as to preclude all possibility of rest or sleep. Morphine gives relief, but should be used with care. Doses of $\frac{1}{8}$–$\frac{1}{4}$ gr. may be repeated as often as required. When it is undesirable to use this drug, antifebrin or phenacetin in gr. v doses, combined with caffeine cit., gr. ij, may be given.

Should the uterus remain lax and soft, an ice-bag should be kept applied to the fundus. Involution may be promoted by friction of the fundus ten minutes two or three times daily, and a pill containing ergot., gr. ij ; quin. sulph., gr. ij ; strych. sulph., gr. $\frac{1}{30}$, may be given twice or thrice in the twenty-four hours.   After the fifth day a hot vaginal douche, night and morning, may prove of value in this condition.

Visits of the physician : The first visit after labor should be made within twelve hours, and afterward one or two visits daily, as the case may require.   While the patient may be allowed "out of bed" when once the uterus has become a pelvic organ, still she should continue under the physician's observation until fully convalescent.

The nurse in charge of the case should record, morning and evening, the temperature, pulse, and respiration, as well as evacuations of the bowels and bladder, and the condition of the lochia.

At each visit the physician should note the record of the pulse, temperature, respiration, etc.   He should also examine the condition of the fundus, the bladder (bearing in mind the danger of distention of the latter), the breasts and nipples, the skin, the digestive apparatus, and the lochia.

The **bowel** having been pretty well cleared at the onset of labor, it is seldom that a purgative is required till the third day.   It is usual to give a dose of castor oil or other laxative so as to operate on the morning of the third day ; after this a daily movement should be obtained, and a mild laxative should be regularly administered if required.

The **infant's temperature** should be taken twice daily until two days after the separation of the cord, which usually takes place in from five to ten days.

It should be a routine practice to make a **bimanual examination** of the pelvic organs in the third or fourth week of the puerperium, with the object of determining the presence or absence of injuries of the vagina and cervix, the degree of uterine involution, and the existence of displacement of the uterus or other abnormal conditions.

PATHOLOGY OF PREGNANCY.

THE DECIDUA.

The **decidual mucous membrane** of the pregnant uterus may be the seat of disease, owing to the enormous hypertrophy of the mucous membrane incident to pregnancy.   These diseased conditions often manifest themselves in exaggerated forms as compared with the non-pregnant state. In consequence of the relation of the decidua to the ovum, diseased conditions of this membrane may have more serious consequences than in the non-gravid state. Most decidual diseases have their origin in either acute or chronic endometritis.

Acute Decidual Endometritis.

Etiology: This is a very rare condition. It may result from trauma, in consequence of attempts to procure abortion ; or from certain infectious diseases. When due to trauma the inflammation is frequently of a septic nature, and is characterized by the presence of an offensive purulent discharge. Deciduitis accompanying the development of infectious diseases during pregnancy usually results in abortion. This result is probably due to the hypertrophied mucosa, because of its vascularity, becoming the seat of an intense inflammation and participating in the eruption which usually affects the mucosa of the body in exanthemata.

The **treatment** in these cases consists in controlling hemorrhage, favoring abortion, and attending to complications as they arise.

Chronic Decidual Endometritis.

Occurrence: Chronic inflammation of the decidua is very common ; and is the cause of a vast majority of early abortions. Usually the inflammation of the endometrium ante-dates the pregnancy.

Two forms are commonly observed, a chronic *diffuse endometritis*, or polypoid degeneration ; and a *catarrhal endometritis*, or hydrorrhœa gravidarum.

In **diffuse endometritis** there is more or less *hyperplasia* of the connective tissue, resulting in great thickening of the decidua.

Should the disease advance with *great rapidity* an abortion will usually result, either from hemorrhages into the mucous membrane, thus separating it from the uterine wall ; or from the death of the embryo owing to crowding of the ovum by the rapidly thickening decidua. In the latter case the embryo may be absorbed, and the decidua afterward cast off as an empty sac with greatly thickened walls, forming what is known as a *fleshy mole.*

If the inflammation of the decidua be of a more *chronic character,* the pregnancy may proceed to term. In this case the parturition is likely to be prolonged by reason of the undue adhesion of the membranes; or great difficulty may be encountered in the third stage from adhesion of the placenta to the uterine wall.

In the **catarrhal form** of chronic deciduitis there is present not only a proliferation of the cellular elements of the decidua, but also increased secretion—*hydrorrhœa gravidarum.* In this form there takes place, every few days, a discharge from the uterus of a greater or less quantity of a clear viscid liquid having a yellowish tinge and containing albumin. Hydrorrhœa occurs more frequently in multiparæ than in primiparæ. The discharges may begin early in the pregnancy, but usually occur toward the end.

The **treatment** consists of keeping the patient as quiet as possible. An anodyne may be administered should uterine contractions accompany the escape of fluid. Vaginal douches are likely to do more harm than good, and should not be employed.

Atrophy of the decidua: Very often the decidua may fail to develop as it should during pregnancy, tending to prolapse of the ovum, and ultimately to abortion.

THE FŒTAL APPENDAGES.

The Amnion.

The amnion, being a serous membrane, is subject to pathological conditions, which may result in alteration of its contained fluid, and in the formation of plastic exudates and bands of adhesion.

Oligohydramnios, or Deficiency of the Amniotic Fluid.

The cause of this condition is unknown; it is usually associated with deformities of the fœtus.

The quantity of fluid may be so much below normal as

seriously to interfere with the growth of the fœtus and thus to cause its premature expulsion.

The condition cannot be **recognized** before labor begins. Labor is apt to be tedious, owing to the absence of the fluid wedge of the "bag of waters."

Hydramnios, or Dropsy of the Amnion.

Definition: The conventional limit of the quantity of liquor amnii is given as from two to four pints. Should this be exceeded the condition of hydramnios exists.

Occurrence: In frequency it is a comparatively rare condition, if the term be restricted to cases in which the quantity of fluid is sufficiently in excess to cause symptoms. It has been stated to occur in about 1 in every 150 to 200 cases; it occurs more frequently in multigravidæ and in twin pregnancies.

Etiology: Until the origin of the liquor amnii has been satisfactorily explained the etiology of this condition must remain a purely hypothetical problem. It may be due to oversecretion or to deficient absorption of the liquor amnii. Some authorities hold that this fluid is derived from the blood-current of the mother through the chorion and the amnion by transudation. Others consider it is produced solely by the fœtus, either as an excretion from the kidney and skin or by a process peculiar to the amnion.

Symptoms: As a rule, hydramnios does not develop before the fifth or sixth month of gestation, though it may occur as early as the tenth week. Usually the first sign to attract the patient's attention is the undue enlargement of the abdomen, which is usually out of proportion to the period of pregnancy. Thus at the sixth month the uterus may reach the diaphragm. This great distention gives rise to œdema of the lower limbs, palpitation of the heart, and dyspnœa. Locomotion becomes difficult, the functions of the liver or kidney may be interfered with, and icterus or albuminuria develop; sleep may also be interfered with, and the patient becomes worn and haggard.

On *palpation* the uterus is tense, and the fœtus, if felt, will be found preternaturally mobile; while on auscultation the heart-sounds may be feeble or inaudible.

Diagnosis: The condition is to be differentiated from twin pregnancy, ascites, and ovarian cysts, as follows:

In *twin pregnancy* the enlargement of the abdomen begins earlier and progresses more slowly; the preternatural mobility of the fœtus is not present. Two fœtal heart-sounds in different parts of the abdomen may be heard. It may be possible to palpate two fœtal heads and bodies.

In *ascites* the symptoms of pregnancy are absent, but it is quite possible that both conditions may be present in the same case. On percussion a dull note is obtained in the flanks, while the central portions of the abdomen are tympanitic. In hydramnios the dulness is in the central region of the abdomen while the flanks are tympanitic. In ascites change in the patient's position alters the location of the tympanitic areas. In ascites organic disease of the heart, liver, or kidneys will be found to exist.

Ovarian cyst is to be distinguished by the history and physical signs; the growth is more gradual and longer in development. Menstruation is generally present. The fluid wave is more pronounced. No fœtal parts can be palpated. A bimanual examination will permit the uterus to be differentiated from the tumor. The enlargement of the abdomen is not, as a rule, as symmetrical as in hydramnios.

Prognosis: For the mother this is usually favorable, but probably one-fourth of the children are born dead or non-viable. The risk to the mother is increased by the tendency to malposition of the child, by overdistention of the uterus leading to changes in its structure which render hemorrhages during and subsequent to labor more frequent, and by the increased liability to collapse following the sudden escape of fluid.

Treatment: The abdomen may be supported by a properly fitting abdominal binder; the patient should be kept at rest as much as possible. When the distention becomes extensive and serious symptoms develop then the membranes should be ruptured. When this is done the liquor amnii should be allowed to escape slowly and precautions should be taken to avoid syncope. Strychnine (gr. $\frac{1}{15}$) and fl. ext. of ergot ($\mathfrak{3}$j) should be administered after the placenta has been delivered, to insure good uterine contraction and to avoid the risks of post-partum hemorrhage.

Other Affections of the Amnion.

Amniotic bands : Early in embryonal life should there not be sufficient liquor amnii present to separate the amnion from the early formed skin of the embryo, adhesions may form between the skin and the amnion. As the amniotic cavity becomes distended the adhesive material becomes stretched, finally forming bands of greater or less length and thickness. No satisfactory theory has been advanced to explain the pathology of this condition. Braun regards the adhesions as resulting from folds of amnion, inflammation of the amnion being impossible, as it contains no bloodvessels.

The bands thus formed result in producing grave deformities in the fœtus, such as eventration, anencephalus, amputation of the limbs, etc. The fœtal cord may be artificially shortened, or even completely severed by such amniotic bands.

Premature rupture of the amnion : Several cases have been reported where later on in pregnancy the amnion has undergone rupture and yet the integrity of the ovum has been preserved by the chorion. The amnion in these cases is usually found rolled upon itself and forming a sort of cuff about the placental end of the cord.

Alterations in the character of the liquor amnii : The liquor amnii is a clear limpid fluid in the earlier months of gestation ; later on it becomes thicker and contains small whitish flakes derived from the vernix caseosa. In cases of death of the fœtus with maceration, the fluid becomes much thickened, of a dirty brownish or greenish color, and occasionally emits a fœtid odor.

The Chorion.

Hydatidiform Degeneration of the Chorion, or Vesicular Mole.

Occurrence : This is a rare disease, occurring once in about 2500 cases.

It is characterized by hypertrophy of the chorionic villi, and by their conversion into cysts varying in size from that of a millet to that of a hen's egg. These cysts are connected to each other and to the base of the chorion by pedicles of various lengths and are filled with a clear viscid fluid (Fig. 77).

Pathology : The degeneration of the chorion usually begins not later than the tenth week ; as a rule the whole membrane is involved and the fœtus perishes ; in fact it is seldom to be found when the mole is expelled.   The epithelium lining the

FIG. 77.

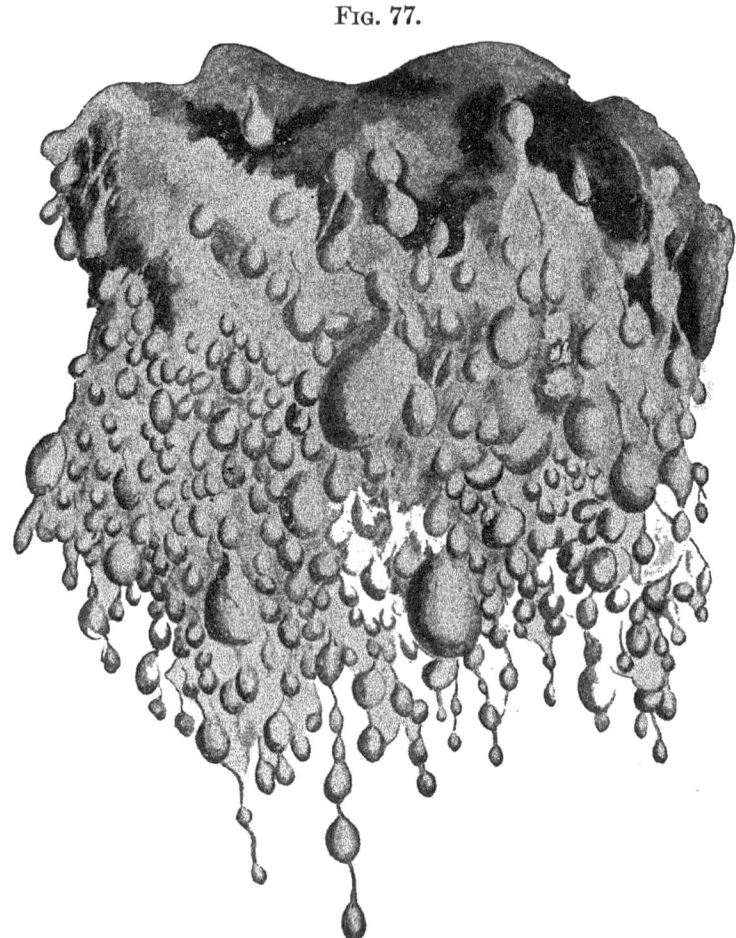

Vesicular mole. (Modified from Ribemont-Dessaignes and Lepage.)

chorionic villi is the part first affected, it undergoes a marked proliferation, which distends each villus, and thus the grape-like bodies are produced.   Occasionally when the disease comes on late it may be limited to the placenta.   In exceptional instances the growth may encroach on the uterine wall and even penetrate the peritoneal covering.

Etiology: Nothing definite is known as to the cause of the disease. The process probably originates primarily in the ovum.

Vesicular mole—symptoms: Three symptoms are available for the diagnosis of this condition :

(*a*) There usually occurs a more or less profuse *serosanguineous discharge* from the uterus resembling red currant-juice. This discharge may be continuous or intermittent.

(*b*) A *sudden and rapid increase in the size of the abdomen*, in which the uterine enlargement does not correspond to the supposed period of gestation.

(*c*) *The expulsion of cysts from the vagina.* This is the only pathognomonic symptom and is comparatively rare. The uterus usually presents a doughy feel and fœtal movements and ballottement are absent. The condition may be confounded with placenta prævia and hydramnios.

Prognosis: The dangers to the mother are sepsis and hemorrhage. This condition may lead to the subsequent development of chorio-epithelioma, hence all cases should be carefully observed for a few months.

Vesicular mole—treatment: The uterus should be emptied as soon as a diagnosis is established. The patient should be anæsthetized, the os dilated, and the growth slowly removed, the hand only being used for this purpose. Should it be impossible completely to clear the uterus in this way, then the blunt curette may be employed ; but it must be borne in mind that the uterine wall may be so thinned out in areas as to be very easily penetrated. This should be followed by a hot uterine douche and, if uterine retraction fails, the cavity of the uterus may be packed with iodoform or plain sterilized gauze.

CHORIO-EPITHELIOMA.

Chorio-epithelioma is a malignant variety of uterine tumor which may develop after any pregnancy. It frequently follows in cases of hydatidiform mole. It rapidly gives rise to abundant metastases, particularly in the vagina, lungs, and brain. The invasion usually follows the venous channels, being carried thus from the primary tumor in the uterus throughout the body. All these tumors, wherever found, consist of protoplasmic masses identical in structure with the syncytial layer of the chorionic epithelium.

Symptoms : When a primary tumor exists in the uterus metrorrhagia is common.   In some cases the first sign of the disease is the development of a soft tumor mass in the vagina or vulva.   When the lungs are infected, cough and bloody expectoration occur.   The uterus may be perforated and intra-abdominal hemorrhage prove fatal.

Diagnosis : Uterine hemorrhage persisting after a pregnancy, and especially after the expulsion of a hydatidiform mole, render imperative a curettage and microscopic examination of the scrapings.

Treatment : Excision of the uterus and all metastases that can be reached.

Prognosis : Most cases have proved fatal, though early diagnosis and prompt surgical treatment may offer a chance of saving life.

Anomalies of the Placenta.

Of **position, size, shape,** and **weight :** Normally the *position* of the placenta is near the fundus uteri, but it may occupy any position on the uterine walls (see *Placenta Prœvia*).

In *size* it may vary considerably.   In conditions of chronic inflammation of the endometrium the placenta may be abnormally thick and enlarged in all directions.   Atrophy of the decidua or interstitial overgrowth followed by retraction may cause the placenta to be abnormally small.   In this case the fœtus will be found ill developed.

The following varieties as to *shape* may be encountered :

Placenta membranacea : The villi may persist over the entire surface of the chorion and may all develop equally.

Crescentic, or horseshoe placenta : This is a very rare form.

Battledore placenta : In this form the cord is inserted at the margin of the placenta.   Occasionally an accentuation of this form is seen, in which the vessels from the cord branch out before reaching the placenta—this is termed a *velamentous* insertion of the cord.

Placentæ succenturiatæ : There may occasionally be found two or more distinct masses of placental tissue produced by the growth of isolated patches of chorionic villi.   The vessels of each patch course along the membranes to unite with those going to the cord. In multiple pregnancies each child may have its own placenta.

Diseases of the Placenta.

Calcareous degeneration of the placenta: Deposits of lime salts in the placenta are not uncommon. These deposits only occur as fine sand-like particles, or as scales. They usually occur at the edges, though they may be found in the substance of the cotyledons; and consist of amorphous phosphates and carbonates of lime and magnesia. They cannot be said to have any pathological significance.

White infarctions: Yellowish or grayish masses of degenerated placental tissue are to be found in nearly every placenta. When small and few in number they have no pathological significance; but if extensive, fœtal death may result.

Fatty degeneration of the placenta may occur as the result of some local obstruction of blood supply to the parts affected. Small areas are commonly observed close to the margin of the placenta. If extensive degeneration occurs the function of the placenta may be interfered with and the fœtus perish.

Placental Apoplexy.

Definition: This is an effusion of blood either within or behind the placenta. If it takes place before the third month the effused blood may force its way between the loose attachments of the decidua and chorion and thus result in abortion, a very common occurrence.

Joncquemin described three well-marked **forms** of placental apoplexy as follows:

(*a*) The effusion takes place directly into one or more placental cotyledons forming here and there small soft clots.

(*b*) The effusion leads to destruction of portions of placenta forming irregular cavities which are surrounded by infiltrated and reddened areas.

(*c*) The effusion may occupy a number of clearly defined irregular cavities of varying sizes, from millet seed to a pigeon's egg, which are not surrounded by areas of infiltration. In time these apoplectic areas lose their color, become denser, and form yellowish-white masses.

Causes: Placental apoplexy is determined by diseased states of either the maternal or the fœtal structures entering into the formation of the placenta. Most commonly the cause is *maternal* in origin, as nephritis and albuminuria, which produce increased arterial tension and venous congestion. Traumatism, as a blow or kick upon the abdomen, may produce it.

Rarely the cause lies in diseased conditions of the *fœtal villi* leading to rupture ; when the umbilical vessels are diseased, rupture of one or more of their branches may result in exsanguination of the fœtus and its death.

The **results of placental apoplexy** depend on the stage of gestation at which the hemorrhage occurs, the number of clots formed, and the extent of placental tissue involved. After the third month placental apoplexy but rarely results in abortion or premature labor. If the effusion is large and the placenta situated low down, the blood may dissect its way down to the os and escape, constituting *accidental hemorrhage*. Large effusions may result in destroying so much of the placenta that the nourishment of the fœtus is impaired to such an extent that it is born feeble and puny.

Placental apoplexy—symptoms: Slight hemorrhage gives rise to no symptoms; large hemorrhages give rise to pain and tenesmus. If these symptoms are produced, then death of the fœtus will probably follow.

Treatment consists in absolute rest and sedatives, such as morphine (gr. ¼), administered every six hours.

Placentitis.

This term is applied to an **inflammation** of the substance of the placenta. The condition is rare.

Pathological changes: Some authorities contend that by reason of the anatomical structure of the placenta a true inflammation cannot occur. But it is certain that a marked *hyperplasia* of the connective-tissue cells entering into the formation of the placenta does sometimes occur. This fibrous change may originate in the decidua serotina, the placental villi or the intervillous spaces. When the decidua serotina is affected the result is firm attachment of the placenta to the uterine wall, the so-called *adherent placenta.*

In the other two forms the placenta will be found to contain a number of firm fibrous masses. Occasionally the central portions of these masses may undergo a cheesy degeneration which appears very like pus.

Tumors of the Placenta.

Rarely either **cystic** or **solid** tumors of the placenta are met with.

Syphilis of the Placenta.

The syphilitic placenta is **characterized** by its thickness and density, while its general color is paler than normal. Scattered over its surface and through its substance are cherry-like nodules. There are present marked fibroid degeneration and great hypertrophy of the villi.

The **seat** and **extent** of the lesions vary with the manner and time of the fœtal infection. It is only by a *microscopical examination* that a placenta can safely be pronounced syphilitic.

Œdema of the Placenta.

A **serous infiltration** of the placenta is often observed with a dead and macerated fœtus. Interference with the fœtal or placental circulation may also produce this condition.

Anomalies of the Umbilical Cord.

Length : The cord may be found abnormally long, measuring as much as seventy inches, or abnormally short, measuring only two to four inches. Anomalies of *insertion* of the cord have already been mentioned.

Coils : The cord, if it be of unusual length, may be found encircling the limbs or neck of the child. It is most frequently coiled about the neck ; in extreme cases as many as six or eight coils may be present. In such cases asphyxia is common.

Knots: When the liquor amnii is excessive and the cord unusually long it may be found to have one or two knots, formed by the passage of the foetus through its loops. Rarely this results in the death of the foetus.

Hernia into the cord: A congenital *protrusion* of some of the abdominal viscera into the sheath of the umbilical cord is occasionally met with. It is due to imperfect development of the abdominal wall at the seat of the hernia.

THE FŒTUS.

Anomalies and Monstrosities.

Teratology, which is the science pertaining to foetal malformations and monstrosities, forms a special branch of pathology, reference to which must be had elsewhere.

Such malformations of the foetus as interfere with the mechanism of labor will be discussed under the heading of **dystocia of fœtal causation.**

DISEASES OF THE FŒTUS.

It is probable that **foetal mortality** exceeds that of any other period of life. It is impossible to say exactly what is the foetal death-rate, as actual statistics are wanting; but that it must be very high the frequency of abortion proves. Whitehead has stated that the ratio of abortions to pregnancies is 1 to 7; while Priestly, from a study of the miscarriage-rate in the well-to-do classes, considered the ratio of abortions to pregnancies as about 1 in $4\frac{1}{3}$.

But a few of the more important pathological conditions affecting the foetus can be referred to in a limited work of this kind.

Idiopathic Diseases.

Those originating, so far as at present known, in the foetus itself:

Congenital cystic elephantiasis: This disease is *characterized* by a great overgrowth of the subcutaneous connective tissue all over the body. At intervals in the hypertrophied tissue cysts are present, which vary greatly in size. As malformations of a grave character are usually associated with this disease, the subjects of it are usually born prematurely and scarcely ever survive the birth.

Anasarca: General anasarca of the fœtus is occasionally seen. The condition is usually associated with collections of fluid in the pleural and abdominal cavities. The subjects of this disease are usually born prematurely and seldom survive.

Ichthyosis: This disease is observed in two forms, the grave and the mild.

The *grave form* is characterized by the existence over the whole surface of the body of horny epidermic plates separated from each other by fissures and furrows, and associated with deformities of the face and extremities which lead to death of the infant soon after birth.

The *mild form* is characterized by the presence of a collodion-like substance over the whole body of the fœtus which later, by a process of desquamation, forms into flakes. It is usually associated with ectropion and eclabium. It does not, as a rule, prove fatal, but may persist more or less throughout life, or may terminate by complete cure.

With regard to the *etiology* but little can be said beyond asserting that heredity is probably the most powerful factor.

Treatment: Warm baths and inunctions with weak antiseptic ointments promote separation of the scales. Perfect cleanliness is necessary to prevent infection of the fissures existing in the skin.

Rachitis: That this disease occasionally occurs during intra-uterine life is believed by many. Children have been born whose bones were still soft and easily distortable ; while in others, in whom the disease had probably pursued a longer course, the bones were thick and hard, and set in the deformed shapes they had acquired in utero. The presence of the disease in the fœtus has been held to account for those rare cases of spontaneous fracture in utero, in which there has been no history of external violence.

Transmitted Diseases.

Those due to diseases in the parents :

Fœtal Syphilis.

This is probably the most important if not the most common disease of intra-uterine life.   Page has reported that 83 per cent. of premature and stillbirths have their cause in syphilis of one or both parents.

Infection: The ovule may be diseased before impregnation, where the woman is a syphilitic.   Infection may occur along with impregnation where the male is a syphilitic.   The fœtus may become infected at any period of intra-uterine life, should the mother contract syphilis while pregnant.   When the infection is directly *paternal* in origin, the syphilitic poison may be conveyed from the fœtus to the mother, and she may thus develop secondary symptoms of the disease without a primary lesion.   It is undoubted that many women give birth to syphilitic offspring without themselves at any time manifesting symptoms of the disease.   The likelihood of development of the disease in the fœtus is undoubtedly affected by the period of time since the acquisition of syphilis by either parent, though as yet no limit of safety has been discovered.   The author has met with a case where the disease had remained latent in the father for twelve years.   The mother at no time gave evidence of syphilitic infection, yet the only child developed well-marked symptoms a few weeks after birth.   Hutchinson has reported cases in which women were infected near term and gave birth to syphilitic infants.

Manifestations of fœtal syphilis: The disease produces a great variety of manifestations, the lesions depending upon the tissues attacked.   Thus there are bullous eruptions of the skin ; inflammations of mucous and serous membranes ; abnormal development of connective tissue in the liver, kidneys, lungs, spleen, etc ; and a characteristic osteitis and osteochondritis.   In some cases the infants are born apparently healthy and only manifest symptoms of the disease within a few weeks of birth.

Diagnosis: Should the fœtus be born dead the diagnosis can be made with certainty by a few perfectly reliable and easily detected signs.

The most certain sign of fœtal syphilis is to be found in the condition of the dividing line between the diaphysis and epiphysis of the long bones—this line instead of being sharp and regular as it is in the healthy infant, will be found to be jagged, broad, and of a yellow color, due to an osteochondritis. This is known as *Wagner's sign* and is determined by making an incision over the trochanter as though for excision of the head of the femur; the end of the bone is then turned out after cutting its ligaments, and a median section of the epiphysis and diaphysis is made with a strong cartilage knife.

The *liver* and *spleen* of a syphilitic infant are always enlarged as a result of connective-tissue overgrowth. For a more detailed diagnosis of syphilis in the infant the reader is referred to other works.

The **treatment** of fœtal syphilis consists in submitting the mother to a thorough course of antisyphilitic treatment throughout pregnancy. If a history of syphilis in either parent be obtained, whether occurring before or subsequent to conception, the woman should receive throughout the pregnancy antisyphilitic treatment as a prophylactic measure.

Other Infectious Diseases.

A large number of cases have been collected by various observers which prove the possibility of **contagious diseases** being transmitted from the mother to the fœtus in utero. Rare cases are recorded where children have been born with unmistakable evidences of variola, scarlatina, measles, erysipelas, malaria, and typhoid.

With regard to **tuberculosis** Hirst states that there is a remote possibility of the passage of the tubercle bacilli from mother to fœtus; but that it must be regarded as a very exceptional occurrence.

Fœtal Death.

The death of the fœtus in utero may be due to many **causes.** Among these may be mentioned syphilis, acute infectious diseases, icterus gravidarum, malnutrition, etc. It is also caused by twisting or knotting of the cord, diseased conditions of the placenta, or by trauma.

Sequelæ: If death occur before the second month the product of conception may be entirely absorbed. In the later months of pregnancy the fœtus may undergo maceration, mummification or calcification. Should putrefaction of the dead fœtus occur, the mother may be involved in sepsis. The dead fœtus is usually cast out of the uterus in a short time, though it may be retained for years.

PATHOLOGY OF THE PREGNANT WOMAN.

The Vulva and Vagina.

Abnormal conditions of the vulva or vagina during pregnancy are generally **due** either to increased blood-supply or to infection.

Varices: Obstruction to the venous return offered by the enlarging uterus frequently results in varicosed conditions about the vulva or vagina; these varices may be ruptured by straining or by a blow or kick; severe hemorrhage may occur and has proved fatal.

Treatment consists in protection by means of a snugly fitting T-bandage, and rest in bed with the hips elevated.

Œdema may occur in normal pregnancy simply from pressure of the uterus. It may result from renal insufficiency or from labial abscess.

Pruritus of the vulva in varying degrees is not uncommon during pregnancy. It may be *caused* by irritating discharges or may be a neurosis.

Treatment: Cleanliness and tepid injections of such solutions as the following: borax, ʒj to Oj; acid. carbolic., 1 : 200; or zinci acetat., ʒss to Oj; an ointment composed of chloral hydrate, camphor, āā ʒss, ung. aq. rosæ, ʒij, may give relief. In severe cases it may be necessary to apply solutions of cocaine, 4 grains to the ounce, in order to obtain any relief.

Vaginal leucorrhœa may be very troublesome during pregnancy. In all cases where the discharge is profuse it should be examined for gonococci. Simple leucorrhœa usually yields to mild antiseptic astringent douches which should be given with great care, *e. g.*, Condy's fluid, ℨj to Oj.

Should *gonococci* be found in the vaginal discharge the treatment should be energetic : bichloride (1 : 2000) or permanganate of potassium (ℨj to Oj) douches should be given twice daily, and an occasional application to the walls of the vagina and urethra of a solution of silver nitrate (gr. x–xx to ℨj) will probably give good results.

Vegetations of the vulva sometimes reach excessive size during pregnancy. The *treatment* consists in washing with liquor sodæ chlorinatæ, afterward dusting with calomel, and keeping them perfectly dry.

The Uterus.

This organ may in pregnancy be **displaced** forward, backward, to either side, or downward.

Retroversion of the Gravid Uterus.

Causation : The displacement is of frequent occurrence and may have existed before the onset of pregnancy ; or it may occur as the result of a fall or sudden jar.

Anatomical results : As long as the uterus is less than four inches in length it may lie across the axis of the pelvis. As its bulk and length increases, it becomes too large for the pelvis. If upward movement be prevented by the projecting promontory incarceration occurs, and pressure symptoms begin to develop. Incarceration usually occurs about the end of the third or the beginning of the fourth month. The distended fundus will on examination be found to occupy the hollow of the sacrum causing a bulging downward of the posterior vaginal wall, while the cervix is pressed upward and forward against the pubes, thus displacing the anterior vaginal wall and urethra. The bladder is thus displaced upward. The uterus may regain its normal position by growing upward in the direction of least resistance ; or it may remain incarcerated and give rise to serious trouble.

Symptoms : The earliest and most distinctive symptom is dysuria, accompanied by sensations of weight and bearing-

12—Obst.

down pains. If the condition be overlooked or neglected the bladder symptoms become rapidly more marked. Retention of urine from pressure on the urethra brings about overdistention of the bladder, and a more or less severe cystitis results.

While the urinary symptoms are the most characteristic, the condition also gives rise to rectal tenesmus and obstinate constipation. Œdema of the vulva and of the uterine walls may develop from interference with the pelvic circulation. The abdomen becomes distended and vomiting may occur.

Diagnosis: Where the retroversion is suspected the bladder must first be catheterized before making a vaginal examination. The condition will then be readily ascertained.

The history of retention of urine and dribbling in a woman who has been pregnant for three or four months, the round doughy-feeling mass occupying the vagina, and the position of the cervix make the diagnosis conclusive.

The condition may be *simulated* by ectopic gestation, subinvolution of the uterus, intraperitoneal hæmatocele, uterine fibroid, and ovarian cyst; but careful examination, if necessary, under an anæsthetic, will clear up the diagnosis.

Treatment of Retroversion.

In **mild cases** the bladder having been catheterized and the patient placed in the knee-chest position, the uterus can be replaced by pressure upward on the fundus in the direction of one or the other sacro-iliac joints, so as to avoid the promontory, two fingers being placed in the posterior vaginal fornix for this purpose. If necessary the cervix may at the same time be drawn down with a tenaculum. If the attempt succeeds, as it usually does, a large tampon should be placed in the posterior vaginal fornix to retain the uterus in position. This may be replaced later by a large-sized pessary. If the attempt fails, the patient should be placed under ether and a second effort made to replace the uterus.

In **severe incarcerated cases** there is occasionally great difficulty in emptying the bladder. If, after drawing down the cervix with a tenaculum, the catheter fails to pass, then the bladder must be aspirated by suprapubic puncture. If all attempts at reduction fail, then abortion must be induced. If the cervix cannot be reached for this purpose then the uterine wall must be punctured through the vaginal vault and the liquor amnii drained away. This may make it possible to draw down the cervix, which should then be dilated and the uterus emptied. Vaginal hysterectomy may be necessary in rare cases where suppuration or gangrene of the uterine wall has occurred.

Prolapse of the Gravid Uterus.

Causation: This condition may occur in the early months of pregnancy as the result of accident or from violent straining when the vaginal walls and outlet are greatly relaxed.

Treatment consists in the replacement of the prolapsed organ and the adjustment of a perfectly fitting pessary to retain it.

Endocervicitis; Tumors.

Endocervicitis: This condition is frequently found during pregnancy. It may be the origin of a leucorrhœa and is frequently associated with hyperemesis.

It is best *treated* with applications of fairly strong solutions of silver nitrate (gr. xx to ℥j) through a cylindrical speculum. The speculum is pushed up against the cervix and the solution then poured in and allowed to remain in contact for at least five minutes.

Uterine fibroids and cancer usually complicate *labor* more than pregnancy, and will therefore be dealt with under that head.

Diseases of the Breasts.

Mammary abscess may occur during pregnancy (see *Diseases of Puerperal Period*).

Excessive secretion: Occasionally during the latter part of pregnancy the breasts secrete excessively, causing a serous flow which gives rise to considerable inconvenience. Applications of belladonna may afford relief.

Eczema of the nipples may require treatment, though the condition is very obstinate.

DISEASES OF THE ALIMENTARY CANAL.

Gingivitis is an unpleasant though somewhat infrequent affection of the pregnant woman. This and other conditions about to be mentioned are due, not so much to uncleanliness, as to an alteration in the secretions of the buccal cavity consequent upon pregnancy. The *gums* become spongy and soft, red or violet in color at the margins, and occasionally ulceration occurs. Pain on eating, foul breath, and bleeding are symptoms of this condition.

Treatment: Sometimes gingivitis is very obstinate and in spite of treatment persists through pregnancy and even lactation. Astringents, locally, and alkaline tonics give the best results. Special attention in the way of cleanliness as regards the mouth and teeth should be observed throughout pregnancy.

Dental caries: There is a common saying among women, " for every child a tooth," so frequent is caries of the teeth during pregnancy. All dental cavities should be cleaned out and filled temporarily, as prolonged and painful dental operations are to be avoided during pregnancy. Syrup of the lactophosphate of lime in doses of ʒj t. i. d. has been recommended.

Parotitis, either unilateral or bilateral, is an infrequent complication of pregnancy.

Ptyalism, or Salivation.

Occurrence: This is a not infrequent complication of pregnancy. It is generally associated with extreme nausea and vomiting in highly neurotic women. It may persist throughout pregnancy, beginning as early as the second month; some cases lose as much as a quart of saliva a day. Ptyalin, and sodium salts are diminished or may be absent from the saliva. Frequently these patients complain of pain on swallowing; and the submaxillary and sublingual glands become swollen and tender.

Treatment is most unsatisfactory in most cases. Copious rinsing of the mouth with weak solutions of potassium chlorate, ash bark, cinchona, etc., may be employed. In the experience of the author, local measures afford but little if any relief. The condition is a *neurosis* and must be treated as such. Therefore chloral and sodium bromide in large doses may be tried; atropine in doses of gr. $\frac{1}{100}$ t. i. d. may give relief. What rarely fails to give temporary relief is morphine (gr. $\frac{1}{4}$) with atropine (gr. $\frac{1}{150}$), these administered together give better results than either alone. The latter must not be given as routine treatment, but only occasionally to permit rest and sleep, while the patient should always be kept in ignorance of what she is given in order to guard against the formation of the morphine habit. Antipyrin (gr. v, t. i. d.) and small doses of cocaine hydrochlorate (gr. $\frac{1}{6}$, t. i. d.) have proved useful in the hands of some physicians.

Indigestion ; Constipation ; Diarrhœa.

Indigestion: Gastric indigestion is very common in the earliest months of pregnancy. If careful feeding and the ordinary remedies fail to give relief, chloral, bromides, and other nerve sedatives should be resorted to. Intestinal indigestion may give rise to severe abdominal pains and may simulate appendicitis or even extra-uterine fœtation. Pil. aloes et asafœtidæ and careful dieting, as a rule, give good results.

Constipation is very frequent in most women at all times. Care should be taken to regulate the bowels by careful dieting and ordering plenty of fluids. Where this condition is chronic the tablet triturate of aloin, belladonna, cascara, and strychnine will be found satisfactory; active purgation is to be avoided.

Diarrhœa as a complication of pregnancy is rare; if persistent in spite of ordinary astringent treatment, nerve sedatives will probably give relief.

Vomiting.

Vomiting is one of the commonest disorders of the digestive tract occurring in pregnancy.

It is met with in **two forms**: A *simple vomiting*, which is physiological; and *pernicious vomiting*, which is pathological.

Simple vomiting of pregnancy has been already referred to. It is usually present during the earlier months and ceases at the end of the fourth month. While causing distress and discomfort, it does not seriously impair the nutrition of pregnant women.

Recently I have advanced the view that probably the **essential exciting cause** of the nausea and vomiting of pregnancy is the *physiological uterine contractions*. It is well known that the uterus is subject to rhythmical contractions throughout the whole period of pregnancy. The purpose of these contractions is probably the acceleration of the circulation of blood through the uterine sinuses. The enormous dilatation of the veins of the uterus which occurs as the result of pregnancy brings about a retardation of the blood flow through them. As the result of contraction of the uterine muscular fibres these sinuses become emptied of blood and thus the uterus may be said to supplement the action of the heart, to which it may be compared, as its nervous supply is very similar in arrangement. The nerve supply of the uterus is chiefly derived from the ovarian and hypogastric plexuses of the sympathetic system, which to a limited extent have an independent action; while in the medulla there exists a centre presiding over uterine contraction. The development of the embryo and its envelopes, as well as the hyperplasia of the uterus and its lining, are accompanied by tremendous chemical changes. It is certainly from the venous sinuses at the placental site that the embryo derives its chief nourishment and into which its effete material is emptied. The ordinary circulation of the blood through the sinuses to a certain extent provides for change in the supply, but owing to the retardation of the blood-current from dilatation of these sinuses there must be a certain residuum, which, as it becomes surcharged with effete material, probably acts as an irritant and stimulates the uterus to contraction, and thus to a certain degree the organ may be said to empty itself.

It is these contractions, so brought about, which probably precipitate the paroxysms of nausea and vomiting. The nausea is seldom constant, but is usually rhythmical in its occurrence. As has already been stated it is usually most severe in the morning when after a long fast the patient assumes the erect position. It is probable that the occurrence of the retching at this time is due to the engorgement of the pelvic circulation consequent on the change of posture. This engorgement leads to excessive uterine contraction, and thus the peripheral irritation is increased. It is commonly noticed that if the patient partakes of food before rising nausea and vomiting are not so likely to ensue. This is due no doubt to the engorgement of the pelvic veins being reduced by the determination of blood to the stomach from the presence of the food in that viscus.

Hemorrhoids.

The pelvic congestion of pregnancy and the pressure of the gravid uterus **predispose** to this troublesome affection.

Treatment can only be palliative. Laxatives, rest in bed, and the frequent assumption of the knee-chest posture will afford relief. Locally, ung. gallæ cum opio, or hot sugar of lead lotions, may be serviceable. Suppositories containing opium (gr. $\frac{1}{2}$) and ext. hamamelidis (gr. j) may be employed if the pain is severe.

DISEASES OF THE URINARY SYSTEM.

The Bladder.

Cystitis, occurring during pregnancy, may be due to colon bacillus infection or to gonorrhœa. Ureteritis or pyelonephritis may result if the condition is not recognized and promptly treated.

Pyelonephritis: This disease is a not infrequent complication of the latter half of pregnancy. Usually the right kidney is affected, though one or both may be attacked.

In an overwhelming proportion of cases the infective agent is the colon bacillus.

Symptoms: The symptoms are bladder irritation, followed by paroxysmal pains, usually in the right lumbar region. The pain often radiates down the groin and thigh. Fever and frequently chills, thirst, and constipation are present.

At first the urine may be clear, but in a short time is found to contain a large amount of pus and occasionally blood. Compression of the ureters by the enlarged uterus is supposed by many to give rise to this condition. The resistance of the mucous membrane becomes impaired by overstretching and infection follows. The latter may result from extension upward from the bladder and from the blood or lymph channels. The condition may be mistaken for appendicitis or salpingitis. It may complicate the puerperium and be mistaken for puerperal infection.

Catheterization of the ureters in suspected cases will make diagnosis certain.

Treatment consists of rest in bed, milk diet, the copious use of fluids, and the administration of urotropin. Should this fail to effect prompt improvement, the affected ureter should be catheterized and the pelvis of the kidney douched daily with a 10 per cent. boric acid solution. Rarely, it may be necessary to terminate the pregnancy.

Diabetes : Sugar is not infrequently present in the urine of pregnant women. It is usually lactose and is of no pathological significance. Should glucose be found, the patient should be watched carefully and dieted if necessary. Should untoward symptoms develop, the pregnancy should be terminated.

Nephritis will be considered in the section on Toxæmias of Pregnancy.

Hæmaturia may occur during pregnancy and is generally associated with vesical hemorrhoids. If severe, the bladder should be washed out daily with a weak solution of silver nitrate (gr. ss–j to ℨj).

Scanty, high-colored urine, having a high specific gravity, results from indiscretion in diet, and is associated with inactivity of the skin and bowels ; this condition of the urine should always receive attention. A non-nitrogenous diet, laxatives, and copious draughts of water should be ordered.

DISEASES OF THE RESPIRATORY SYSTEM.

Cough, with or without evidence of bronchial catarrh, is a very common and occasionally troublesome affection during pregnancy. The reflex cough of pregnancy may be very persistent, and when the paroxysms are severe and continuous may lead to abortion. In its *treatment* antispasmodics and sedatives are indicated rather than expectorants. Bromide of sodium and tr. belladonnæ in combination give good results, as do also drachm doses of the linctus codeia.

Dyspnœa occasionally occurs as a reflex, and may cause the patient considerable distress. It is more frequent in the later months of pregnancy, when it is generally due to over-distention of the abdomen and mechanical pressure of the uterus upon the diaphragm. In the former class of cases sedatives are indicated; while in the latter relief may be obtained by avoiding tight clothing, and having the patient sleep with the head and shoulders elevated.

Pneumonia is a disease much to be dreaded when complicated by pregnancy. The *symptoms* are always aggravated and the mortality for both mother and fœtus is high.

Phthisis pulmonalis: Pregnancy has a most unfavorable influence on this disease. Rarely, patients suffering from phthisis seem to improve during pregnancy; but the disease only advances the more rapidly after delivery has occurred. Women already affected and predisposed to tuberculosis should be strongly advised against maternity.

DISEASES OF THE CIRCULATORY SYSTEM.

Cardiac diseases in pregnancy are not rare; the danger of the heart lesions is increased by pregnancy; abortion is apt to occur from the formation of infarctions in the placenta; not infrequently the child is born badly nourished.

The *complications* to be dreaded are failure of compensation due to fatty degeneration; and pulmonary congestion. If compensation is good, no untoward symptoms are likely to develop, beyond œdema and albuminuria, the latter being due to renal congestion. Hirst states that with proper treatment he has no fear of heart disease in pregnancy.

Treatment: All women suffering from cardiac disease should be kept under constant observation throughout gestation. The urine should be frequently examined. Should symptoms of failure of compensation arise, digitalis and strophanthus should be exhibited, combined with strychnine; the bowels should be kept open and rest and moderate exercise ordered.

Many consider that pregnancy should not be allowed to continue longer than the thirty-sixth week in a woman who exhibits any symptoms of imperfect compensation. Cardiac diseases do not contraindicate the employment of anæsthetics during labor. These benefit by preventing the injurious effects of straining and by quieting the action of the heart during parturition.

Functional heart-murmurs in pregnancy : In the later months of pregnancy soft, blowing murmurs can occasionally be heard, both over the mitral and aortic areas ; these are usually systolic in rhythm, but may also be diastolic. They may in part be due to a certain amount of displacement of the organ resulting from overdistention of the abdomen. They disappear completely shortly after labor.

The bloodvessels : Varicose conditions of the veins of the pelvis, abdominal walls, and lower limbs are frequent during pregnancy. They result in part from changes in the vessels themselves, and in part from the mechanical obstruction to the circulation offered by the increasing bulk of the uterus. *Treatment* consists of elastic support where this is possible, and in the avoidance of constipation.

Enlargement of the thyroid gland : The fact that there exists a peculiar relationship between the thyroid gland and the uterus and general circulation is well known. Usually a sympathetic growth of this gland occurs at the same time as enlargement of the uterus ; hence the fulness of the neck so often noticed in pregnant women. Thus in simple and in exophthalmic goitre pregnancy exerts a very unfavorable influence. The growth of the gland may progress to such a degree as to cause pressure upon the trachea resulting in dyspnœa, and even threatening maternal death from asphyxia. In rare cases tracheotomy has been resorted to in order to save the patient's life.

DISEASES OF THE NERVOUS SYSTEM.

Neuralgia in various portions of the body is a frequent af-fection of the pregnant woman. The most common situations are the head, hands, face, teeth, and breasts. Pelvic neuralgia is usually due to pressure of the growing uterus upon the pelvic nerves; occasionally neuralgia occurs in the uterus.

In the *treatment* of these troublesome neuralgias, tonics containing iron, quinine, and arsenic are particularly valuable. Attention should always be paid to the matter of diet, sleep, and the state of the emunctories in these cases. Any of the coal-tar derivatives, combined with the citrate of caffeine to prevent depression, usually promptly relieve the severe pain. All sources of local irritation should be sought for and removed.

Neuroses.

Chorea : Mild grades of chorea cannot be said to be uncommon in pregnancy. Chorea is more common in primiparæ. Rheumatism, chlorosis, heredity, and the previous occurrence of the disease in childhood are considered as predisposing causes. It usually appears early in pregnancy and is apt to persist throughout its course. As a rule, in the milder cases it does not manifest itself during sleep. In the grave form it may result in the patient's death, after causing premature expulsion of the ovum.

The *treatment* is the same as when not complicated by pregnancy.

Epilepsy is a rare complication of pregnancy. It does not, as a rule, exert an unfavorable influence upon the course of gestation, and it can usually be controlled by the free administration of potassium iodide.

Hysteria is frequent during pregnancy.

Vomiting and **coughing** occur as neuroses during pregnancy, and have already been referred to.

Psychical disturbances : Not uncommonly a complete change in the disposition and mental character of the woman may occur during pregnancy.

Insomnia may be troublesome toward the close of pregnancy. A warm bath on retiring, a glass of milk, or a cup of warm broth, taken at the same hour, may be sufficient to induce sleep; sulphonal or trional in 10- to 15-grain doses may be resorted to if required.

Insanity is of but rare occurrence during gestation, being much more likely to develop during the puerperal period. Melancholia and mania are the more usual forms, the former being more frequent.

The *prognosis* in the maniacal form is more grave than in the melancholic. Insanity may recur in successive pregnancies. It may be stated that gravidity exerts usually an unfavorable influence upon insanity.

The *treatment* can only be expectant and symptomatic; induction of labor, when marked symptoms have developed, only tends to aggravate the condition.

Temporary delirium may occur during labor, and is far from common. A woman rendered delirious from acute suffering in labor may do serious injury to her child, for which she cannot be held responsible.

DISEASES OF THE CUTANEOUS SYSTEM.

Herpes gestationis is a peculiar neurotic skin affection usually met with in early pregnancy. It generally persists throughout gestation in spite of treatment. The eruption is multiform, exhibiting erythema vesicles and bullæ. Its treatment consists in the administration of nerve sedatives and the regulation of the diet and mode of life of the patient.

Impetigo herpetiformis is rare. It usually occurs toward the close of pregnancy. It generally locates itself in the folds of the body around the groins, the umbilicus and axillæ, and under the mammæ. It occurs as small pustules forming crusts; it tends to spread rapidly and may cover the whole body. It is generally accompanied by marked symptoms of systemic disturbance, high fever, chills, vomiting, and severe prostration. Hirst states that of twelve cases ten terminated fatally. The disease did not terminate gestation prior to the maternal death.

The *treatment* is symptomatic, with the application of soothing remedies locally.

Pruritus is usually a local affection limited to the vulva;

but it may occur as a general affection. It may cause intense suffering to the patient, and cases have been reported in which it was necessary to induce labor in order to relieve the patient.

Treatment consists in alkaline baths (5 ounces of bicarbonate of sodium to the bath), and frictions with sedative lotions, as the camphor or chloroform liniment. Usually this treatment must be combined with the internal administration of chloral and bromide.

Exaggerated pigmentation : Dark spots of pigmentation may appear on the breasts, thighs, and abdomen, and occasionally on the face. The condition is not amenable to treatment, and usually disappears shortly after labor.

Infectious Diseases.

Certain of the infectious diseases are more prone to attack the pregnant woman than are others.

Variola is probably the most virulent of the infectious diseases attacking the pregnant woman. It generally results speedily in both fœtal and maternal death.

Scarlatina is apt to be exceedingly virulent, but it is more prone to attack the puerperal woman.

Measles in the pregnant woman usually assumes a severe type and generally leads to abortion. The patient exhibits a marked tendency to develop pneumonia as a complication.

Typhoid fever does not, as a rule, tend to assume an unusually severe type when it attacks the pregnant woman. The prolonged elevation of temperature tends to bring about abortion.

TOXÆMIAS OF PREGNANCY.

Certain disturbances of health of a toxic nature seem to depend primarily on pregnancy itself, and to these we apply the term " toxæmias of pregnancy."

The causation is obscure and at present is the subject of much discussion. Certain it is that during pregnancy the general metabolism becomes profoundly modified. The excretory functions are strained to the utmost in the endeavor to eliminate the waste products of the fœtal, as well as the maternal, organism. This strain renders certain organs, as the liver and kidneys, liable to serious derangements.

Certain European, as well as certain American, observers state that hepatic insufficiency, resulting from the retention of metabolic products, gives rise to a definite series of clinical phenomena, varying from headache, malaise, and salivation, on the one hand, to stupor, coma, and convulsions on the other.

Others state that the initial cause is the development of abnomal products of a toxic nature in the placenta, which, entering the maternal circulation, bring about pathological changes in the liver and kidneys.

Veit and others advance the view that cytolytic processes, depending upon the entrance of chorionic tissue and fœtal ectoderm into the maternal circulation, are responsible for the pathological changes in the maternal excretory organs.

Williams opposes these views, and states that " chemical analysis of the urine, as well as the histological study of the tissues obtained at autopsy, clearly indicates that essential and characteristic differences exist between the various conditions grouped together," as the toxæmias of pregnancy.

For the full discussion of the state of our knowledge of this subject, the reader is referred to the larger text-books and recent monographs.

Certain groups of the toxæmia of pregnancy will be briefly discussed, and no other attempt made to classify or deal with them other than from the practical standpoint.

PERNICIOUS VOMITING OF PREGNANCY.

Mention has already been made of the ordinary nausea and vomiting incident to the early weeks of pregnancy, and the theory advanced that the essential causative factor is uterine contractions possibly setting up reflex irritation.

When the vomiting becomes so severe that the patient is unable to retain nutriment of any kind and rapidly loses flesh, the condition is then designated *pernicious vomiting.*

It is more frequently encountered in the so-called neurotic type of individual, and is met with in its severer forms but rarely.

Etiology : Many factors seem to contribute to the production of this condition.   Certain it is that in many cases the removal of some pathological condition, such as an ovarian tumor or the replacement of a retroverted uterus, has been followed by immediate improvement in the symptoms. In other cases, hypnotism or " mental influence has been sufficient to bring about a cure."

Williams, in his monograph published in 1906, has stated that " the evidence at present available justifies the differentiation of three types of serious vomiting of pregnancy; namely, reflex, neurotic, and toxæmic."

The reflex and neurotic forms have been already referred to. The toxæmic form is associated with profound metabolic disturbances manifested by characteristic changes in the urine and definite lesions in the liver and kidneys. Williams states that in this form the urine presents a high ammonia coefficient, indicating that a much greater proportion of the total nitrogen is excreted in the form of ammonia than usual. Normally, the ammonia coefficient varies between 4 and 5 per cent., while in toxæmic vomiting it varies between 10 and 40 per cent.

The liver changes in fatal cases of toxæmic vomiting are identical with those of acute yellow atrophy of this organ. There is a " profound necrosis of the central portion of the lobules, while the periphery remains intact." The kidney changes are degenerative in character and are limited to the secretory portions.

These tissue changes are undoubtedly due to some underlying toxæmic process.

Symptoms: These usually develop gradually, as the vomiting, at first infrequent, becomes more constant and more violent, till ultimately nothing can be retained in the stomach. The patient becomes emaciated, rapidly loses strength, and her movements become languid, the face pale, the voice weak, and the pulse increases in rapidity. Constipation or diarrhœa may be present. Salivation is not infrequent in the early stage; later the mouth may become dry and the tongue heavily coated.

In the most severe form the symptoms of toxæmia develop, often appearing suddenly. These are, vomiting of a coffee-ground material, torpor, delirium, and possibly convulsions. Jaundice may develop and the temperature rise, though this is not usually the case.

The urine at this stage becomes scanty and contains albumin, casts, and more or less blood- and bile-pigment.

Death may follow convulsions or coma, though the mind remain practically clear till the last.

Diagnosis: As soon as vomiting becomes severe enough to lead to loss of weight in a pregnant woman, a careful general examination should be made. Attention should be given to the condition of the genital organs, stomach, kidneys, and brain, and any pathological condition noted should be corrected if possible.

As Williams has stated, the neurotic and reflex form of vomiting yield more or less readily to treatment, but in the toxæmic form arrest of the pregnancy before organic lesions have become pronounced is of supreme importance if the patient's life is to be saved.

Careful examination of the urine by a competent chemist to determine the ratio which the amount of nitrogen contained in the ammonia bears to the total nitrogen, is the course recommended by Williams. By this means only can the toxæmic form be distinguished from the other varieties of vomiting in the pregnant woman.

He states that if the ammonia coefficient be found to be normal, the vomiting is due either to reflex or neurotic influences; whereas, if it be increased, and particularly if it much exceeds 10 per cent., a diagnosis of toxæmic vomiting should be made.

Treatment: All reflex causes of irritation should be removed. Neurotic cases should be isolated, with a competent nurse. Treatment consists of rectal salines in large amount, and for forty-eight hours nothing whatever should be given by mouth. Then fluids may be given in small quantities at short intervals, and as the stomach tolerates it the amount and quality of the diet augmented.

In the toxæmic form abortion should be induced as soon as the diagnosis is clear. A general anæsthetic should be avoided if possible, and the operation performed with the least disturbance of the patient possible. Following the operation, large quantities of a 1 per cent. solution of sodium bicarbonate should be given, and also free use should be made of high rectal salines. Strychnin and other stimulants should be given by hypodermic if required.

Prognosis: This is very satisfactory in the reflex or neurotic forms, but is always very grave in the toxæmic form, as recovery depends upon the extent and severity of the organic lesions.

TOXÆMIA IN THE LATER MONTHS OF PREGNANCY.

The toxæmia most frequently encountered is that associated with the later months of pregnancy. It may become evident in rare cases before the sixth month, but is most commonly met with after the thirtieth week of pregnancy. As it leads up to a definite outbreak of eclampsia, it is designated by many *pre-eclamptic toxæmia.*

The clinical manifestations of this toxæmia are so varied, the etiology and pathology as yet so obscure, that it is impossible at present to classify or define the varied forms that have been met with.

Two more or less well-defined types of this toxæmia may be mentioned. These are the nephritic and the cholæmic or eclamptic.

The NEPHRITIC TYPE of toxæmia, in which the clinical manifestations resemble those of uremia, is most commonly met with in multiparæ, and it not infrequently results in chronic renal disease.

The CHOLÆMIC TYPE of toxæmia is the more common, and is most frequent in prima gravidæ. Its onset is more sudden, its course more rapid, and recovery from it more complete, as it is rarely followed by renal disease. It is extremely rare for it to recur in subsequent pregnancies.

Diagnosis: The clinical differentiation of these forms is not always easy, but, fortunately, the treatment of both is practically the same, and the prognosis, if the cases are carefully guarded, is usually fair.

Generally speaking, the urinary findings differ in these forms of toxæmia, but scarcely sufficiently to be depended upon for a differential diagnosis.

In the nephritic form the urine may be normal in amount, albumin is present in large quantity, while the total nitrogen and the urea are usually only slightly diminished.

13—Obst.

In the cholæmic form the output of the urine is greatly reduced, albumin, though almost always present, is rarely abundant, but the total nitrogen and the urea are markedly diminished. In both forms casts and blood may be present in varying amounts in the urine. The severity of the toxæmia usually is manifested by the degree of the urinary alterations.

Symptoms: The symptoms are rarely well marked in the early stages or in the mild forms. They may vary from malaise and lassitude to those indicating grave toxæmia. Headache, disturbance of vision, vomiting, epigastric pain, and occurrence of edema may herald the onset of toxæmia. Associated with these we have possibly diminished output of urine, which usually contains albumin and numerous casts. The chemical examination varies with the degree of intoxication, though usually the total nitrogen and urea are reduced.

The visual disturbance may be so great as to produce complete amaurosis. Hallucinations may develop or even insanity, or somnolence, leading to coma or convulsions, may ensue.

Treatment: The routine examination of the urine of the pregnant woman every two weeks after she has reached the sixth month must be insisted upon if the onset of toxæmia is to be recognized early.

If the albumin is detected, a twenty-four hours' specimen must be obtained, measured, and a careful chemical study made of it. The quantity of albumin and urea present should be noted. If the latter is below 12 gm., the toxæmia is grave, and the patient must be carefully guarded. Daily chemical examination of the urine is demanded once symptoms of toxæmia have been discovered.

If the urinary findings are not momentous, the patient should be moderately purged and placed on restricted diet, meat and soups being withdrawn. Milk, soft puddings, cereals, and green vegetables may be permitted. The patient should be ordered to drink a definite quantity of water and milk per day, and the total intake and output of fluid should be estimated in order that the functioning power of the kidneys may be recognized.

If this treatment fails to bring about improvement, the patient must be put to bed and restricted to milk and water diet.

At the same time the bowels must be kept active by means of regular doses of Epsom salts, and, if the skin is dry and sluggish, she may be given hot baths or, better, a bed sweat.

Prognosis: Should the condition yield to treatment, the outlook is favorable, but should there be little if any response, the uterus should be promptly emptied.

Usually, the introduction of bougies within the uterus is sufficient to bring on labor, but if the condition of the patient is serious, accouchement forcé must be resorted to.

ECLAMPSIA.

Definition: The term eclampsia is derived from the Greek $\epsilon\chi\lambda\alpha\mu\varphi\iota s$ = a shining forth, and is applied to an acute disorder occurring in the pregnant, parturient, or puerperal woman, characterized usually by clonic and tonic convulsions, associated with loss of consciousness and followed by more or less prolonged coma.

Frequency: Hospital records show that eclampsia occurs about once in one hundred and sixty cases. As these cases are usually sent to the hospital for treatment when possible, such records tend greatly to exaggerate the apparent frequency of the condition. It is probable that it is met with in one case in every four hundred, though its frequency seems to vary in different localities. It is somewhat more frequently met with in primiparæ.

Etiology: Zweifel has designated eclampsia "the disease of theories." Theories without number have been advanced to account for the onset of the eclamptic state, and to the larger text-books the student of obstetrics is referred for a full discussion of these varied theories.

At present the generally accepted view is that eclampsia is due to some ferment or toxin circulating in the maternal blood, which brings about degenerative and necrotic changes, chiefly in the liver and kidneys, in consequence of the occurrence of thrombosis in many of the smaller vessels.

Ignorance prevails as to the true nature or source of the toxic material. Observations have been advanced to prove that it is of fœtal origin, others that it is of placental origin, and others that the condition is due to an autointoxication which is metabolic in character.

Pathology: The main lesions are found in the liver, kidneys, heart, and brain, though those most constant in their character are the hepatic lesions.

The HEPATIC LESIONS may be apparent to the naked eye, and appear as mottled areas irregularly shaped, reddish-gray in color, scattered throughout the organ in the neighborhood of the smaller portal vessels. Microscopically, these are recognized as necrotic areas infiltrated with blood-cells.

The KIDNEY LESIONS may be very marked or only slight in character. They are usually those of acute nephritis, with more or less degeneration and necrosis of the renal epithelium.

The brain lesions consist of œdema, hyperæmia, thrombosis, and embolism. Small areas of necrosis, in consequence of the presence of thrombi in the smaller cerebral vessels, are frequently found.

The CARDIAC LESIONS consist of degeneration of the myocardium.

Clinical Course: Most commonly the toxic condition of the patient is heralded by the symptoms previously described, though occasionally convulsions may occur without any premonitory signs of the intoxication.

Headache, disturbance of vision, and severe epigastric pain, with which may be associated more or less œdema, particularly of the lower limbs and of the face, are the most marked symptoms heralding an attack of eclampsia. At the same time constipation is usually present, and the urine is found to contain albumin and casts and to be deficient in urea.

The **eclamptic fit** usually begins with a fixed expression of the eyes, the head being turned to one side; the eyelids twitch rapidly, the pupils contract, and the eyeballs roll. The spasm of the muscles then spreads rapidly, the mouth is drawn to one side, the jaws clench, often causing severe injury to the tongue, which may be caught between the teeth; the head is rolled rapidly from side to side and then drawn back; as the muscles of the trunk and limbs become affected the whole body is thrown into a condition of tonic spasm. As respiration is interfered with the face becomes livid and bloody froth issues from the mouth.

This condition is rapidly succeeded by a series of *clonic spasms*, in which all the muscles are thrown into violent contractions, causing quick jerky movements of the limbs and head. In severe cases the woman may be thrown into a position of opisthotonos.

CONSCIOUSNESS is lost during the attack, and the patient usually remains in a condition of coma, breathing stertorously for some time after.

The DURATION of the fit is seldom longer than a minute, while the coma lasts a variable time, from a few minutes to several hours. The paroxysms are repeated at varying intervals, in which the patient may regain consciousness. In some cases the patient remains in a condition of coma, with or without restlessness. Sometimes restlessness precedes another paroxysm. As many as one hundred and sixty fits have been counted in one case.

The arterial blood-pressure is always elevated in toxæmia cases, and may reach well over 200 mm. of Hg. It is well to test the blood-pressure by means of a suitable apparatus for this purpose, for an arterial blood-pressure of over 150 mm. of Hg. is always of serious import in these cases.

The pulse is usually full and bounding, and the rate varies between 120–180 per minute.

The temperature frequently becomes elevated, particularly if the convulsive seizures are frequent, 103°–105° F. being commonly recorded. It usually falls as the patient improves.

The convulsions may occur before, during, or after labor. Opinions vary as to the relative frequency of these forms, though, generally speaking, antepartum and intrapartum eclampsia are most frequently encountered.

Antepartum eclampsia usually results in labor setting in, when the uterus may be emptied either spontaneously or by operative means. The patient may die undelivered or the eclampsia may subside and the woman recover, later giving birth to a dead and macerated child ; or, in rare instances, the child may survive the attack and be born in good condition.

Intrapartum eclampsia usually results in rapid delivery of the child, as the pains commonly increase in frequency and severity.

Postpartum eclampsia develops shortly after delivery, and is commonly described as the mildest form, though in the experience of the author this has not proved to be the case.

Recovery may be complicated by temporary insanity, which

is usually quite transient. Again, cerebral hemorrhage may result in hemiplegia. Occasionally jaundice of varying intensity may develop.

The *urine* during eclampsia usually shows that the kidneys are more or less seriously damaged; it is always diminished in amount or anuria may exist; it may be very dark colored from containing blood; casts are found in great abundance, chiefly of the hyaline and granular variety. Albumin is almost always present, usually in the proportion of about 1 per cent. This is temporary and usually rapidly disappears as the condition of the patient improves. Williams states that in eclampsia the ammonia coefficient of the urine is diminished, and that its increase is of good prognostic import. Urea is reduced to one-half the usual quantity and there is an increase of the amido acids.

The urine rapidly returns to a normal condition as the patient improves.

True eclampsia ends in death or recovery usually within forty-eight hours.

Treatment: It is doubtful if eclampsia is always preventable, for in rare cases of toxæmia, giving every evidence of satisfactory response to treatment, eclampsia may suddenly appear. At the same time careful examination of the urine, proper dieting, and eliminative treatment, as previously outlined, usually prevent the actual development of convulsions.

Experience teaches that those cases associated with œdema, the nephritic type, are most amenable to treatment.

During an actual convulsion but little can be done for the patient beyond placing a cork or folded napkin between the teeth to prevent injury of the tongue.

Many advise the administration of chloroform or the hypodermic injection of a full dose of morphin. Others recommend that chloral hydrate be given per rectum in doses of between 30 and 60 grains.

Believing that fresh air and quiet are essential in the treatment of eclampsia, the author endeavors to secure these by placing the patient, wrapped in blankets, in bed in a large room, with the windows wide open. The attendants are instructed to make as little noise and disturbance as possible. During the convulsion oxygen may be administered and a hypodermic containing $\frac{1}{2}$ grain of morphin be given.

As soon as the convulsion has subsided, chloroform may be lightly administered to dull the sensibility, while the stomach is washed out by means of a tube, and 2 ounces of a saturated solution of Epsom salts and 2 drops of croton oil are introduced. The lower bowel is then emptied by means of a continuous hot saline irrigation, the tube being introduced as high as possible. A pint of normal saline solution should then be injected, by means of a large needle, beneath each breast. Hot air is then introduced by means of a suitable apparatus under the blankets and the patient given a good sweat-bath. Should hot air not be available, the patient may be wrapped in blankets wrung out of hot water. By these means purging and diuresis are induced.

The chloroform may now be stopped.

The patient's mouth should be kept clear of mucus by an attendant, and as soon as she can swallow she should be given as much of a 1 per cent. solution of sodium bicarbonate as she can be induced to take.

If the pulse is full and rapid, 5 minims of tincture of veratrum viridi may be injected hypodermically, and repeated at intervals of half an hour till the pulse-rate is reduced to below 70 per minute; or, better, a 500 cc. of blood may be withdrawn from the median basilic vein of the arm.

Should the convulsions recur and the coma persist, then delivery should be effected with the least disturbance of the patient possible. Fortunately, in a large proportion of the cases, labor sets in shortly after the convulsions begin. In these cases delivery should be accomplished, under an anæsthetic, by means of forceps or version as soon as the dilatation of the os uteri will permit.

When it is desirable to empty the uterus and labor has not set in, then vaginal or the classical Cæsarean section should be resorted to, provided the circumstances permit.

In private practice, when such operations are not possible, then manual dilatation of the os uteri or the employment of the Pomeroy or Champetier de Ribes bags may be resorted to for this object. The Bossi dilator, a many branched metal instrument, may be employed for this purpose, but is a very dangerous instrument, and is liable to cause serious lacerations even in skilled hands.

Following delivery by whatever means effected, bleeding

from the uterus should be encouraged. Then saline enemata should be given, and also subcutaneous injections used should the patient not be able to swallow.

Salines, sweat-baths, fresh air, and perfect quiet constitute the treatment of puerperal eclampsia. Sedatives should be employed as may be required, and bleeding resorted to when the coma persists.

The intake and output of fluids should be carefully measured, and thus the activity of the kidneys estimated.

Should anuria persist for eighteen hours at any time after delivery, the operation of decapsulation of the kidneys, as first recommended by Edebohls, may be considered.

Conditions of toxæmia may arise during pregnancy dependent upon a preëxisting *chronic nephritis,* or on an *acute nephritis* pure and simple. These are simple cases of uræmia complicated by pregnancy. Edema, headache, pallor, and disturbance of vision, due to the occurrence of albuminuric retinitis, are the most frequent symptoms.

This form of toxæmia is frequently attended by pathological lesions in the placenta, which may be so extensive as to interfere with the development or even cause the death of the child.

These cases usually respond to treatment, but the ultimate prognosis is bad, as the original morbid condition of the kidneys is accentuated. In such cases subsequent pregnancy should be avoided.

The treatment is the same as that of ordinary toxæmia of pregnancy and eclampsia.

Certain cases of *neuritis* met with in pregnant women are undoubtedly due to toxæmia, and yield only to eliminative treatment and suitable dieting.

Again, various *psychoses* occurring during pregnancy are of toxæmic origin. Rarely, one meets with cases of severe jaundice arising during pregnancy associated with *acute yellow atrophy of the liver.*

Prognosis: Maternal mortality is about 30 per cent., while the fœtal mortality is about 50 per cent. The earlier in pregnancy the eclamptic condition occurs, the worse is the prognosis.

Prognosis is *favorable* when :

The attacks are infrequent and mild ;

The patient regains consciousness between the attacks;

The skin, bowels, and kidneys can be stimulated to functionate freely.

Prognosis is *unfavorable* when :

The attacks become progressively more severe in spite of treatment and coma persists ;

The urine is completely suppressed and purgation cannot be induced.

Pathology of Abortion.

As the result of uterine contractions, or from degeneration of the vessels, **blood is effused** from the ruptured vessels into the decidua vera, and forces its way between the decidua and chorion, stripping off the ovum, which is then expelled entire. If the ovum be floated in water, it presents very much the appearance of a chestnut-burr.

Occasionally the **decidua is cast off entire** along with the ovum, which it completely envelops.

Occasionally also blood is extravasated into the membranes, at intervals. This coagulates in strata, and leads to the formation of what is known as a **blood-mole.**

In some cases the abortion may not be completed for some time, and the coloring-matter of the effused blood may be absorbed, while the strata undergo partial organization and a **fleshy mole** results. This may form a connection with the uterine wall, and be retained indefinitely.

In those cases in which portions of placenta are retained these masses may form **polypi**, remaining in the uterus for weeks or months, causing a fetid discharge and an elevation of temperature.

Etiology.

The causes of abortion may be **divided** into those of *paternal*, of *maternal*, or of *)fœtal* origin.

Paternal: Syphilis is probably the most common paternal influence in causing abortion. Other causes which may be mentioned under this heading are alcoholism, debility, tuberculosis, lead-poisoning, advanced age, and excessive venery.

Maternal: *General:* Similar causes to those mentioned in the father act in the mother.

Acute and chronic diseases cause abortion by excess of temperature, or by blood-changes, or by producing alterations in the placenta. Traumatism and severe emotional disturbances may produce abortion. Certain drugs, as quinine, savin, ergot, and a host of others, are said to cause abortion; but it is doubtful if this is the case when the uterus is in a normal condition.

Local: Displacements of the uterus, pelvic inflammations or adhesions, cervical lacerations, endometritis, metritis, fibromyomata, and abnormal development of the uterus may be mentioned as conditions which predispose to abortion.

There are women who abort constantly in whom no reasonable cause can be found; to this condition the term " *habitual abortion* " is applied.

Foetal: Syphilis, which acts by producing changes in the ovum or in the placenta, leading to the death of the foetus, is probably the most common foetal cause of abortion.

Degeneration of the chorion, hydramnios, and vicious insertion of the placenta frequently result in abortion.

Diagnosis.

In cases of suspected abortion it is necessary to determine the existence of pregnancy. The abortion may be *threatened; inevitable;* or wholly, or partially *accomplished.*

Threatened abortion: If the patient has been exposed to the possibility of impregnation and the menses have been suppressed; if a hemorrhage from the uterus occur, associated with more or less pain; then it is probable that an abortion is threatened.

Dysmenorrhœa may be mistaken for impending abortion; but in this case the cervix is closed and firm to the feel. Hemorrhage, associated with the presence of a *soft polypoid tumor* in the uterus, may simulate the condition of threatened abortion very closely; but a careful local examination will generally establish the nature of the condition present.

Inevitable abortion: When the membranes have ruptured, or the foetus is dead, or when any foetal part is engaged in the cervix, the abortion may be said to be *inevitable.* Cases have occurred in which large portions of decidua have escaped from the uterus, associated with considerable hemorrhage, and yet have afterward gone on to full term. Again the os may open sufficiently to admit the finger, yet close again, and the pregnancy continue. It is, therefore, sometimes a difficult matter to say that an abortion is "inevitable."

Complete, or partial, abortion: It is important always to determine whether a part of, or the whole uterine contents have been expelled. To make a diagnosis, everything discharged from the uterus must be carefully examined; when any doubt remains a digital exploration of the uterine cavity must be made; when anything is retained, the cervix usually remains patulous so that the finger can be inserted without much difficulty.

In cases of complete abortion in the first two months of pregnancy there is functionally no lochial discharge. Should the hemorrhage continue it is probable that portions of the decidua have been retained.

In incomplete abortions at the third month, or later, the lochial discharge remains free and bloody, instead of gradually subsiding, as it should when the uterus has been emptied and is involuting properly.

Prognosis.

The prognosis of abortion depends upon the treatment.

If the **uterus has been carefully emptied** under aseptic precautions, then the mortality from abortion should be *nil.*

Retained masses of decidua or of placenta are followed by decomposition of these substances in utero, and acute or chronic septic infection is the result.

Hemorrhage very rarely leads to a fatal result in cases of abortion.

When neglected, abortion may be the starting-point of various uterine diseases, as subinvolution, metritis, etc., which may lead to invalidism.

Treatment of Abortion.

Prophylactic: When any of the conditions are present which may tend to premature expulsion of the ovum, all precautions must be taken to prevent such an accident. Appropriate systemic treatment should be undertaken when indicated, and at the same time the patient should be instructed to observe special precautions, such as the avoidance of overexertion by lifting or reaching, particularly at the menstrual periods. The use of strong purgatives should be avoided. At each menstrual epoch the patient should remain in bed for several days. Abnormal uterine conditions, such as displacements, metritis, and lacerations of cervix, should receive appropriate treatment. Sexual intercourse should be avoided, especially at or about the menstrual epochs.

Threatened abortion : The main principle of treatment is to secure for the patient absolute rest, mental and physical. This is obtained by putting her to bed, in a cool, darkened room, where she can be kept in absolute quietness; and by the free use of opium, bromide, and chloral.

Opium is best administered by the rectum. A suppository containing opium, gr. ss, should be gently inserted every eight hours, or at least sufficiently often to keep the patient well under the influence of the drug. At the same time a mixture containing sodium bromide, gr. xxx, and chloral hydrate, gr. xv, may be given three times daily. Many prefer the fluid extract of viburnum prunifolium in drachm doses, t. i. d., instead of the bromide and chloral mixture.

Inevitable abortion : Two methods of treatment are available, the expectant and the active :

The expectant treatment : Should the bleeding be severe before the os is dilated, it must be controlled by means of a vaginal tampon of sterile or iodoform gauze. To apply vaginal tamponage properly the patient should be placed in the left semiprone position, with the hips resting on a rubber sheet or Kelly pad at the edge of the bed. The vulva and vagina should then be washed with spirits of green soap and hot water, and then swabbed with a 1 : 500 formalin solution. If the vulvar hair is long, it should be clipped. The only instruments required are a Sims speculum, a pair of uterine forceps, and a pair of scissors, which may be sterilized while the patient is being prepared.

The speculum is then inserted and the perineum retracted so as to expose the cervix to view. A strip of gauze (sterile or iodoform), about two inches wide and a yard long, is then seized above by means of the uterine forceps and packed firmly around the cervix. As the gauze is being inserted the speculum is gradually withdrawn. A sufficient quantity of gauze should be introduced to distend the vagina. The patient is then made comfortable, and should remain in bed.

To facilitate the emptying of the uterus, the fluid extract of ergot may be administered in half-drachm doses three times daily. If the uterine contractions are painful, an opiate may be combined with the ergot. The vaginal tampon should be removed in twenty-four hours, and replaced by a fresh one if necessary. A close watch should be kept over the patient's temperature. Often when the first tampon is removed the ovum comes with it, or the cervix will be found softened and the os sufficiently dilated to permit the introduction of the finger, with which the ovum may be extracted. If the ovum rupture and a part be retained in the uterus, the woman must be kept in bed, the ergot continued, and the vagina daily douched with a solution of formalin, 1 : 500. In many cases this treatment will be sufficient; but in spite of every precaution the discharges may become foul and the temperature rise, in which case the uterine cavity must be thoroughly curetted.

Active treatment : This is the treatment to be recommended, in preference to the expectant plan, in the large proportion of cases. The vaginal tampon may be employed, as recommended above. If at the end of twenty-four hours the os is not patulous, the patient should be anæsthetized, and the cervix dilated with Hegar's or Barnes's dilators, and the uterus emptied, as recommended below.

As soon as the os is sufficiently dilated to permit the introduction of the forefinger the ovum should be swept out and the decidua or placenta removed by scraping. The forefinger of the right hand is the best instrument for this purpose. It can be made to reach all parts of the uterus, with the assistance of the left hand pressing on the fundus through the abdominal wall. When the secundines cannot all be removed in this manner the interior of the uterus may be gently scraped with a blunt curette. In all cases, after emptying the uterus its cavity should be thoroughly douched with plain sterilized water or formalin solution, used hot. For this purpose the Fritsch-Bozeman uterine catheter is by far the best instrument. The Emmet curette forceps will be found to be a very valuable adjuvant to the curette in removing shreds from the uterine cavity.

After-treatment of abortion: The woman should be kept in bed for at least a week or ten days, the temperature should be watched, and, if necessary, appropriate treatment to prevent the onset of lactation should be applied.

Missed Abortion.

It occasionally happens that the fœtus perishes, symptoms of impending abortion develop only to disappear, and the ovum is retained in the uterus for weeks, or even months. To this condition the term "missed abortion" is applied. No *treatment* is indicated, provided the condition does not affect the general health of the patient, for sooner or later contractions will occur and the uterus empty itself of its contents.

Premature Labor and Miscarriage.

The phenomena of premature labor are very much the same as of labor at term, with the exception that the placenta is more frequently adherent to the uterine wall. When such is the case the uterus must be entered and the placenta stripped off and removed, after which a hot uterine douche should be given.

Missed Labor.

In this condition, which is very rare, the woman may exhibit a few ineffectual signs of labor at term; these disappear, and the product of conception is retained in utero for months, or even years. The fœtus in these cases always perishes, and either macerates or mummifies. The soft parts of the fœtus may be absorbed, and the bones may be discharged at intervals for a long time afterward, or they may find their way through the uterus into the bladder or rectum. It is a *good general rule* to induce labor in all cases in which the patient is known to have gone two weeks beyond the normal period of pregnancy.

ECTOPIC GESTATION.

Definition: When the impregnated ovum becomes attached, and develops outside the uterine cavity, the pregnancy is termed ectopic, or extra-uterine.

Frequency: Ectopic gestation occurs probably about once in 500 cases of pregnancy.

Varieties: There are *three primary forms of ectopic gestation:* (1) *tubal;* (2) *ovarian;* and (3) *abdominal.*

Many authorities classify the various terminations of these primary forms of ectopic gestation as *secondary forms,* each being designated according to the location of the displaced ovum. The term "secondary" as thus employed simply means *subsequent to rupture* or displacement.

While primary ovarian and abdominal pregnancies do occur, they are undoubtedly extremely rare, and are difficult of absolute demonstration ; as a general rule, ectopic gestations are *tubal.*

Tubal pregnancies are classified according to the site of the attachment of the ovum, as:

(1) *Interstitial* when the ovum develops in that portion of the tube which passes through the wall of the uterus, or in a diverticulum of this portion of the tube.

(2) *True tubal,* or ampullar, when the ovum develops in the free portion of the tube.

(3) *Infundibular* when the ovum develops in the infundibulum of the tube, and prevents the closure of the abdominal ostium. Cases of this variety are also termed *tubo-ovarian.*

Terminations of Ectopic Gestation.

Interstitial pregnancies usually terminate about the third month by rupture into the peritoneal sac. The patient generally succumbs to hemorrhage and shock. Rupture into the uterine cavity, with expulsion of the fœtus through the cervix, is possible, as is also rupture into the base of the broad ligaments.

True tubal pregnancies terminate by rupture either (*a*) upward into the abdominal cavity, or (*b*) downward between the layers of the broad ligament. When the rupture occurs *into the abdominal cavity* the hemorrhage is usually severe, and may be fatal in from sixteen hours to three or four days. When rupture occurs early and the hemorrhage is not severe, the fœtus may be absorbed, as the embryonic sac usually ruptures at the same time as the tube.

When the rupture *occurs downward*, between the layers of the broad ligament, the ovum may perish and all trace of it disappear, while the blood effused may be retained, forming a pelvic hæmatocele. The ovum may develop for a time, and then burst into the peritoneal cavity, or continue to full term by stripping the peritoneum from the pelvic wall as it enlarges. In either case the ovum develops for a time and then perishes, and is either absorbed or macerated, when it may ulcerate through into the bowel, bladder, or vagina, and escape.

In still other cases the gestation-sac may undergo putrefaction from access of bacteria from the bowel, and be converted into a broad-ligament abscess, which may rupture into the peritoneal cavity, or into the bladder, rectum, or vagina. In other cases the fœtus after death may be converted into a lithopædion or may be mummified, and thus remain for years.

Infundibular pregnancies may either rupture into the peritoneal cavity or develop to full term.

Ovarian pregnancies may terminate by rupture of the sac and profuse hemorrhage; or arrest of development may occur at an early period and the sac remain a cystic tumor. Advance to full term is possible, but not probable.

Abdominal pregnancies may advance to full term; or the sac may rupture early, and the fœtus be either absorbed or mummify.

Tubal abortion: This term is applied to a certain rare condition in which blood is effused into the ovum, destroying it and its attachments to the tube-walls. The ovum may remain as a *tubal mole*, forming a solid tumor of the tube; or it may escape with the blood from the fimbriated extremity of the tube into the abdominal cavity.

Etiology of Ectopic Gestation.

As has been stated, the ovum usually becomes impregnated while still in the Fallopian tube. If the tube is in a normal condition, the impregnated ovum is moved along it until it finds its resting-place in the uterine cavity. It is therefore probable that the most important factor in producing ectopic gestation is some **abnormal condition of the tubes.**

Such abnormal conditions may arise either from *inflammation* of the tissues of the tubes or from parametritic exudations, which lead to their constriction or destruction. *Malformations* of the tubes are not infrequent, such as diverticula, accessory tubal canals, etc., and have been noticed in connection with ectopic gestation.

Any diseased condition of the **mucous membrane** of the tubes, or any condition which interferes with their normal peristaltic action, may be said to favor the development of ectopic gestation.

The condition is generally encountered in women who present a history of a **protracted period of sterility.**

Pathology of Ectopic Gestation.

The uterus: With the establishment of pregnancy the uterus begins to enlarge; the enlargement continues throughout the pregnancy, though at a much slower rate than is the case in intra-uterine gestation. As a rule, this organ begins to involute when the fœtus perishes. A decidua forms in all cases of ectopic gestation, which is quite similar to the decidua vera of normal pregnancy. It is cast off either complete or in shreds, at the time of the primary tubal rupture, whether the ovum perishes or not. The shredding of the decidua is invariably accompanied with metrorrhagia. The decidua varies in thickness from one-eighth to one-fourth of an inch; it is shaggy on its uterine side, while its inner surface is quite smooth and shows no trace of either the decidua serotina or reflexa.

Changes in the tube and ovum: As the tube enlarges its relation to surrounding parts becomes greatly modified. The first change in the tube is a turgescence, due to increase in size of the vessels, the result of the stimulus of pregnancy.

14—Obst.

The muscle-fibres of the tube's walls then increase in size, but later atrophy as the result of minute ruptures due to small hemorrhages into their substance. Then follows free development of connective tissue, which replaces in great part the muscle-fibres. As the ovum enlarges the tube-walls become thinned out, the thickest part being at the site of the placental attachment, and the thinnest directly opposite. Closure of the abdominal ostium usually takes place at the sixth or seventh week; rupture of the tube takes place before the end of the second month in probably two-thirds of the cases.

The tube *is movable* to a limited degree until fixed by peritonitis. From its increased weight it tends to fall below its normal level, and it may be found in Douglas's pouch. As the ovum enlarges the uterus is pushed to one side. In some cases the tube remains closely attached to the uterus, while in others it forms a distinct mass.

In the pregnant tube a *decidua* is formed which is composed of the usual two layers, a superficial compact and a spongy lower layer. That portion of the decidua which is to form the maternal placenta, and which corresponds to the serotina, grows more rapidly than that in the rest of the tube. A decidua reflexa is also formed, but it tends to degenerate rapidly, and gives rise to hemorrhages very early in the pregnancy. These hemorrhages result in inflammatory changes which alter the general texture of the mass.

The **placenta** is formed in the same way as in intra-uterine gestation, but the lack of space in the tube results in traumatisms which altogether change its character, converting it into a liver-like mass. When the tube ruptures the torn walls of the tube spread out, and should the ovum survive, the placenta forms attachments to neighboring structures and continues its growth.

The **amnion** and **chorion** are only altered from their usual conditions by the results of trauma and sepsis.

Symptoms of Ectopic Gestation.

The phenomena which indicate the existence of ectopic gestation are: *irregular hemorrhages* from the vagina accompanied with *more or less severe pelvic pain;* and the *presence of a mass close to* and *often associated with the uterus.*

In a **typical case** the patient has been regular in menstruation for some time, when she misses a period. Shortly after this she has irregular attacks of bleeding, accompanied with sharp, cutting pelvic pain. These symptoms may lead to the suspicion of abortion, which is strengthened by the passage of portions of decidua. One of these attacks may be excessively severe and cause collapse. Not infrequently these attacks are accompanied by dysuria and rectal tenesmus.

The **amount of blood** lost varies from a mere show to a severe hemorrhage; with the blood may be found small shreds of mucosa, or even a complete cast of the decidual lining of the uterus.

The **pelvic pain** is usually of a sharp, tearing character; when excruciating, and accompanied with collapse, it indicates a serious rupture.

A vaginal examination in such a case will reveal the **presence of a mass** in close proximity to the uterus, which may be found somewhat enlarged. The character of the mass depends upon the situation of the ovum and whether it has ruptured or not. In cases in which rupture has taken place early into the general peritoneal cavity no mass may be felt.

If the **first attack be survived,** other similar attacks may follow and the internal hemorrhages be fatal. In other cases the effused blood may be absorbed after the perishing of the ovum.

The ovum **if it survive** may go on developing, in which case signs of pregnancy will continue, an abdominal tumor develop, and finally evidences of a living fœtus will manifest themselves. Such cases may go on to full term and a spurious labor occur.

In other cases **secondary rupture** takes place at a later period when the patient usually dies of hemorrhage or peritonitis; or if the patient survive, the fœtus becomes mummified or forms a lithopædion, being retained for some time, and finally is cast out piecemeal through a fistulous opening.

Diagnosis.

To make a positive diagnosis of ectopic gestation **previous to rupture** of the sac, while possible in a large majority of cases, is always a matter of difficulty.   The history of the signs of early pregnancy, associated with aggravated reflex nervous phenomena ; the early appearance of sharp, cramp-like pelvic pain increasing in severity, make a diagnosis possible.

Usually the condition is not recognized until **rupture has taken place.**   At this time the history of delayed menstrua-- tion, the occurrence of a paroxysm of frightful pain, sudden collapse, and symptoms of internal hemorrhage make the diagnosis very simple.

A **microscopical examination** of the shreds contained in the vaginal blood will reveal their decidual character, and make a differential diagnosis from abortion possible, as no chorionic villi will be found unless the pregnancy is intra-uterine.

In cases of **advanced ectopic gestation** the diagnosis is, as a rule, not difficult.   Owing to the great displacement of contiguous organs, abdominal pain is often excessive.   This pain is due in part to pressure, and in part to the development of peritonitis of a chronic type.

Prognosis.

Ectopic gestation is one of the most serious obstetrical conditions.   If **left to nature,** the mortality is over 60 per cent., the remainder recovering by death of the ovum and absorption of the contents of the gestation-sac.

When **treated by abdominal section,** Hirst states the mortality should be about 5 per cent. or lower, if the operator sees the patient in time.

Treatment.

As soon as a diagnosis of ectopic gestation is established the only rational treatment consists in the **immediate removal of the gestation-sac,** whether it has ruptured or not.

Abdominal section is the most satisfactory method of operating, though some operators prefer the vaginal route.   The latter method has many disadvantages, and should only be resorted to by those operators having special experience in operating by the vaginal route.

As it is a matter of considerable difficulty in many cases to control the hemorrhage and to separate the gestation-sac, the operation of *abdominal section* for the removal of an ectopic gestation should not be undertaken by an unskilled operator.

The technique of the operation: Though the operation has frequently to be performed in an emergency, plenty of time should be taken to secure an aseptic condition of the abdomen of the patient, of the operator, of the assistants, and of the instruments and dressings.

The operator, having opened the abdomen by a median incision, should at once insert his hand and seize the affected tube at its uterine end, so as to control the hemorrhage. The broad ligament should then be transfixed by a pedicle-needle to the inner side of the round ligament, and the tube ligated *en masse*. After the tube and ovary have been cut away, the abdominal cavity should be cleared of clots, if necessary flushing it with a large quantity of warm sterile water. The incision may then be closed without the insertion of a drainage-tube, unless a considerable number of adhesions have been encountered. The subsequent treatment is the same as for an uncomplicated ovariotomy.

When the hemorrhage has been very considerable a quantity of sterile salt solution should be injected under each breast, during the operation, by an assistant. After the operation it is advisable in all cases to inject at least a quart of the same solution into the bowel, by means of a long rubber tube and gravity syringe.

In **advanced ectopic pregnancy** many advise that interference be delayed until just short of term. In this case effort should be made to enucleate the fœtal sac whole.

When this is found to be impossible, after the fœtus has been removed the cord should be cut as close as possible to the placenta and the edges of the sac stitched to the edge of the abdominal wall, and the sac drained by packing it lightly with iodoform gauze.

The **after-treatment** in such cases consists in daily irrigation of the sac with antiseptic solutions, dusting it well with an antiseptic powder, and introducing fresh packing.

For further information on this subject reference should be had to standard gynæcological works, as ectopic gestation has passed from the domain of obstetrics to that of gynæcology, since the treatment of the condition is purely surgical.

PATHOLOGY OF LABOR.

The term **eutocia** is applied to normal labor which terminates easily without serious damage to mother or fœtus and without artificial aid.

Dystocia is the term applied to abnormal labor. If the abnormality of the labor depends upon some form of fœtal irregularity, the condition is termed *fœtal dystocia;* while if it be dependent upon some abnormal condition in the mother it is known as *maternal dystocia.*

The **cause of the dystocia** may be in any of the three factors which constitute the mechanical problem of labor. The *fœtus* or its appendages may be abnormal in size, shape, or position ; the *expelling forces* may be insufficient or excessive ; or the resistance offered by the *maternal passages* may be too great or too little.

When called upon to render assistance in a case of dystocia the physician should first ascertain which of the factors is at fault. The recognition of the disturbing cause forms the basis of rational treatment.

DYSTOCIA DUE TO MALPOSITIONS OF THE FŒTUS.

OCCIPITOPOSTERIOR CASES.

Occipitoposterior positions of the head are *primary* or *acquired.*

Primary, if the head enters the brim of the pelvis with the occiput posterior.

Acquired, if the occiput rotates from an anterior position at the beginning of labor to a posterior at its close ; the latter is very rare.

Diagnosis of Occipitoposterior Cases.

Abdominal examination: The back of the fœtus may be felt in the maternal flank ; but is frequently difficult to outline. The fœtal members may be felt over the whole anterior aspect of the abdomen. The head can be felt at the pelvic brim, while the anterior shoulder can easily be distinguished at a point about midway between the middle of Poupart's ligament and the umbilicus. The fœtal heart-sounds may be heard in the flank at about the level of the umbilicus.

Vaginal examination: If the cervix is dilated sufficiently, the sagittal suture may be felt in the line of the oblique diameter of the pelvis, while the posterior fontanelle is directed toward the right or left sacro-iliac joint. Labor in occipitoposterior positions is generally tedious, due to the irregular and ineffectual pains which characterize the first stage in these cases, and also because of the long internal rotation which must take place before the occiput is directed under the pubic arch.

Mechanism of Occipitoposterior Cases.

In **normal cases** the mechanism is much the same as in *anterior* positions of the occiput. Flexion is more difficult on account of the maladaptation of the head to the pelvis in these posterior positions, as the widest part of the head, the biparietal, is in relation with the narrowest part of the inlet, the diameter between the iliopectineal prominence and the

FIG. 78.

FIG. 79.

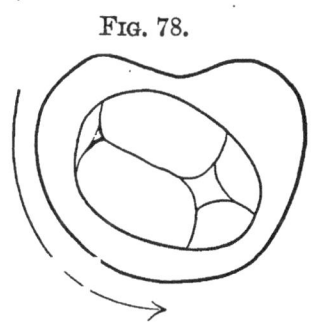
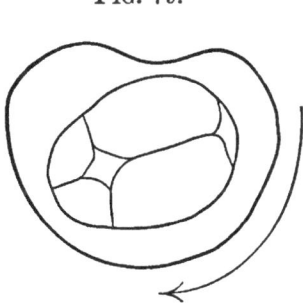

Right occipitoposterior position of head. The arrow shows the direction of the long internal rotation made by the occiput in delivery. (Jewett.)

Left occipitoposterior position of head. The arrow shows the direction of the long internal rotation made by the occiput in delivery. (Jewett.)

promontory. When flexion is complete and the head descends to the pelvic floor, internal rotation is prolonged on account of the great distance the occiput must traverse to come under the pubes; hence there is greater pain, and the labor is prolonged (Figs. 78 and 79).

Abnormal Mechanism.

(1) **Extended position of head**: The disproportion between the occipital end of the head and that portion of the brim in relation to it already referred to, may result in interference with flexion to such an extent that the head may enter the pelvis in an extended position, as in brow or face presentations.

(2) **Face to pubes**: When the head enters the pelvis imperfectly flexed the sinciput may reach the pelvic floor first, and is then directed toward the pubic arch, while the occiput

FIG. 80.

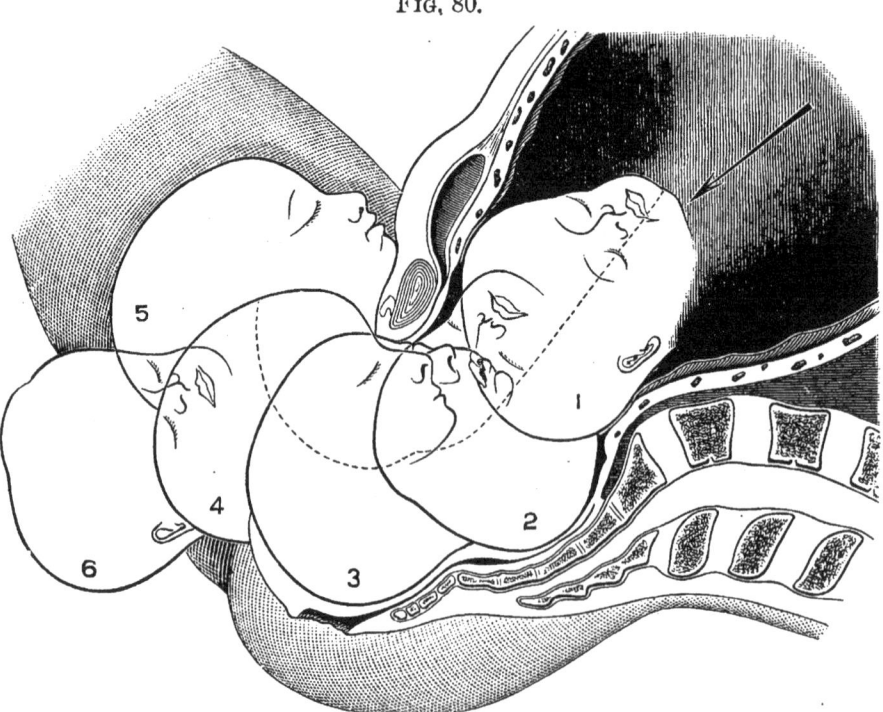

Faulty mechanism in a right occipitoposterior case. The occiput is shown rotating to the back. (After Schultze.)

rotates into the hollow of the sacrum. This mechanism results in delivery "face to pubes."

In such persistent occipitoposterior cases the head continues to descend until the glabella (the root of the nose) pivots under the pubes, when flexion takes place to permit the escape of the occiput over the perineum. When the occiput is delivered the head extends and the face escapes from under the pubes (Fig. 80). Spontaneous delivery in a face to pubes case is only accomplished with difficulty, and requires strong pains, lax maternal parts, and not too large a head. After the birth of the head the mechanism is the same as in other cases.

(3) In other cases the head may enter the pelvis poorly flexed, descend until it reaches the pelvic floor, and there remain fixed with its *long diameter* (O. F.) *transverse in the pelvic cavity*, generally at the level of the ischial spines, between which it becomes impacted.

Moulding of head in face to pubes cases: The occipitomental and occipitofrontal diameters of the fœtal head are shortened and the suboccipitobregmatic lengthened, as a result of the head pivoting at the glabella (Fig. 81).

Management of Labor in Occipitoposterior Cases.

Prophylaxis: Attention has been drawn to the desirability of making an abdominal examination to determine the position of the fœtus some time before the expected onset of labor. If at this examination the fœtus be found to occupy a posterior position, it is possible to rectify it by postural treatment in many cases. The woman should be instructed to assume the knee-chest position as frequently as possible, and to remain in this position for some time before turning upon the side to which it is desired to direct the occiput. In this posture the tendency is for the child to sag away from the brim under the influence of gravity, as the fundus and anterior uterine wall become the lowest portions of the uterus. The

Fig. 81.

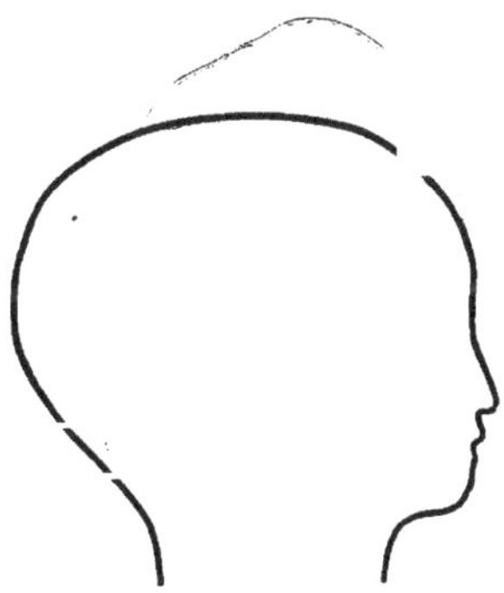

Diagram showing head unmoulded and moulded in a persistent occipitoposterior case. Black, moulded. Red, unmoulded.

child thus becomes free to rotate upon its own axis, and as its dorsum is heavier from the presence of the spinal column it is brought into apposition with the anterior wall of the uterus. Hence as the woman assumes the erect position the child's head tends to settle down against the brim in an anterior position.

At the Pelvic Inlet.

Frequent examinations should be made to ascertain whether flexion is being maintained as the head descends into the brim. Should extension of the head take place without descent, interference is demanded, as there is but little likelihood that the head will pass the brim by natural efforts.

Three methods of delivery are possible :

1st. **Version** : This is probably the most popular as well as the easiest method of dealing with these cases, because, as a rule, the general practitioner can perform this operation with greater ease to himself and less danger to the patient than either of the other methods.

2d. **Normal restoration of flexion and rotation of the fœtal head and body to an anterior position, with the subsequent application of the forceps** : This is a rather difficult operation, and should only be undertaken by those who are thoroughly skilful in the use of forceps. To perform this operation properly the patient should be placed under the influence of chloroform, so as to relax thoroughly the uterus. The operator, after the usual antiseptic precautions have been observed, should then pass his whole hand into the uterus so as firmly to grasp the brow and face of the child. The head having been raised slightly, so as to free it from the brim, is then gently rotated to an anterior position. The external hand of the operator should be used to promote rotation of the trunk, which should accompany rotation of the head. The rotation should be carried out slowly and with the utmost gentleness. After this has been accomplished the head should be urged into the brim by external pressure, and should be maintained in position by an assistant while forceps application is made. As in all high operations, only the axis-traction forceps should be used.

3d. **Application of the forceps without alteration of position** : This operation should only be undertaken as a last resort, as it is very dangerous both to mother and child. As a preliminary to this operation the head should be flexed.

In the Pelvic Cavity.

As in all posterior positions the head tends to pass the brim in a somewhat extended position, it is important to secure a speedy **restoration of flexion,** in order that the labor may be accomplished as easily and rapidly as possible, and to spare the patient unnecessary suffering.

Flexion may be restored by pressure upward upon the sinciput with two fingers during the intervals between the pains. During the pains the descent of the sinciput may be retarded by maintaining this pressure from below. Occasionally it is possible to hook the finger of the other hand over the occiput and draw it down, while at the same time the sinciput is being pressed up; but to do this the head must be very low and the parts lax.

When rotation fails and signs of exhaustion occur, then the **forceps must be applied.** During this operation care should be taken to prevent the blades slipping, as this accident is very liable to occur. Between the tractions the blades should be separated, because sometimes the occiput tends to rotate spontaneously. As the head emerges it should flex and the root of the nose pivot under the pelvic arch. It should be delivered slowly and with extreme caution, so as to favor moulding and to control the extent of perineal laceration. In many cases it is necessary to perform episiotomy, in order to prevent the laceration of the perineum extending into the rectum.

Prognosis.

The prognosis for both mother and child is not so favorable as in anterior positions. Backward rotation of the occiput takes place in about $1\frac{1}{2}$ per cent. of all cases of labor.

Laceration of the maternal soft parts is frequent and often extensive. The mortality of the fœtus is somewhat over 9 per cent., as compared with 5 per cent. in anterior positions.

FACE PRESENTATIONS.

Occurrence : Face presentations rarely exist prior to the onset of labor; they may be considered as altered vertex presentations. Presentation of the face cannot be said to be common, for it occurs once in about every 250 cases of labor.

Positions : The chin is the denominator, as it replaces the occiput in the mechanism when compared to vertex presentations, for the head is extended instead of being flexed.

The long diameter of the face, the frontomental, usually occupies the right oblique diameter of the pelvic brim ; hence the most common positions are : R. M. P. and L. M. A.; rarely, R. M. A. and L. M. P. positions may be met with.

Causes : Any condition which tends to interfere with proper flexion of the head may be set down as a cause of face presentation. The most common causes are :

1. Obliquity of the uterus, which acts by altering the line of fœtal-axis pressure.

2. Tumors of the fœtal neck, thyroid, or thymus.

3. Coils of thick cord around the neck.

4. Dead fœtus.

5. Excessive liquor amnii.

6. Small size of fœtus.

7. Deformed pelvis.

8. Tumors of uterus or neighboring structures.

9. Tumors upon the back, as meningocele.

10. Dolichocephalic head.

11. Occipitoposterior positions, in which there is a tight fit at the brim.

Diagnosis of Face Presentations.

Abdominal examination : It is sometimes a matter of difficulty to make a diagnosis of face presentation when the abdominal wall is thick or tense. Usually the bulky cranial vault can be felt in one hypogastric region, and a deep groove may be made out between it and the fœtal back. On the opposite side of the abdomen the fœtal members may be distinguished (Fig. 82). As the fœtal back is displaced from the uterine wall by the extended head, the *heart-sounds* are to be heard most distinctly on the same side of the abdomen upon which the fœtal extremities are felt.

Vaginal examination: Early in labor before rupture of the membranes, the rounded head to be felt in the vertex

Fig. 82.

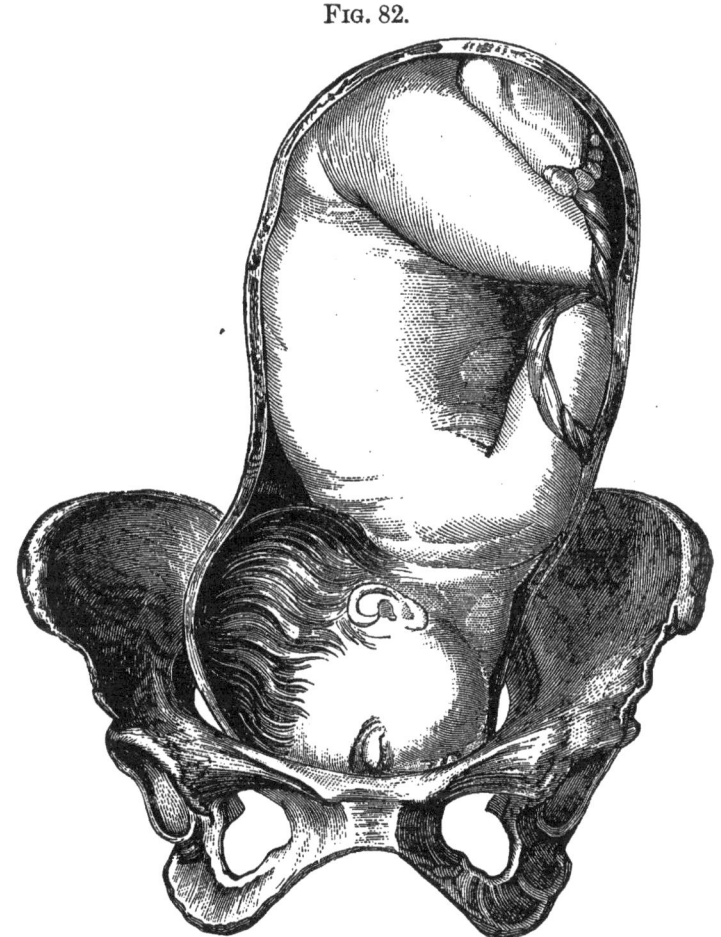

Transverse position of face at superior strait.

cases is wanting, and usually nothing can be reached but the bulky bag of waters, as the face is arrested high up. Care should be taken not to rupture the membranes in attempting to reach the presenting part of the fœtus. Should the bag of waters be ruptured, then it may be possible to distinguish the superciliary ridges, the eyes, the nose, and especially the mouth. The latter is distinguished by feeling the tongue and the alveolar margins. If the caput succedaneum has formed over the face, it may be mistaken for a breech, unless care be taken to distinguish clearly the relationship of the parts within reach of the finger.

Mechanism of Face Presentations.

The first stage of labor is delayed because the head does not fit the lower uterine segment so well as in vertex presentations.

The mechanism of face cases **differs** from that of the vertex in that:

1. The chin takes the place of the occiput in being the leading part of the head in descent. It does not come down so far in advance of the rest of the head as the occiput in vertex cases, so that internal rotation of the chin forward to the pubic arch occurs rather late and is slow.

2. Moulding takes place with more difficulty than in vertex cases.

3. The head is delayed longer at the brim, as extension has to be very marked before descent can begin; hence, as a rule, labor is delayed.

R. M. P.: As this is probably the commonest position, its mechanism will be described in detail.

The long diameter of the face, the frontomental, descends through the inlet in the right oblique diameter of the pelvic brim. The chin descends, strikes the pelvic floor, then rotates forward through three-eighths of a circle on the right side of the pelvis till it comes under the pubic arch. The brow rotates into the hollow of the sacrum, and the frontomental diameter thus corresponds to the anteroposterior diameter of the outlet. The chin then appears at the vulva and escapes beneath the pubic arch. The movement of flexion then begins, the chin pivoting under the pubic arch, and the face, forehead, vertex, and occiput successively clear the perineum (Fig. 83). The head now being free assumes its relationship to the shoulders, which occupy the right oblique diameter of the pelvis; the rest of the mechanism is the same as in a case of L. O. A.

L. M. A.: The mechanism is the same as in a vertex case, except that the occiput is replaced by the chin, which pivots

FIG. 83.

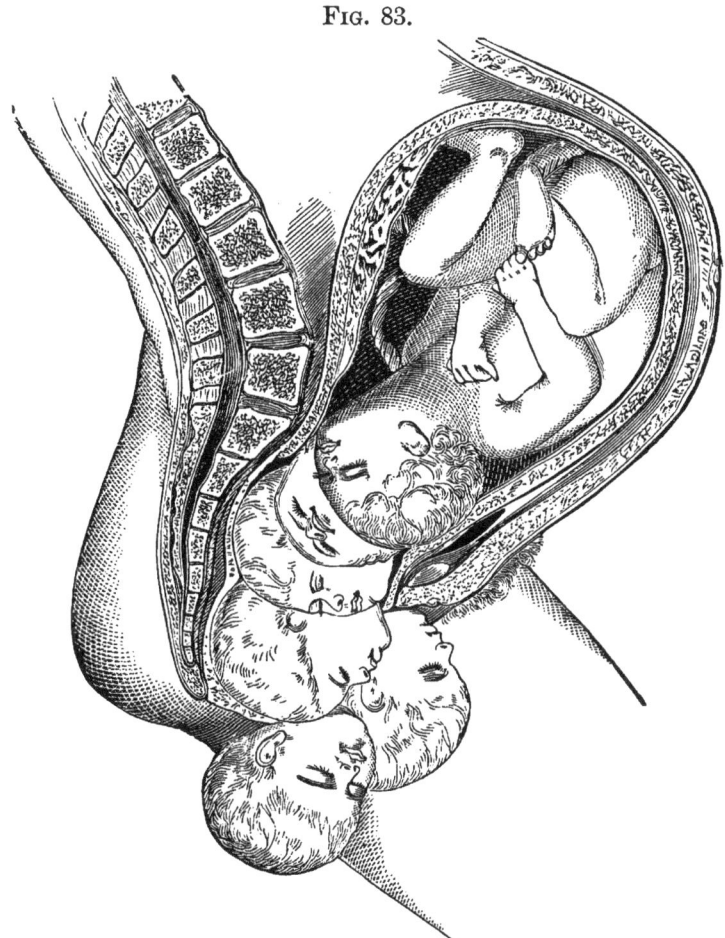

Diagrammatic view of mechanism in a right mentoposterior *position* of a face *presentation*, chin rotating to pubes.

under the pubes; then the head is delivered by flexion. Sometimes in a large pelvis the head may be pushed through in extension without any special mechanism.

In **mentoposterior** positions the head may descend into the pelvis sufficiently far to prevent completely the anterior rotation of the chin, which is then forced into the hollow of the sacrum. This condition is practically fatal to the child.

Head-moulding: The vault of the head becomes flattened and pushed backward; the diameters lengthened are the occipitofrontal and the occipitomental; the diameters shortened are the suboccipitobregmatic and the cervicobregmatic.

The **caput succedaneum** is found on the face, chiefly around the eye which lies anterior when the face is at the brim; owing to the laxity of the tissues of the face the swelling is often very great and the discoloration considerable. The eye may be closed for days, and the child may be unable to suckle from the swelling of the lips.

Prognosis.

The fœtal mortality in face cases is about 15 per cent.; the maternal mortality is given as being over 6 per cent., for these cases are frequently mismanaged. The labor is tedious, as a rule. Anterior positions of the chin are better than posterior, as the labor is quicker. There is usually more or less serious laceration of the perineum.

Management of Face Presentations.

The important point in the first stage is to **preserve the bag of waters** intact as long as possible, because the face is a poor dilator of the cervix. The patient should therefore be kept in bed all through this stage.

Flexion by Schatz's method: If the chin is posterior an attempt should be made to restore flexion and thus convert the position into a vertex anterior. This may be accomplished by gentle external manipulations according to the method recommended by Schatz (Fig. 84). The woman is placed in the Trendelenburg position, which may be accomplished by arranging an ordinary wooden chair (first sawing off the legs close to the wooden seat) on the bed so that its back forms an inclined plane, covering it with a folded blanket and drawing the patient up over it so that her buttocks rest on the back edge of the seat. The operator then presses on the occiput of the child with one hand, so as to force it into the pelvis, while he presses the other against the child's neck on the opposite side, thus flexing the head and straightening the vertebral column of the fœtus. When flexion has thus been accomplished, pressure is then maintained upon the fundus, so as to force the head into the pelvic brim in the flexed position.

If this be found impossible, the case may be left until the os has dilated, when, after rupturing the membranes, an effort

FIG 84.

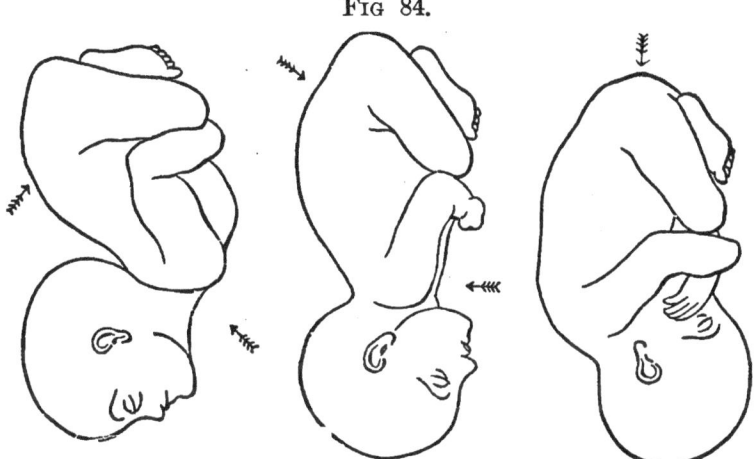

Schatz's method of rectification by external manipulation.

may be made to restore flexion by **introducing the hand into the uterus.**

If it be found impossible to maintain the head in the flexed position after this manœuvre, the **forceps should be applied** and the head drawn down into the cavity in a flexed position, when the blades may be withdrawn and the delivery left to nature.

If the patient is a **multipara** with lax parts and the uterine contractions are powerful, the case may be left to nature; but care should be exercised to secure good extension as the head descends, in order that the chin may reach the pelvic floor in advance of the rest of the head.

In a **primipara** in whom the presentation is posterior and it

15—Obst.

is found impossible to restore flexion, *internal version* may
be employed.

Forceps: If version be impossible in anterior positions
where delay occurs at the brim, then forceps may be applied;
but the operation is difficult and dangerous, as the blades
tend to slip off the head when traction is made.

If all these efforts fail and the child has perished, then
craniotomy must be performed to secure delivery

When the head has passed the brim and **fails to advance
further,** there is danger to the child from the tension on the
vessels of the neck causing engorgement of the cerebral circulation. In such cases the forceps should be employed to
hasten delivery.

Brow Presentations.

Many authorities describe a **half-way stage** in the development of face presentations. It can scarcely be classified as a
special presentation, but should be considered as simply a displacement of the vertex.

Should such a presentation be met with, it can only be **diagnosed** by vaginal examination. The extension of the head is
recognized by the fact that, instead of the vertex, the finger
comes in contact with the brow; possibly the anterior fontanelle may be distinguished, as well as the supra-orbital ridges.

Treatment consists in the manual restoration of flexion;
and if this be impossible, version must be resorted to in order
to effect delivery with a minimum of risk to the mother and
child. In rare instances in which the brow is directed anteriorly the head may descend to the pelvic floor in this partially
extended condition; in such cases the sinciput, being in
advance of the rest of the head, is directed to the pubes,
the root of the nose pivots under the pubic arch, and the head
is delivered in flexion, precisely the same as has been described in speaking of " face to pubes " cases.

BREECH PRESENTATIONS.

Definition: The presentation of any part of the pelvic pole
of the fœtal ovoid at the inlet is termed a breech presenta-

tion. The term, therefore, includes a presentation of the *buttocks, knees,* or *feet.* The denomination is taken from the position of the sacrum.

Frequency : Breech presentations occur in the proportion of 1 in 30 labors; if premature births be excluded, then the

FIG. 85.

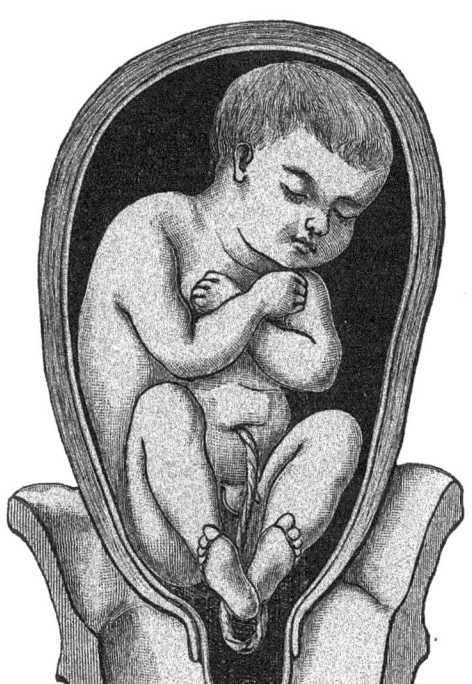

Breech presentation. Right sacroposterior. Feet and cord in relation to os internum. (After A. R. Simpson.)

proportion is about 1 in 60. The positions in order of frequency are : L. S. A.; R. S. P.; R. S. A.; L. S. P. (Figs. 85 and 86).

Causes : Certain conditions favor presentation of the breech. These are : lax uterine or abdominal walls, excessive liquor amnii, uterine obliquity, multiple pregnancy, death or prematurity of the fœtus, placenta prævia, contracted pelvis, tumors of the uterus or neighboring structures, monstrosity, and hydrocephalus.

FIG. 86.

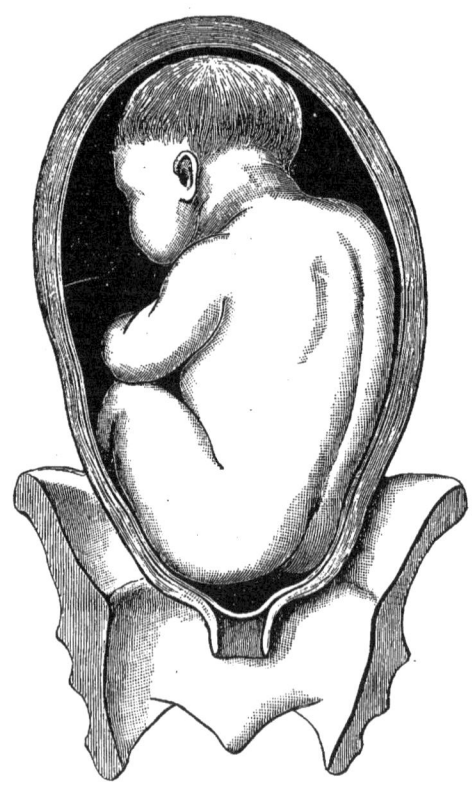

Breech presentation.   Left sacro-anterior position.   (After A. R. Simpson.)

Diagnosis of Breech Presentations.

Abdominal examination: On exploring the excavation of the pelvis it will be found empty, while at the brim a large, bulky, irregular, movable mass may be distinguished, which is not engaged unless labor has well advanced.   At the fundus the hard, well-defined contour of the head will be easily recognized.   The fœtal heart-sounds will be heard on the side to which the back is directed, at or above the level of the umbilicus.

Vaginal examination: Care must be taken not to rupture the membranes if they be found intact, in making the vaginal examination. Generally the breech is situated so high up that it cannot be reached without risk of rupturing the bag of waters if the examination is made early in labor. After labor has advanced and the membranes have ruptured the breech may be recognized by feeling the sacrum, coccyx, and ischial tuberosities of the foetus. The anus may be recognized by the grasp of the sphincter ani, and by the presence of meconium on the examining finger. If the child is a male, the scrotum and penis may be felt. Occasionally the former may be œdematous and may then be mistaken for the bag of waters. One or both feet may be felt; the foot may be distinguished from the hand by the projections of the heel and the malleoli. The knee may be distinguished from the elbow by the presence of the patella and by the larger size. Care must be taken to distinguish the breech from the face, for which it is often mistaken.

Mechanism of Breech Presentations.

The **first stage** of labor is very prolonged, for the breech forms a poor dilator of the cervix, and on account of its softness acts imperfectly as an irritator of reflex uterine contractions.

The breech descends generally with the **anterior hip** slightly in advance of the other. The anterior hip in striking the pelvic floor is rotated forward to the pubic arch, where it becomes fixed, while the trunk is driven down and the posterior hip moves forward over the perineum (Fig. 87). Generally both hips emerge through the vulva at the same time, then follow the thighs and trunk. If the legs are flexed properly, they generally escape with the thighs and breech.

The **shoulders** pass the brim with their long diameter transverse; they then turn into the oblique, and finally, at the outlet, into the anteroposterior diameter. The anterior shoulder is generally delivered first, followed by the posterior.

The **head** by this time, if flexion has been maintained, has entered the brim with its long diameter in the opposite oblique diameter of the pelvis to that in which the shoulders engaged.

The occiput usually strikes the pelvic floor first and rotates to the front, while the face is directed to the hollow of the sacrum. The face and forehead are then born, followed by the rest of the head.

Abnormalities in the mechanism: 1. The *breech* may be arrested at the brim or may not engage. This may be due either to pelvic contraction or to excessive size of the fœtus.

2. The *breech* may descend into the cavity of the pelvis and there be arrested. This may be due to excessive size of the fœtus, to imperfect dilatation of the external os, to pelvic deformity, or to the extended position of the limbs along the body of the child preventing its lateral flexion.

FIG. 87.

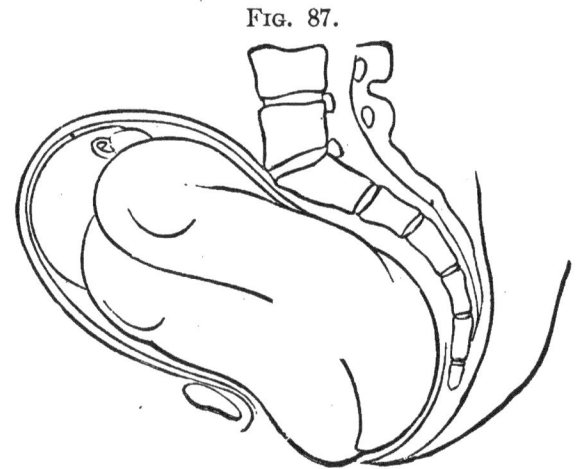

Passage of buttocks over perineum in a breech case. (After Barnes.)

3. The *arms* may become extended and cause arrest of the head at the pelvic brim. This accident may be due to an imperfectly dilated os or to pelvic contraction. It is very apt to occur if traction is made upon the body of the fœtus to accelerate delivery.

4. The *head* may become arrested at the brim or in the pelvic cavity, as a result of extension or from pelvic deformity. Occasionally when the face is directed anteriorly the chin may catch on the upper border of the pubes and cause delay.

Moulding of the fœtus: The breech is generally swollen and often discolored from ecchymoses; the discoloration is generally more marked over the anterior hip. If the child is a male, the scrotum is generally œdematous.

Prognosis of Breech Presentations.

The **fœtal mortality** varies from 10 to 30 per cent., depending upon the skill of the physician. The risks to the child are great, due to the prolapse of the cord and the pressure of the after-coming head upon it. Fractures and dislocations may be caused by efforts at rapid delivery.

The **risks to the mother** are increased only by the tendency to laceration and to bruising of the soft parts on account of the necessity for rapid and sometimes violent extraction of the after-coming head.

Management of Labor in Breech Presentations.

General: Very early in labor, before the membranes have ruptured or the breech has become engaged in the brim, it may be possible to perform an external version. The operation is not always practicable, and therefore should not be attempted unless there is certainty that it can be successfully accomplished.

The position of the physician in charge of a breech case should be one of armed expectancy. As long as the natural processes are progressing satisfactorily he should be watchful but inactive, and should be prepared to interfere promptly on the appearance of danger to the child.

When possible a skilled assistant should be obtained, whose duty it is to give the anæsthetic and attend to the maintenance of pressure upon the fundus, so as to prevent extension of the head during the delivery.

Preparations should be made for treating asphyxia of the newborn infant. At hand should be placed, sterilized and ready for use, the ligatures for the cord, scissors, two pairs of artery-forceps (to be used instead of ligatures in cases in which speed is demanded), a basin containing warm sterile water in which are a couple of sterile towels for wrapping around the child's body during delivery, and the ordinary obstetric forceps.

Throughout labor the patient should be kept in bed, and should be cautioned against straining during the first stage, as it is desirable to retain the membranes without rupture as long as possible, to favor complete dilatation of the os uteri. The fœtal heart-sounds should be frequently auscultated during the second stage of labor, since there is always danger of compression of the cord. Irregularity of the heart-beats is sufficient cause for interference.

When **delivery is imminent** the patient should lie in the dorsal position, with the thighs flexed. In cases in which it is necessary to effect a speedy delivery the patient should be placed across the bed in the lithotomy position. As soon as the buttocks emerge they should be wrapped in a warm sterile towel, to prevent the child making efforts at respiration. From the moment the buttocks appear at the vulva till the placenta is delivered the fundus uteri should be *constantly* under the control of an assistant. The trunk, as it emerges, should be supported, so as to prevent undue strain upon the perineum and traction upon the after-coming head. As soon as the feet appear the legs may be gently drawn down in such a way as to make no traction upon the body of the child.

As soon as the umbilicus comes within reach of the finger, a **loop of cord** may be gently drawn down and examined. If it is pulsating well, the case may be allowed to deliver slowly ; but should there be evidence of compression upon it, then the delivered portion of the child's body should be pressed backward and upward, and an attempt made to loosen the cord and to place it in one or other iliac fossa out of harm's way ; if this effort fails, then delivery should be accomplished as speedily as possible.

As the **elbows appear** at the vulva the arms should be drawn down, and then the child's body should be well elevated, so as to prevent the escape of the head.

In the delivery of **the head** there is no need for rapidity in normal cases, when once the mouth and nostrils have cleared the perineum. These must be wiped off to prevent aspiration of mucus should the child attempt to breathe. Then the head should be delivered slowly and carefully, so as to avoid rupturing the perineum.

Treatment of Arrest of Breech at the Brim.

Arrest of the breech at the brim may be due to the excessive size of the child or to pelvic deformity. The precaution should always be taken of measuring the mother's pelvis, unless this has been done, before any operative measures are adopted.

To secure descent five methods are available : (1) by bringing down the anterior leg ; (2) traction with a finger in the groin ; (3) the blunt hook ; (4) the fillet ; and (5) application of forceps.

Traction after bringing down a leg: The hand, the palm of which corresponds to the abdominal aspect of the child, is

FIG. 88.

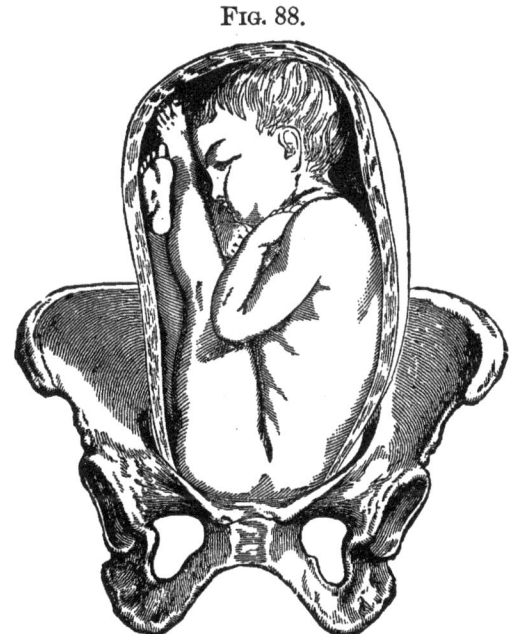

Breech presentation—legs extended.

slowly introduced in the uterus, care being taken to ascertain the position of the fœtal cord so as to avoid dragging it down. It is well also to press gently back the breech, so as to disengage it from the brim before seizing a foot. The anterior foot should always be selected, and when firmly grasped may be gently drawn through the os and vagina. Occasionally the legs may be found extended along the chest of the child (Fig. 88). In such a case the foot may be brought within reach by passing two fingers along the back of the thigh, at the same time abducting it so as to press the knee to one side; thus the foot tends to drop down in the median line of the chest, and may be grasped by slipping the fingers down along the leg. Provided there are no indications necessitating speedy delivery, the case may be left to nature as soon as the foot has been drawn down to the vulva.

Should the patient be exhausted, delivery may be hastened by combined traction on the foot which has been brought down, and pressure on the fundus from above. The latter should be managed by the assistant, so that the operator may give his whole attention to the child. When it is desired to effect a speedy delivery the patient should be placed in the Walcher position, and when possible on a table. The foot should be grasped between the first and second fingers, and the line of traction should be downward and backward in the axis of the pelvic brim. When the leg is beyond the vulva it should be wrapped in a warm sterile towel, and then as much of the limb as possible should be grasped in the whole hand. The operator should introduce the forefinger of his free hand into the vagina and hook it into the posterior groin as soon as it comes within reach, in order to distribute the tractive force as widely as possible, and thus reduce the risks of injury to the child. As the breech distends the perineum it should be drawn forward against the pubes, so as to avoid laceration. As soon as possible the posterior limb should be gently drawn out, in doing this, pressure on the thigh should be avoided, care being taken to seize the foot and draw down the leg in such a way that the knee comes down in the median line of the child's body.

When it is impossible to bring down a foot it may be possible **to hook the forefinger in the groin**, which may be done in any manner convenient to the operator. Traction may then be made downward and backward, care being taken to avoid pressure on the shaft of the femur, on account of the danger of its snapping.

The **blunt hook** or **fillet** may be used as a tractor. The latter should be used by preference as much less liable to do damage to mother or child.

The **fillet** is usually composed of a strip of sterilized cotton or gauze bandage. The best instrument for placing the fillet is a gum elastic catheter. The catheter should be threaded with a loop of string and then, with its stilet, should be bent so as to form a large hook. After it has been sterilized the hook should be guided over the anterior hip and rotated so that its point passes between the child's thigh and abdomen. The finger should then be passed between the thighs, and the loop of string dragged down until the fillet can be threaded through it, when by withdrawing the catheter and string the fillet can be drawn into place. The line of traction should then be toward the child's sacrum, so as to avoid breaking the femur.

As a last resort, should all other means fail, **the forceps** should be applied to the breech.

Impaction in the Pelvic Cavity.

When the **breech becomes impacted in the pelvic cavity** (Fig. 89) it is generally impossible to draw down a leg.

Traction may be exerted by hooking an index-finger into the groin ; or the fillet may be used. When these means fail forceps may be employed. If the child is alive and moderate traction with the forceps fails, then pubiotomy may be resorted to. When the child has perished embryotomy is necessary.

Rapid Extraction of the Trunk.

As soon as the **legs and the pelvis** of the child have escaped from the vulva they should be wrapped in a warm towel and grasped with both hands in such a way that the thumbs of the operator lie along the sacrum, while the fingers seize the thighs. This gives the most secure grasp. Traction is then made downward and backward with both hands, while the assistant presses firmly on the fundus. As soon as the cord can be reached a loop should be drawn down, as is done in normal delivery of the breech.

When the **angles of the scapulæ** come into view the delivery of the arms should be attempted. To do this, two fingers of the operator's hand which corresponds to the arm it is desired to reach, should be passed up over the shoulder and down the arm to the elbow, which may then be swept across the chest so as to bring down the forearm and hand, the child's body being held in such a position as to give the greatest freedom

FIG. 89.

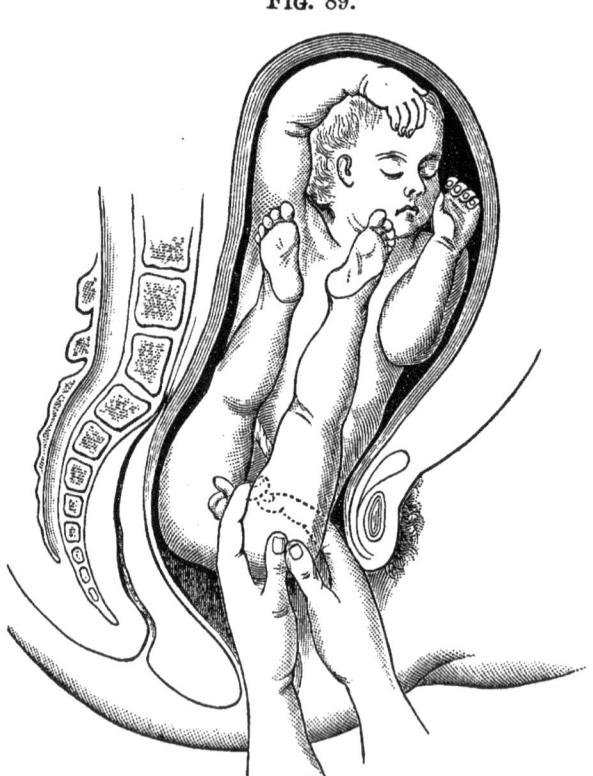

Delivery of child in a breech case by traction made with fingers placed in groin. (After A. R. Simpson.)

of movement possible to the operator. Having released one arm, the operator should then change hands and deliver the other arm by a similar manœuvre.

Upward displacement of the arms: Not infrequently the arms are found to be displaced upward alongside the head. This is generally indicated by greater resistance to traction after the scapulæ have come into view. When this complication is found the body of the fœtus should be pushed up in the axis of the brim, so as to diminish the pressure on the arms at that level. The body should then be rotated until its back is directed to one or other side of the mother. Usually the posterior arm is most accessible, and is therefore brought down first. Holding the child's body up against the pubes the operator presses two fingers up over the posterior shoulder to the elbow, and sweeps the arm down across the face and chest, as directed above. Having released the posterior arm, the child's body is pressed over against the perineum, and the anterior arm is brought down by a similar manœuvre.

The **anterior arm** may be so firmly caught between the head and the pubes that it may be impossible to dislodge it. In this case it should be rotated so as to come into a posterior position. This rotation is accomplished by grasping the trunk of the child's body firmly with both hands, lowering it so as to bring its long axis to correspond to that of the pelvic brim, and then shoving it up so as to release the anterior arm from pressure. As soon as the arm is loose alongside of the head, the child is rotated about its long axis, so that the arm which has been anterior passes along the same side of the pelvis backward and rests in front of the sacro-iliac synchondrosis. By this manipulation the back is moved from one side to the front, and then to the opposite side. The arm is then delivered as was the posterior arm in the first instance. Occasionally the anterior arm may be folded behind the occiput. In this case the revolution of the body must be made in the opposite direction. First turn the abdomen of the child forward and then to the opposite side, thus causing the shoulder to rotate through three-quarters of a circle.

Constriction of the head by the cervix: Occasionally the cervix may become tightly constricted about the child's neck ; a condition which generally endangers the life of the child. The patient should be deeply anæsthetized, and traction made on the shoulders with one hand, while the fingers of the other, placed in the child's mouth, give what assistance is possible.

Delivery of the After-coming Head.

Deventer's method : Probably the easiest method of effecting a speedy delivery in a case in which the pelvis permits the
descent of the head with the arms extended alongside is
Deventer's.　　The body of the child is dropped downward,
the feet are grasped with one hand, while the other presses
upon the upper surface of the shoulders, the neck being between the first and second fingers.　Traction is made downward
toward the floor, the patient being in the lithotomy position.

Fig. 90.

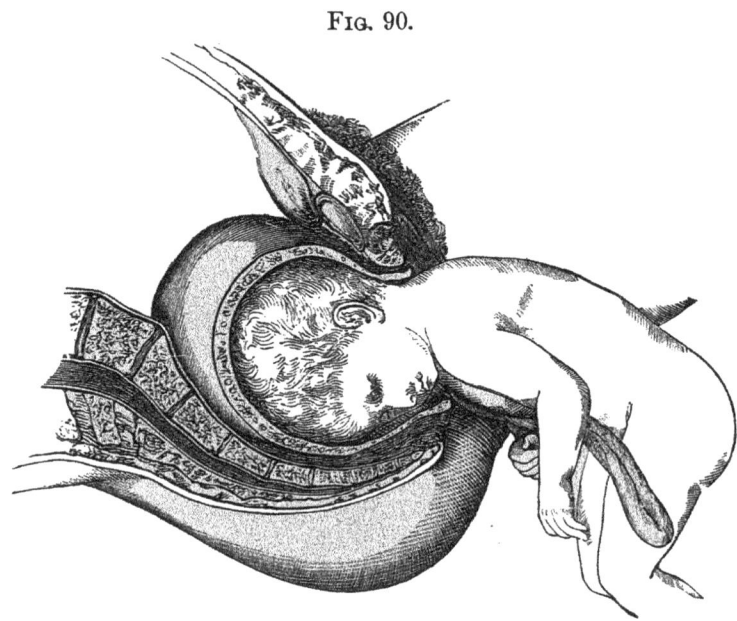

Anterior rotation of occiput.

Thus the occiput appears at the vulva, the vertex slips under
the pelvic arch, and the head is delivered in extension, being
followed by the arms.　This method is applicable only in cases
in which the pelvic space is sufficient to permit the descent
of the head and arms together.　When the fœtus is small, as
in premature cases, this, in the experience of the writer, is
the easiest and most rapid method of delivery.　Contrary to
expectation, laceration of the perineum is rare in cases in
which this method of delivery is possible.

Arms Delivered—Head Still Retained.

Having delivered the arms, the head being still retained, the operator has five methods of delivery at his disposal.

1. The Smellie method: The body of the child having been wrapped in a warm towel, is placed on the flexor surface of the operator's left arm, the legs hanging on either side. The fingers of this hand are passed into the vagina, so that the

FIG. 91.

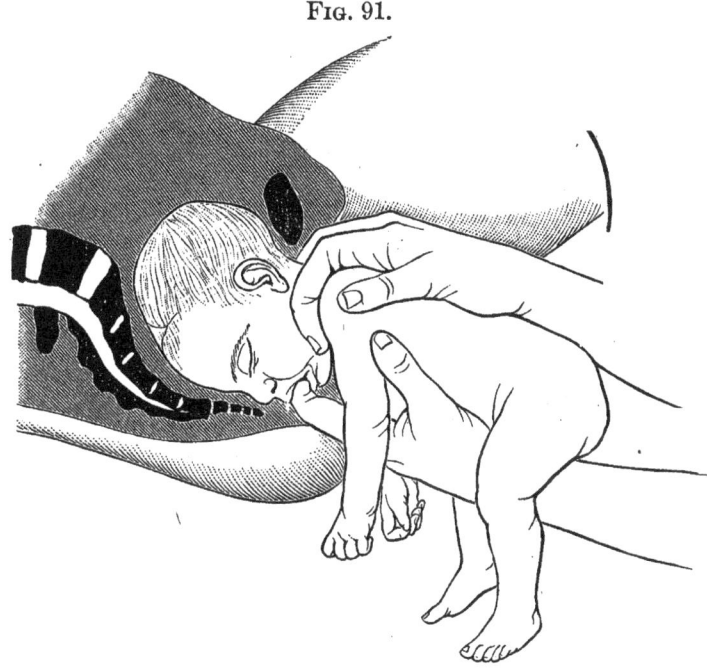

The Smellie-Veit method of extracting the after-coming head. (Döderlein.)

tips rest on the fossa on either side of the child's nose. The finger-tips of the right hand are then placed on the child's occiput. Before making efforts at extraction the head is well flexed by pushing upward with the fingers on the occiput, and at the same time pulling down with the fingers on the face. Having secured good flexion, the operator pulls downward until the occiput is well under the pubic arch (Fig. 90), and then, but not till then, the trunk is raised, at the same time that traction is made so as to pivot the occiput under the pubic arch, and thus the face sweeps over the perineum and the head is delivered. Care must be exerted not to make traction with any degree of force once the head distends the perineum, otherwise the head will deliver with a snap and the result will probably be an extensive laceration.

2. **The Smellie-Veit or Mauriceau method**: The child's body is placed on the operator's arm as described above, but one or two fingers are inserted into the mouth instead of on either side of the nose. The other hand is passed along the child's back until the middle finger rests on the occipital protuberance, while the index and ring fingers are flexed over the

Fig. 92.

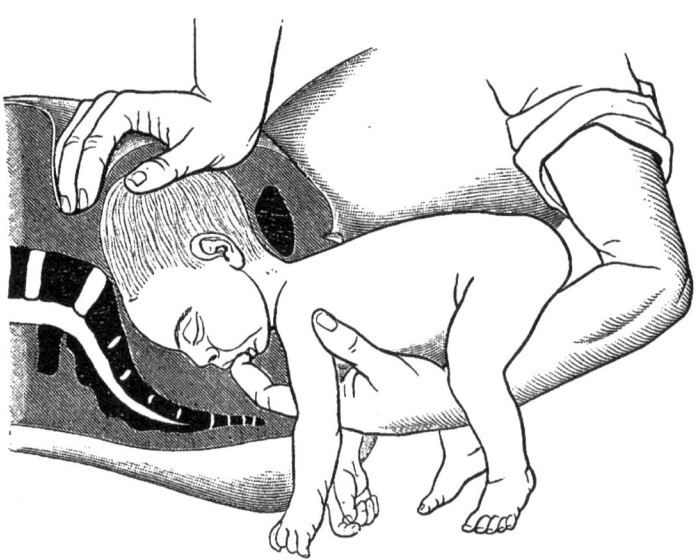

The Wigand-Martin method of delivering the after-coming head. (Döderlein.)

shoulders on either side of the neck (Fig. 91). Having loosened the head and secured good flexion, traction is then made with both hands at once, in the axis of the pelvic outlet, until the occiput pivots under the pubes; then the child's body is carried upward toward the mother's abdomen, this movement being made very slowly and deliberately, to avoid laceration of the perineum. Care must be taken not to fracture or dislocate the lower jaw.

3. **Wigand-Martin method:** The child's body is held on the left arm, the index-finger of the left hand being inserted into the mouth in order to flex the head. The right hand is then placed on the mother's abdomen over the pubes, so as to secure a firm grasp of the head (Fig. 92). Firm pressure is then made with the right hand in the axis of the parturient canal; at the same time traction is made with the left hand, and as the head descends the child's body is elevated toward the mother's abdomen.

FIG. 93.

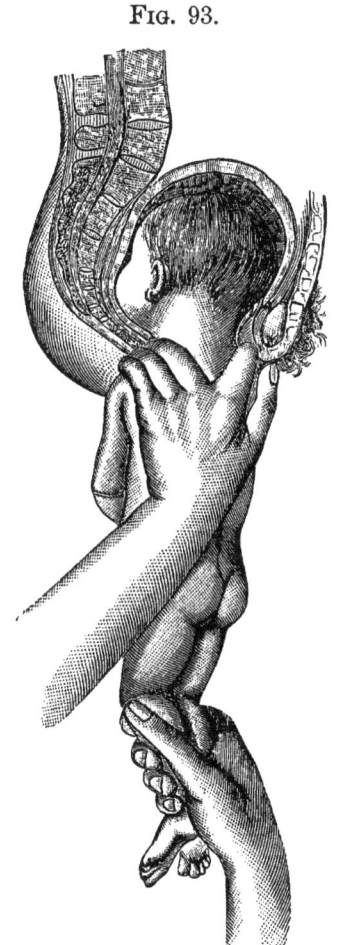

Prague grasp.

4. **Prague method:** Having wrapped the body in a warm towel, the operator seizes the child's feet with the right hand, the middle finger being placed between the internal malleoli, the index and ring fingers being above the external malleoli. The left hand is then placed on the child's shoulders in such a way as to secure a firm grasp (Fig. 93). Traction is then made downward *with both hands* until the head has entered the pelvic cavity. Then the right hand swings the body upward, at the same time making traction, while the left hand is held firmly in position, being used as a fulcrum around which the head moves, until it is finally forced out of the parturient canal by this lever-like movement of the body.

The force exerted by this method is very considerable, and therefore it should be used only after the foregoing methods have been attempted.

5. **Forceps:** Manual efforts at extraction having failed, the forceps may be used. To permit the application of the blades,

16—Obst.

the child's head must be held up toward the mother's abdomen by an assistant.   Properly directed suprapubic pressure by an assistant increases the efficacy of all methods of delivering the after-coming head.   Six minutes is the maximum time at the operator's disposal once the placental circulation has been completely cut off.   Therefore it is advisable to have the assistant call off the minutes as the time passes, so that the last two may be utilized for the application of the forceps should recourse to these instruments be required.

TRANSVERSE PRESENTATIONS.

Definition: Any presentation of the trunk of the child's body is termed a transverse presentation.   As the result of uterine action after the onset of labor transverse presentations resolve into *shoulder presentations*.   The term *cross-birth* is frequently applied to a transverse presentation.

Frequency: Less than 0.5 per cent. of all cases of labor present transverse presentations.

Causes: The same causes that result in breech presentations also act in producing transverse presentations.

Varieties: The long axis of the trunk is very rarely transverse, but is usually obliquely placed as regards the long axis of the uterus; thus any part of the fœtus may present at the brim.

Positions: Some writers classify transverse presentations according to the position of the lowest shoulder, making use of the scapula as the denominator; *e. g.*, S. L. A.; S. R. P., etc.   It is generally sufficient to classify the positions as follows:

  1. *Dorso-anterior:*
    (*a*) Head on the right side of mother.
    (*b*) Head on left side (Fig. 94). .
  2. *Dorsoposterior:*
    (*a*) Head on right side.
    (*b*) Head on left side.

The *most frequent position* is dorso-anterior, head to the right side of the mother.

Diagnosis of Transverse Presentations.

Abdominal examination: On inspection the shape of the uterine tumor will be noticed to be abnormal. The longest diameter, instead of being vertical, will be found to be oblique,

FIG. 94.

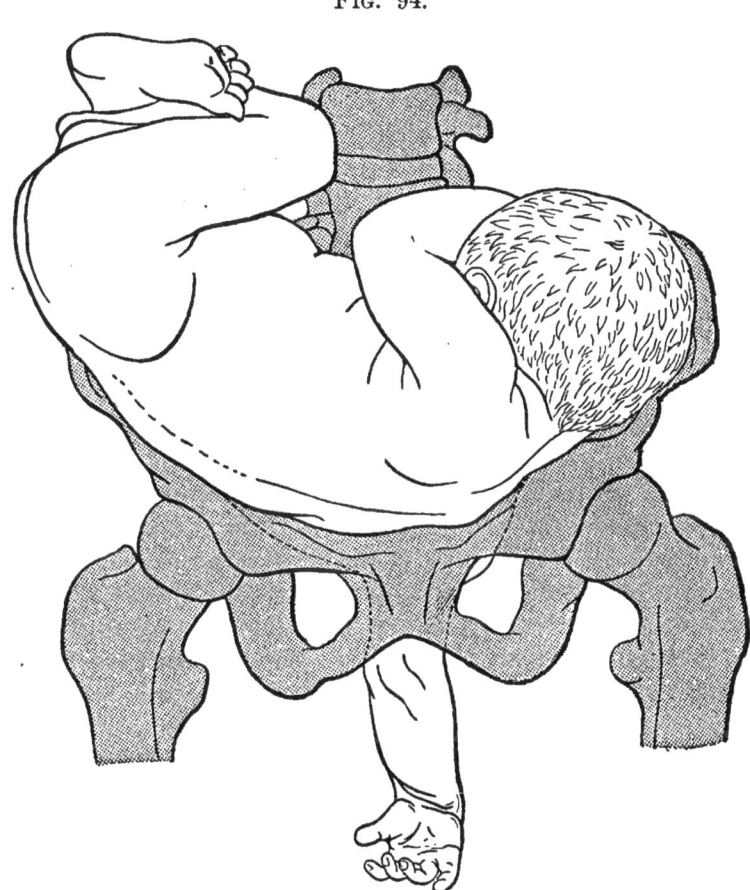

Transverse presentation.   Dorso-anterior, head on left side, arm prolapsed.
(Farabeuf.)

or even transverse. The head will generally be found in one or other iliac fossa, while it is impossible to explore the pelvic excavation from above, for the trunk, as a rule, completely fills the false pelvis. If the back is to the front, its smooth surface can be felt across the lower zone of the mother's abdomen. If the back is directed posteriorly, the fœtal limbs can be felt in front. The fœtal heart-sounds are heard below the umbilicus, plainly when the back is to the front; faintly, if at all, when the limbs are anterior.

Vaginal examination: If the membranes are unruptured, no part of the fœtus can be reached by the examining finger without great difficulty. Occasionally a limb or the prolapsed cord may be felt within the bag of waters. When the membranes have ruptured the finger may come in contact with an arm or the shoulder. The landmarks to be felt are the clavicle, the humerus, and the spine of the scapula. The finger may be forced into the axilla and the ribs felt, thus distinguishing it from the groin. Very frequently in transverse presentations a hand is found prolapsed, which hand it is being distinguished by shaking hands with it.

Prognosis.

As spontaneous delivery is very rare in transverse presentations, the prognosis in cases left to Nature is very grave, both for the mother and the child. As artificial delivery is the rule in these cases, the prognosis depends on the length of time the case has been allowed to go on without treatment and the nature of the operative interference.

The **dangers to the mother** are exhaustion, rupture of the uterus from thinning out of the lower uterine segment, risks of operative interference and of subsequent sepsis.

Mechanism of Transverse Presentations.

As a rule, natural delivery is impossible in transverse presentations, but in extremely rare instances Nature may effect delivery by one of *three* methods:

1. Spontaneous version: Uterine contractions may result in displacement of the fœtus and its gradual version, so that its long axis finally corresponds to the long axis of the uterus. Thus the transverse presentation becomes altered to that of the breech or the head, the delivery then taking place according to the new presentation. Spontaneous version may take place before or after rupture of the membranes, and is more likely to occur in multiparæ and when the child is living.

2. **Spontaneous evolution**: This mechanism is favored by excessively strong uterine contractions, a roomy pelvis, and a small fœtus.

By the strong uterine contractions the anterior shoulder is forced down into the pelvis, and rotates to the front, while the head lies above the brim and over the pubes; the breech and trunk are then compressed, and gradually forced past the head and anterior shoulder, which pivots on the pubic arch.

FIG. 95.

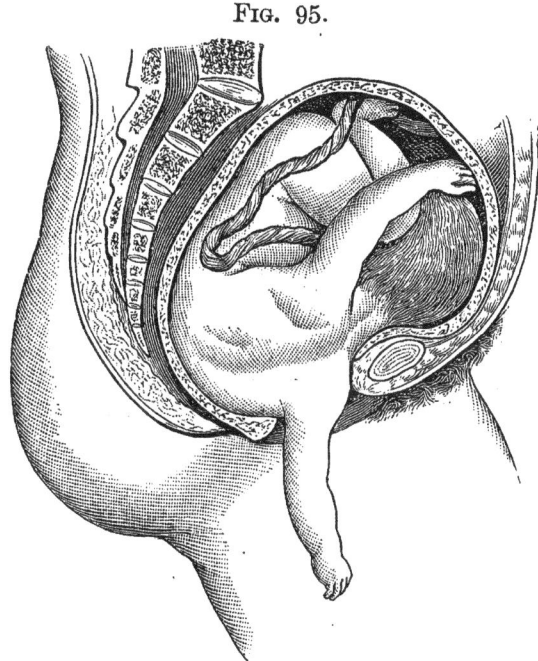

Spontaneous evolution.   First stage.

Thus the chest and breech slip past the shoulder, over the perineum, and are delivered.   Finally the head enters the pelvis and rotates, so that the occiput pivots under the pubic arch and the face sweeps over the perineum, thus completing the delivery (Figs. 95–99).

3. **Delivery with the body doubled up** (*Evolutio con duplicato corpore*): The conditions favoring this mechanism are strong

FIG. 96.

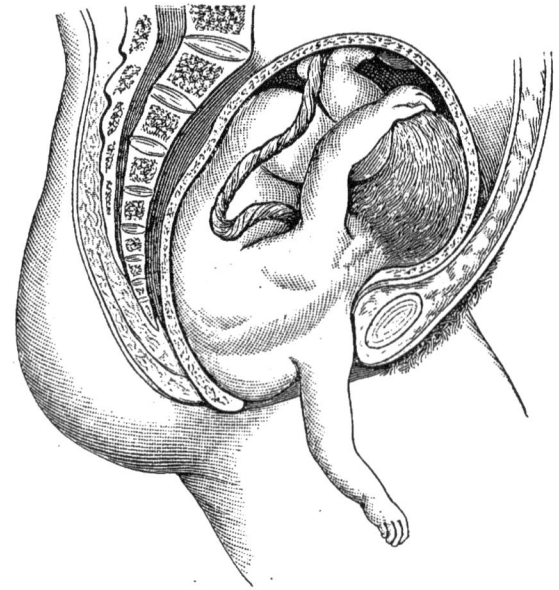

Spontaneous evolution.   Second stage.

FIG. 97.

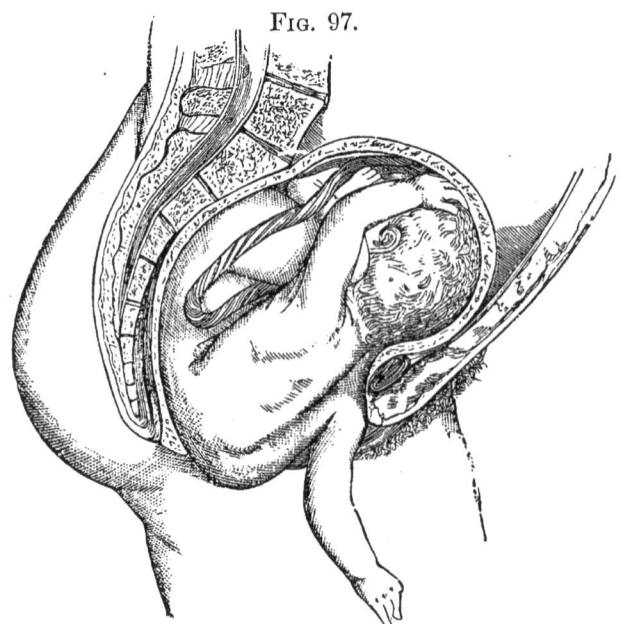

Spontaneous evolution   Third stage.

FIG. 98.

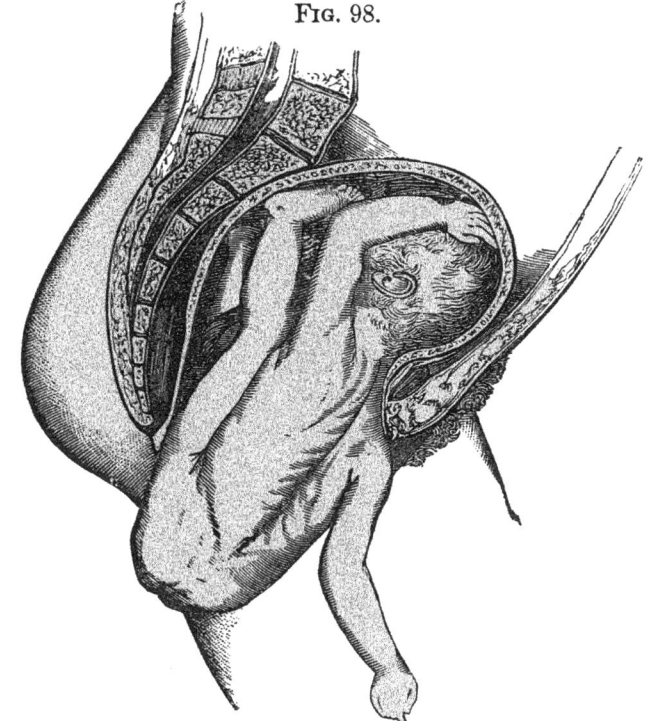

Spontaneous evolution.   Fourth stage.

FIG. 99.

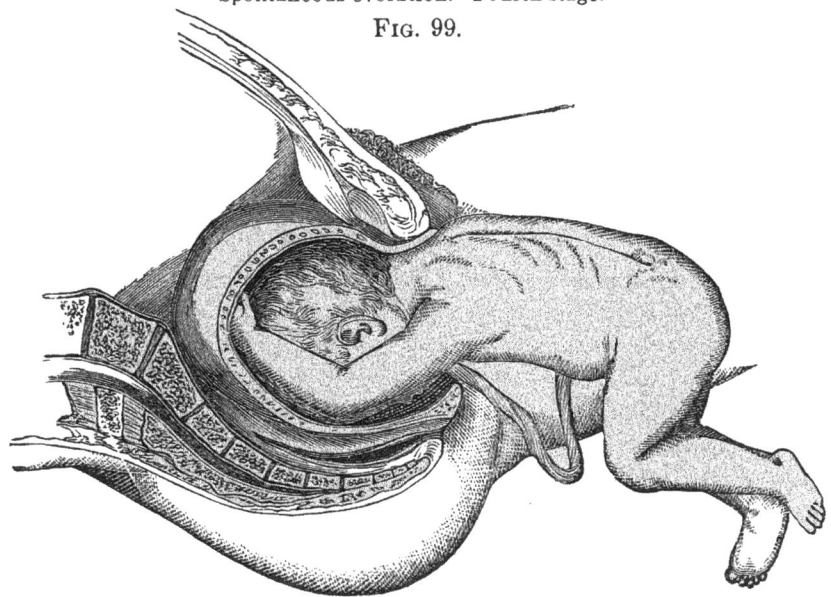

Spontaneous evolution   Fifth stage.

uterine contractions, a roomy pelvis, and a small dead fœtus.
The presenting shoulder is driven down into the pelvis and is

FIG. 100.

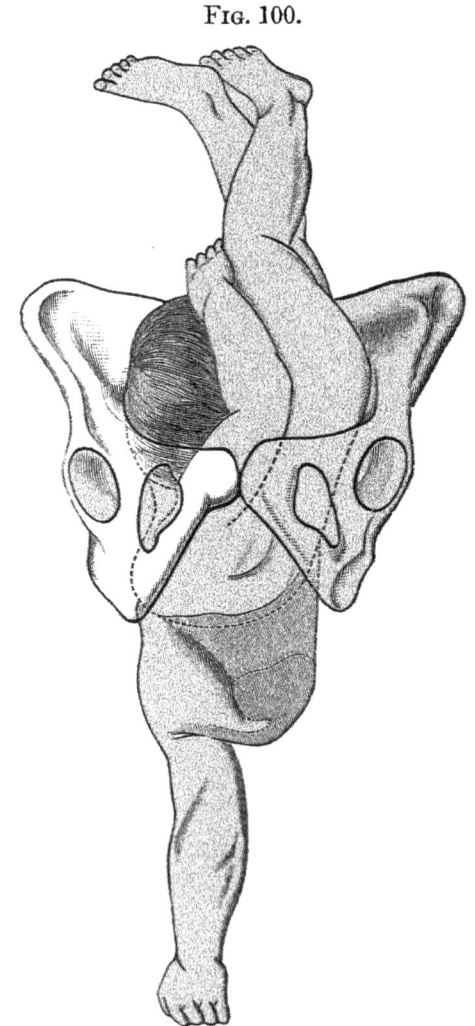

Birth of child doubled. Evolutio con duplicato corpore. (Kleinwächter.)

delivered first, the head and chest of the fœtus are compressed
together and forced through the canal, being thus delivered,
and are followed by the breech and legs (Fig. 100).

Management.

Transverse presentations should never be left to Nature to deliver. If seen early and the fœtus is alive, **version** should be performed.

If seen late, when impaction has taken place and the fœtus has perished, then, if version cannot be easily performed, **decapitation** and **evisceration** should be done, so as to reduce the risk to the mother to the smallest possible limit.

PROLAPSE OF THE FŒTAL LIMBS.

In Head Presentations.

Any or all of the fœtal extremities may **prolapse** alongside the head.

The most common form of this accident is a prolapse of a **hand,** which, when it occurs, is found close to the temporal region. The worst form is when an arm lies across the back of the neck.

Treatment.

If the condition is discovered **before the rupture** of the membranes, an attempt should be made to overcome the difficulty by *postural treatment.* The woman should lie on the side *opposite* the prolapsed extremity, with the hips slightly elevated.

After the **membranes have ruptured** an attempt should be made to dislodge and push up the prolapsed extremity. To do this the woman should be placed as recommended above. Should the attempt fail the *forceps* may be applied, care being taken to avoid including the hand in the grasp of the blades, and the head drawn down to the outlet. This very often causes the arm to slip up out of the way. Should it be found impossible to dislodge the arm sufficiently to apply the forceps, *version* may be carried out.

When the condition is not discovered till the **head is low down** in the cavity, the forceps should be applied and the case terminated as rapidly as is possible.

In Breech Presentations.

The prolapse of the hand is of no importance in breech presentations, and no attention need be paid to it.

In Transverse Presentations.

The prolapse of **a foot** is, of course, favorable.

Should **a hand** or **arm** be found prolapsed, if it cannot be pushed up out of the way, it may be drawn down sufficiently to fasten a broad piece of tape about the wrist. After version has been performed the tape may be held so as to prevent the arm from rising alongside the head and complicating its descent.

PLURAL BIRTHS.

Twin Labors.

These are usually easy and uncomplicated.

Twin pregnancy **occurs** about once in 130 cases of gestation; while triplets occur about once in 5088 cases.

The **tendency** to twin pregnancy is very frequently *hereditary*. The greatest number of reported cases have occurred in *first pregnancies*.

According to the **origin of the ova** will arise the various peculiarities in the development of the placentæ and membranes.

If the two ova have been derived from separate Graafian follicles, each will have its own placenta, cord, chorion, and amnion, each being independent of the other.

Should the two ova have been derived from a single Graafian follicle, the amniotic sacs will be distinct, but the chorion and placenta will be in common, the two cords arising from the same placenta.

Usually twins arising from ova from a single Graafian follicle, are of the same sex; while when the original ova are distinct each is of an opposite sex. *Male* twins are slightly more common than female twins.

Diagnosis: Very frequently the diagnosis of twins is not made until after the birth of the first child. The only *certain* *signs* of twin pregnancy are the presence of two fœtal heart-sounds, heard at different points over the abdominal surface, and having a different rhythm; and the palpation of two dis-tinct heads.

Other signs are, excessive size of the abdomen, with in-creased uterine distention, irregularity of the uterine outline, and the presence of a number of fœtal extremities.

Prognosis: The *maternal* prognosis is somewhat graver than in single births. The *dangers* are: *uterine inertia* due to overdistention of the uterine walls; *abnormal presentation; albuminuria* and *eclampsia,* more frequent in plural preg-nancies; *hemorrhage* in the third stage of labor from trouble in the delivery of the placenta.

The *fœtal prognosis* is always more serious than in single births. The *dangers* are: deficient development from over-crowding in the uterus; *malposition and malpresentation;* and *hydramnios.*

Mechanism: The following table from Spiegelberg, based on 1138 labors, gives the combined presentations in their order of frequency.

Both heads presenting	. 49.00 per cent.
Head and breech	. 31.70 "
Both pelvic presentations	. 8.60 "
Head and transverse	. 6.18
Breech and transverse	. 4.14 "
Both transverse	. 0.37 "

The *order of delivery* varies. When both heads present, usually the larger is delivered first. If one twin presents by the breech and the other by the head, usually the latter is delivered first; if one presents transversely and the other longitudinally, the latter is usually expelled first.

Management of labor: When the presentation of the first child is normal no special treatment is indicated. When the first child has been delivered and its respiratory function well established, before cutting the cord the physician should pal-pate the mother's abdomen to ascertain the position of the second child. If any abnormality exists, it should be at once corrected by external manipulations and the fundus uteri gently kneaded to stimulate retraction. The fundus may then be placed in charge of the nurse or assistant while the physician attends to the cord of the first child. This should be tied in two places and then divided between the ligatures, in case there should be communication between the placental circulations and the second child bleed to death.

Friction on the fundus should be sustained until the uterine contractions are firmly established. It is not advisable to wait more than half an hour for the birth of the second child. The second amniotic sac should then be ruptured and the uterine contractions reinforced by firm pressure on the fundus so as to expedite the delivery of the second child.

From this time until retraction has been firmly established, after the complete emptying of the uterus, the fundus should be kept constantly under control in order to prevent its relaxation and the occurrence of hemorrhage.

Should hemorrhage follow the delivery of the first child, the second should be delivered as rapidly as possible, either by forceps or version, and the uterus emptied artificially. It is not advisable to inform the mother during labor, should a diagnosis of twins be established, as the shock may inhibit uterine action.

Complications of Twin Births.

Compound presentations : Occasionally both fœtuses tend to engage simultaneously in the brim. When *both heads* tend to present at the same time, the highest should if possible be pushed up, and the forceps then applied to the lower head and traction exerted until it is firmly engaged. During the traction an assistant may be able to hold the head of the other child out of the way, by pressure on the abdominal wall of the mother.

When the head of one child and the breech of the other tend to engage at the same time, the breech should be pushed up and the head drawn down.

When fœtal extremities are found to present along with a head, they should be replaced and the head drawn down by means of the forceps.

Interlocking twins : Occasionally both heads enter the pelvis, one being generally well in advance of the other. The upper head then becomes jammed against the neck and thorax of the first child.

Treatment: The most advanced head should be delivered by forceps, as unlocking is generally out of the question. The second head should then be delivered, and when this is done the body of the first child may be extracted, the head of the second being held out of the way by an assistant.

Sometimes it is necessary to perforate one of the heads in order to permit the delivery of the other. When this operation is required it should be performed on the head of the first child, because the second is more likely to be alive, there being less risk of compression of its cord.

In cases in which the breech of one child and the head of the other become impacted in the pelvis an endeavor should be made to push up the head and deliver the breech. The body of the child presenting by the breech should only be delivered as far as the neck, as the two heads usually become locked at the brim by the overlapping of the chins or of the occiputs, or by the face of one child being pressed against the back of the other child's neck.

Should it be impossible to push back the head of the second child or to apply forceps and deliver it, the head of the breech child should be perforated and extracted before attempting to deliver the other.

Triplets.

As a rule **no difficulty** is encountered in the delivery of triplets, as the greater the number of fœtuses the greater the tendency to prematurity of delivery.

The labor is generally prolonged on account of delay in the **first stage** from imperfect uterine contractions.

The **third stage** must be very carefully managed, and it is advisable to empty the uterus artificially in order to insure that no portions of placenta are retained.

DYSTOCIA DUE TO ANOMALIES OF FŒTAL DEVELOPMENT.

Overgrowth of the Fœtus.

Definition: A child may be said to be overgrown when it weighs eleven pounds, or over, at the time of birth. It is but very seldom that a child is born weighing twelve pounds; but cases are recorded in which the birth-weight was over twenty pounds.

Cause : Nothing definite is known as to the cause of this overgrowth. Multiparity, advanced age of one or both parents, and prolongation of pregnancy are generally regarded as the probable causes.

Mechanism : When the head presents in these cases it generally enters the pelvis in extreme flexion. Moulding is generally very marked as the result of a prolonged second stage.

Treatment.

The best treatment is **prophylactic**. When the condition is suspected, which is rare, a careful palpation should be made and the size of the head estimated. The head should then be forced into the brim by the pressure from above, to give one an approximate idea of the relative size of the pelvis. If it be found that it is a tight fit, then labor should be at once induced, as no advantage can be gained by waiting on nature.

When the condition is not discovered until labor, then the proper course to pursue is to support the patient's strength and control the pains by means of hypodermics of morphine as often as required, until the head has had time to mould thoroughly, when *forceps* may be applied and an attempt made to deliver the child. Care should be taken to avoid excessive force in traction.

If no advance is made, and the child is alive, pubiotomy or Cæsarean section is to be performed.

When the condition is recognized early and the disproportion between the head and the pelvis is not marked, *internal version* may offer the child a greater chance of life than a high forceps operation. The choice of operation depends in great measure on the skill of the operator in performing the one or the other.

If the child has perished, *embryotomy* should be the operation of choice.

Premature Ossification of the Skull.

Premature ossification of the bones of the skull, causing more or less obliteration of the sutures and fontanelles, greatly modifies the moldability of the head, and may thus lead to delay in labor.

·Position : The head may be arrested· at the brim or in the cavity.

Treatment: Forceps or pubiotomy may be necessary to secure delivery of a living child.

Hydrocephalus.

This is probably the **commonest cause** of excessive size of the fœtal head.

Etiology: The condition is due to the *accumulation of the serum* in the ventricles of the brain. The accumulation of fluid may be so great as to cause obliteration of the cerebral convolutions and excessive thinning of the cranial bones, which become widely separated. From the excessive size of the vault the face appears small. Spina bifida or some other malformation is generally present in these cases.

Diagnosis : In about a third of all cases of hydrocephalus the breech presents. The condition should always be suspected when in vertex presentations the head fails to engage in the brim, although the pelvis is normal in size and no good reason can be found for the delay.

By *abdominal examination* the gaping fontanelles and sutures may be made out and fluctuation may be obtained in these regions. The cranial bones may be felt to be excessively thin, and pressure on them may give the sensation of crepitation. The head is felt to be enlarged and soft.

These conditions may be better felt by a *bimanual examination* when this is possible.

Prognosis : The life of the child is to be considered as of little moment, for should it survive birth death generally takes place shortly after.

Death of the mother may result from exhaustion or from rupture of the uterus. The rupture generally occurs in the lower segment, which becomes greatly stretched and thinned.

Treatment: When the *head presents* (Fig. 101), it should be perforated and the fluid permitted to drain away. When the head collapses delivery may be effected either by version or by means of a cranioclast.

Forceps should never be applied to a hydrocephalic head if the condition is at all marked, as it is impossible to secure a good grasp on account of its compressibility.

When the *breech presents*, the trunk and arms may be extracted and an attempt made to perforate the cranial vault by

Fig. 101.

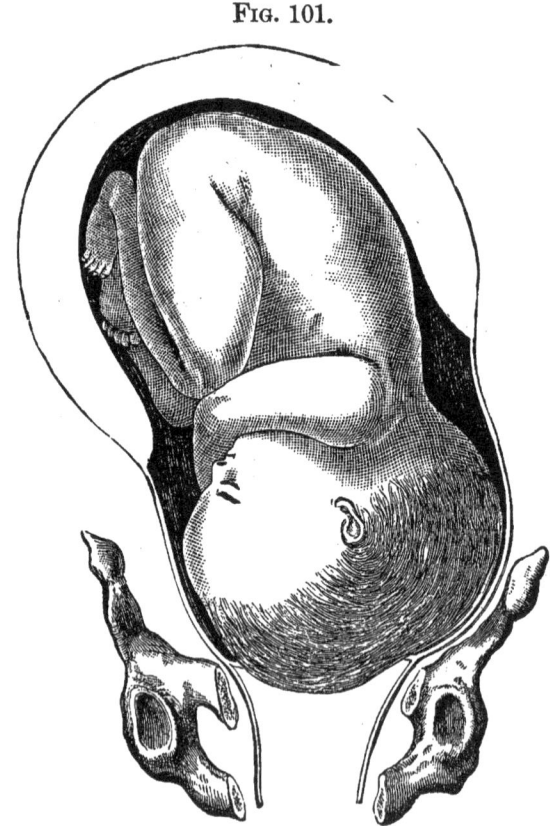

Thinning of lower segment of uterus in obstruction from hydrocephalus.
(After Bandl.)

the temporal fontanelle. If this cannot be reached, then the spinal canal should be opened in the dorsal region by means of a pair of scissors, and a catheter passed through it into the cranial cavity and the fluid thus evacuated (Van Huevel's method : Fig. 102).

Fɪɢ. 102.

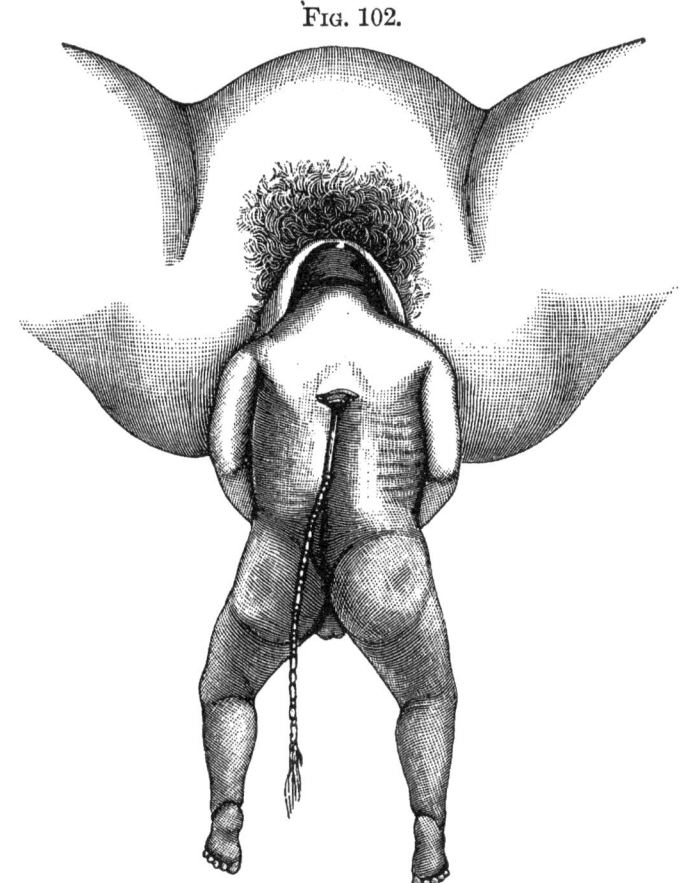

Puncture of spinal canal in a case of hydrocephalus obstructing labor.
(After Herrgot.)

Encephalocele ; Meningocele ; Hydrencephalus.

These conditions when present do not often seriously complicate labor, as the tumors are either small or are so situated that they fail to affect materially the progress of the case. If obstruction to labor occur, the growth should be perforated, when its contents will drain away and make delivery possible.

Tumors of the Fœtal Trunk.

Certain tumors arising in connection with the fœtal trunk may by their bulk or situation induce dystocia.

17—Obst.

Varieties: Spina bifida; teratomata situated on the spine, jaw, or orbit; hydrothorax; ascites; cystic degeneration of the kidneys; malignant conditions of the liver, spleen, or pancreas; distention of the urinary bladder, and hernia of viscera through clefts in the abdominal or thoracic walls, may be mentioned under this heading.

Treatment: Should delivery be delayed, forceps or version may be resorted to, or some form of embryotomy. Tumors with fluid contents should be evacuated.

Monstrosities.

Anencephalus or **hemicephalus** is the form most commonly met with. Delay is generally caused in the first stage by the absence of the head as a dilator. When the diagnosis is made, version, if possible, should be performed.

Double monsters: These may very seriously complicate labor; but, as a rule, the fœtuses are small and delivery occurs naturally. In difficult cases craniotomy or some other form of embryotomy is necessary to effect delivery.

DYSTOCIA DUE TO ABNORMALITIES OF THE FŒTAL APPENDAGES.

Short cord: Cases have been recorded in which the cord has not measured more than two inches in length. Relative shortness of the cord may occur from its coiling around the neck and limbs of the fœtus.

The condition may lead to premature detachment of the placenta, rupture of the cord, or compression of its vessels from stretching, which results in death of the fœtus.

The *diagnosis* is difficult. Sometimes the patient complains of marked pain at the placental site during each contraction. Occasionally a portion of the uterine wall may be felt to be drawn downward and inward during each contraction. Frequently the presenting part is retracted rapidly as the uterine contraction subsides.

Treatment consists in rapid delivery with the forceps or by version.

Prolapse of the Cord.

A loop of the umbilical cord **may prolapse** alongside or in front of the presenting part. As labor progresses the cord is exposed to pressure between the presenting part and the pelvic wall, which results in interruption of the fœtoplacental circulation, and possibly in the death of the fœtus.

Prolapse of the cord may **occur** either before or after rupture of the membranes.

Frequency: This accident occurs once in about 250 cases of labor. It is met with most frequently in presentations of the pelvic pole of the fœtus.

Etiology: The essential cause of prolapse of the cord is failure of the presenting part of the fœtus to fill, completely and continuously, the lower segment of the uterus.

The *fœtal conditions* which predispose to this accident are: malpositions and malpresentations; small size and increased mobility of the fœtus; anomalies of other fœtal appendages, as marginal insertion or excessive length of the cord, hydramnios, placenta prævia; and sudden escape of the liquor amnii with the patient in the erect position.

The predisposing *maternal conditions* are: pelvic deformity; relaxed abdominal wall, as in some multiparæ; uterine and other tumors; uterine obliquity.

The accident is also more liable to occur in cases of multiple pregnancy.

Diagnosis.

Before the rupture of the membranes it is a somewhat difficult matter, as a rule, to recognize a prolapse of the cord on account of its non-resisting nature and the ease with which it recedes before the examining finger.

After rupture of the membranes it may be generally recognized without difficulty, on account of its twists and the pulsations of its vessels.

It has been not infrequently **mistaken for** a prolapsed loop of intestine; and occasionally a portion of intestine has been mistaken for the cord. Care in examination should make such an error in diagnosis impossible.

The **position** the cord usually occupies is at one or other side of the pelvis somewhat posteriorly ; rarely it may lie either in front of the promontory or behind the symphysis pubis.

When the foetal heart-sounds grow progressively weaker and no cause is apparent, prolapse of the cord should be suspected and appropriate treatment inaugurated.

Prognosis.

This complication rarely influences the prognosis for the mother, save in so far as the operative treatment exposes her to risks of shock and sepsis.

For the child the prognosis is somewhat grave, the mortality rising to somewhat over 50 per cent. The cause of foetal death is occlusion of the foetoplacental circulation from pressure on the cord. This pressure results in asphyxiation of the child. Should the prolapsed portion of the cord show an absence of pulsation for ten or fifteen minutes, and abdominal auscultation fail to permit the detection of heart-sounds, the death of the foetus is assured.

Treatment.

If the child has perished, no treatment is indicated, and the case may be left to Nature.

Before rupture of the membranes : The indications for treatment are to prevent rupture of the membranes as long as possible, and to favor the replacement of the cord by appropriate posturing of the patient. The woman should be made to adopt the genupectoral posture (Fig. 103). While the patient is in this position the influence of gravity causes the cord to settle slowly toward the fundus, and thus the prolapsed loop is gradually withdrawn. *During the intervals* between the pains this may be gently pushed back with the hand, care being taken not to rupture the membranes. When the *condition has been corrected*, the patient may be permitted to recline on the side *opposite* to that occupied by the cord. The change of position should be made slowly and carefully, so as to avoid forcing the cord down again. The membranes may then be ruptured, care being taken to force the head down by pressure from above while this is being done.

After rupture of the membranes : Before attempting to re-place the prolapsed loop of cord after rupture of the membranes, care should be taken to find out whether the child is alive. If pulsation has ceased in the cord, the heart may still be beating ; if this is the case, the presenting part should be pushed up, and the cord replaced after pulsation returns.

The woman should be placed in the Sims position on the side opposite to the prolapsed cord. The hips should be elevated by means of a folded pillow. The operator should then push back the presenting part so as to release the cord. This

FIG. 103.

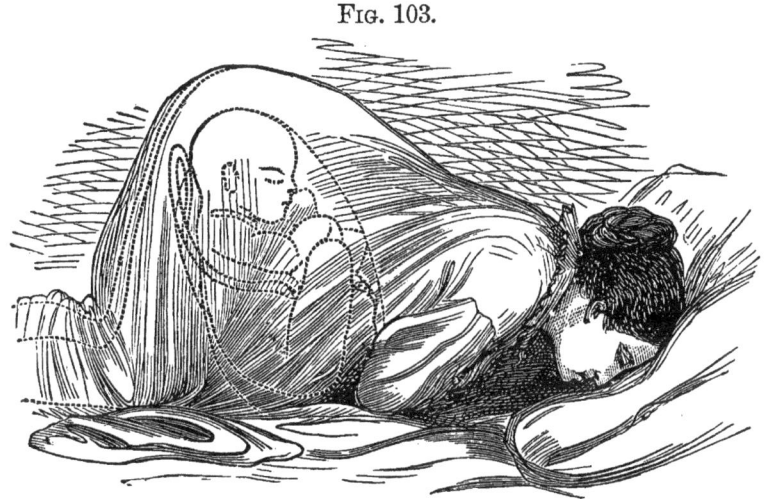

Postural treatment of prolapse of the cord.

may then be loosely twisted, care being taken not to interfere with its pulsations, and the twisted mass gently pushed up beyond the presenting part.

If it be found impossible to replace the cord with the woman in the Sims position, she should be placed on her knees and chest and another attempt made, if necessary giving an anæsthetic so as to relax the uterus completely. The objection to the knee-chest position is the tendency for air to enter the uterine cavity ; if this accident occurs, the subsequent labor should not be unduly prolonged.

Should manual efforts fail, a suitable instrument for replacing the cord may be improvised with a No. 10 or No. 12 gum elastic catheter and some tape. A loop of tape is made to encircle the cord loosely, and its free ends are attached to the tip of the catheter. The catheter, with its stylet inserted, is then pushed well up into the uterus, carrying the cord with it (Figs. 104, 105, and 106). The stylet is then withdrawn and the

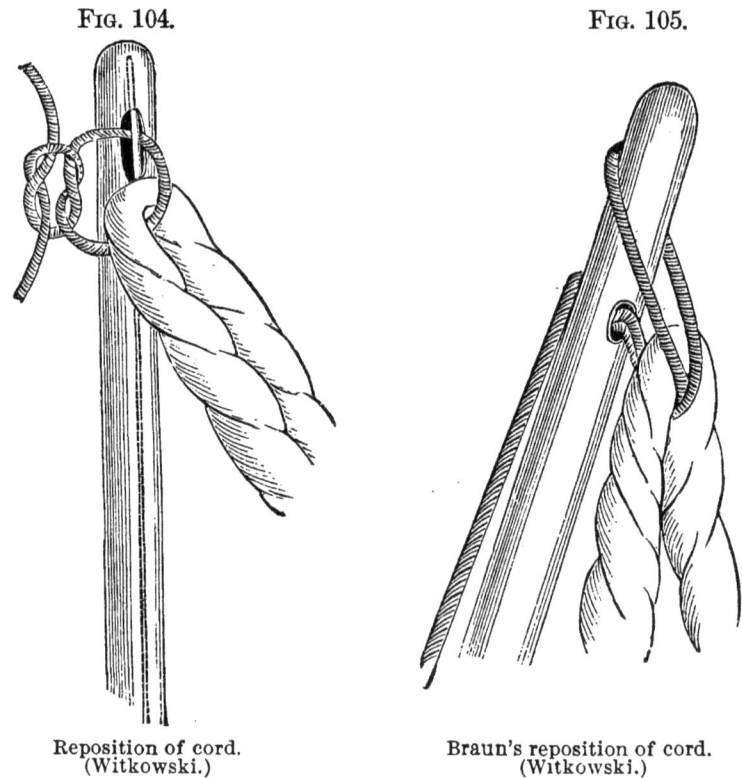

Fig. 104.

Fig. 105.

Reposition of cord.
(Witkowski.)

Braun's reposition of cord.
(Witkowski.)

catheter left in the uterus to come away with the child. Care should be taken to remove the bone button from the end of the catheter.

If all attempts at reposition of the cord fail, then either *version* or *forceps*, with rapid delivery, must be resorted to in order to save the life of the child. Before either of these operations the loop of the cord should be placed opposite the sacro-iliac joint, where it will be least pressed upon.

Coiling of the Cord about the Fœtal Neck.

Quite frequently the fœtal cord is found to be coiled about the neck of the child. It may encircle the neck several times, and thus produce a relative shortening of the cord.

The condition is difficult to **diagnose** before delivery of the head. It may be suspected if the head descends well with each pain, but rapidly recedes in the interval between the contractions.

Results: Occasionally the traction is so severe as to interfere with the fœto-placental circulation; and has been known to cause premature detachment of the placenta.

The only **treatment** that can be suggested is the application of the forceps and the rapid delivery of the head; when the cord may be cut and uncoiled from the neck before the birth of the trunk takes place.

FIG. 106.

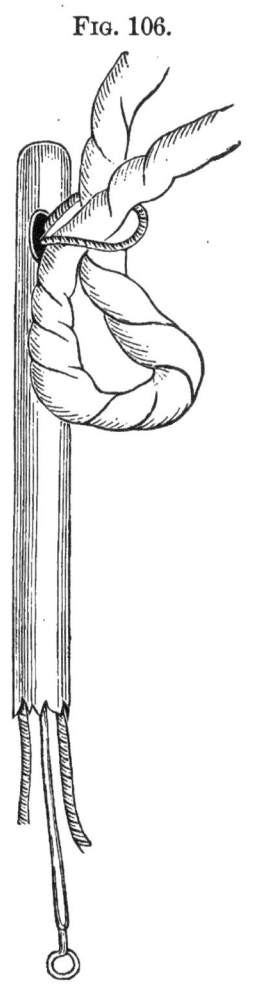

Another method of reposition of cord.

Placenta Prævia.

The placenta is **normally** implanted entirely within the upper uterine segment.

When it is implanted, in whole or in part, upon the lower uterine segment the condition is known as **placenta prævia.**

Varieties: Three varieties are described:

(1) Placenta prævia centralis: The placenta is so situated that its centre corresponds with the internal os (Fig. 107).

(2) Placenta prævia marginalis: The placenta is situated so that but a portion of its margin overlaps the internal os (Fig. 108).

(3) Placenta prævia lateralis: The placenta is situated on

the lateral wall of the uterus, extending well down into the lower segment, but not reaching as far as the internal os (Fig. 109).

In the central and marginal varieties the hemorrhage may begin early in pregnancy; it is repeated frequently, and in labor is much more serious than in the lateral variety.

FIG. 107.   FIG. 108.

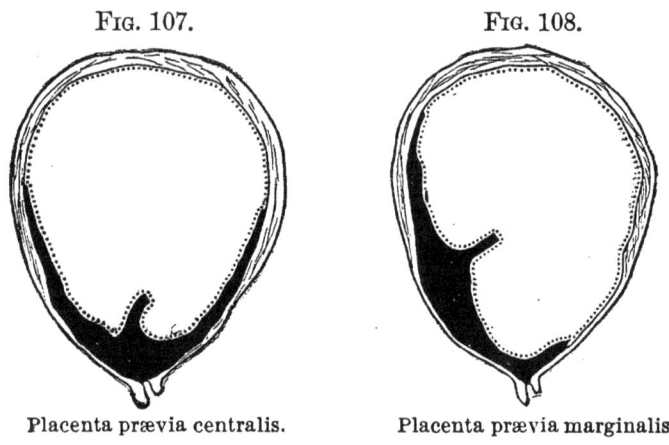

Placenta prævia centralis.   Placenta prævia marginalis.

FIG. 109.

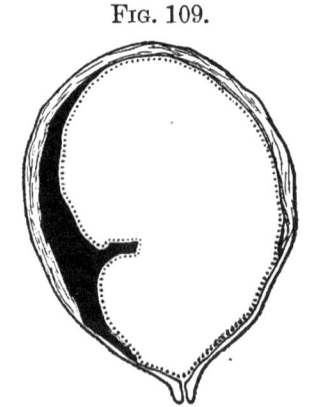

Placenta prævia lateralis.   (After Dakin.)

Frequency: Placenta prævia centralis is very rare; lateral and marginal placenta prævia are the commonest varieties. Placenta prævia occurs about once in 1000 cases. It is more frequently met with in multiparæ than in primiparæ.

Etiology: A satisfactory explanation of the occurrence of placenta prævia has never been advanced. Chronic inflammatory changes in the mucous membrane certainly predispose to its occurrence. Other probable causes are: subinvolution, atrophy of the decidua, new growths, and malformations of the uterus.

Symptoms and Physical Signs.

The **symptoms** of placenta prævia do not usually present themselves until after the sixth month of pregnancy.

The first indication of the condition is **a sudden gush of blood** from the genitals, usually without apparent cause and without pain. The bleeding then recurs at intervals as pregnancy advances. The amount of blood lost is proportionate to the extent of the placental separation. When hemorrhage takes place during pregnancy it is probably due to a partial separation of the placenta in the lower uterine segment, where its attachment is imperfect. This separation is caused by the normal uterine contractions which constantly occur throughout pregnancy.

The first hemorrhage when it occurs during labor may be so severe as to threaten the patient's life. As a rule, the bleeding is most profuse in the intervals between the pains; but this cannot be said to be diagnostic of the condition.

By **abdominal examination** the location of the placenta may be recognized, when the implantation is on the anterior uterine wall, by feeling its edge, which presents as a resisting ring. Below this point the uterus feels soft and boggy, and the fœtal parts can only be felt indistinctly, while elsewhere they may be readily made out. Over this boggy area the placental bruit is to be heard with great distinctness. If the larger portion of the placenta occupies the lower uterine segment, malpresentations of the fœtus may occur, as the presenting part is thus prevented entering the pelvic brim.

By **vaginal examination** the cervix and lower uterine segment are found to be softer than usual. If the insertion of the placenta is marginal, one side of the cervix and lower segment may be softer and more boggy than the other. Pulsating vessels may be felt around the cervix.

The **external os** is usually patulous, and through it the finger may be pushed till the internal os is reached, where the maternal surface of the placenta may be felt, a gritty feel distinguishing it from a blood-clot or the membranes.

Diagnosis.

When hemorrhage takes place in the later months of pregnancy a careful examination should be made to ascertain its cause. The rupture of a varicosed vein in the vagina and premature detachment of the normally situated placenta may lead to severe hemorrhage in the later months of pregnancy. A careful and systematic examination will generally permit a diagnosis to be made.

Treatment of Placenta Prævia.

The **control of hemorrhage** is the principal indication of treatment.

In the rare cases in which the condition of placenta prævia is recognized before the fœtus is viable it may be possible to carry out an **expectant plan of treatment** until the seventh month of the pregnancy is reached. The patient must be kept in bed, not being permitted to rise for any purpose. It may be well to administer chloral (gr. xv) or liq. opii sed. (℥xv) two or three times daily to control the nervous system.

When the seventh month has been reached **labor** should be induced, as after this period the woman may bleed to death before medical aid can reach her.

Being satisfied that the condition of placenta prævia is present, it is the duty of the physician at once to **empty the uterus** if the child is viable.

The patient should be anæsthetized and placed in the lithotomy position, with her hips at the edge of the bed. A Kelly pad should be placed under her. The vulva and vagina should then be scrubbed and douched with formalin or bichloride solution. The operator having sterilized his hands and arms, should then dilate the cervix by inserting one finger, then a second, and then the thumb of the right hand. Search should then be made for the edge of the placenta. If the placenta is lateral or marginal, it may be sufficient to rupture the membranes, tearing them freely, and to sweep the fingers round under the margin of the placenta so as to separate it from the uterus for a short distance. The fingers may then be withdrawn if the head of the fœtus is presenting. Firm pressure on the fundus, so as to crowd the head into the pelvis, may then be sufficient to control the hemorrhage; if so, the case may now be left to Nature. If the os has been sufficiently dilated, the forceps may be applied and the head drawn down, after which the case may be left to Nature to deliver.

If the **placenta is central**, or if a considerable portion of the placenta is found over the internal os, the proper treatment is to perform internal version. A foot is seized and drawn down until the hemorrhage is checked. From time to time the protruding leg may be drawn upon to hasten dilatation of the cervix. Plenty of time must be allowed for the cervix to dilate completely, otherwise there will be difficulty in extracting the after-coming head.

If there has been a great loss of blood and **the cervix is found to be rigid**, it is better to pack the cervix and vagina with sterile iodoform gauze, which may be left in place until the patient has had time to rally under appropriate treatment (see Post-partum Hemorrhage). The gauze tampon not only checks the hemorrhage, but also assists in softening and dilating the cervix and os.

Many authors recommend the employment of **hydrostatic dilators** instead of the gauze tampon. The Champetier de Ribes bag is the best for this purpose. It is claimed that the bag controls the hemorrhage and dilates the cervix more effectnally than does the vaginal packing, while it as a rule causes less discomfort to the patient. For the introduction of the bag the patient is placed in the lithotomy position, the anterior lip of the cervix is seized with a tenaculum and drawn well forward, being then held by an assistant. The dilating bag is folded into a cylinder, grasped with a pair of forceps, and guided carefully into the cervix and through the internal os. The bag should always be placed within the amniotic sac, which should previously be ruptured. Before withdrawing the forceps the distention of the bag should be commenced by injecting into it boiled water by means of a syringe attached to the tube of the bag. Then as the bag distends the forceps may be unlocked and carefully withdrawn. As a precaution against rupture of the bag, the operator should ascertain beforehand how many bulbfuls of water are required to dilate it completely.

The most rigid precautions as regards **asepsis** should be observed in the treatment of placenta prævia, as the risk of infection is greater than in ordinary cases, on account of the low position of the placental site.

After the child has been delivered the operator should introduce his hand into the uterus to remove the placenta and any clots that may be found there. This should be followed by a prolonged hot intra-uterine douche of sterile salt solution or 1 : 500 formalin. A full dose of the fluid extract of ergot should be administered as soon as the uterus is emptied, or else a hypodermic of ergotin.

Prognosis: Placenta prævia constitutes a most serious complication of pregnancy or labor for both mother or child. Under prompt and aseptic treatment the maternal mortality should be practically *nil*. As premature delivery is frequent, the infant mortality-rate is high.

Premature Separation of a Normally Situated Placenta ; Accidental Hemorrhage.

The hemorrhage associated with premature detachment of a normally situated placenta is termed "**accidental**," to distinguish it from the "unavoidable" hemorrhage of placenta prævia.

Varieties: Accidental hemorrhage may be *apparent* or *concealed.*

In **apparent accidental hemorrhage** the blood dissects its way between the membranes and decidua, and escapes through the cervix.

In **concealed accidental hemorrhage** the blood fails to find a way of escape, and may collect within the uterus in sufficient quantity to cause serious symptoms, or even death of the patient.

In this form any of the following conditions may obtain and *prevent the escape of blood :*

1. The placenta may be detached only at the centre, the margin remaining adherent;

2. The upper margin may be detached, so that blood accumulates between the membranes and the uterine wall.

3. A portion of the edge of the placenta and of the adjacent membranes may be detached; the latter may rupture and permit the blood to mingle with the liquor amnii in the sac.

4. The cervix may be obstructed by a clot, the detached membranes, or the presenting part of the foetus (Fig. 110).

Etiology: The predisposing causes may be given as, tubercular and syphilitic degeneration of the decidua, placental degenerations, nephritis, anæmia, and the acute infectious diseases. In the presence of these but a trivial exciting cause is required to produce separation of the placenta. A sudden jar, a blow on the abdomen, or violent muscular exertion may be all that is required to bring about such a separation.

FIG. 110.

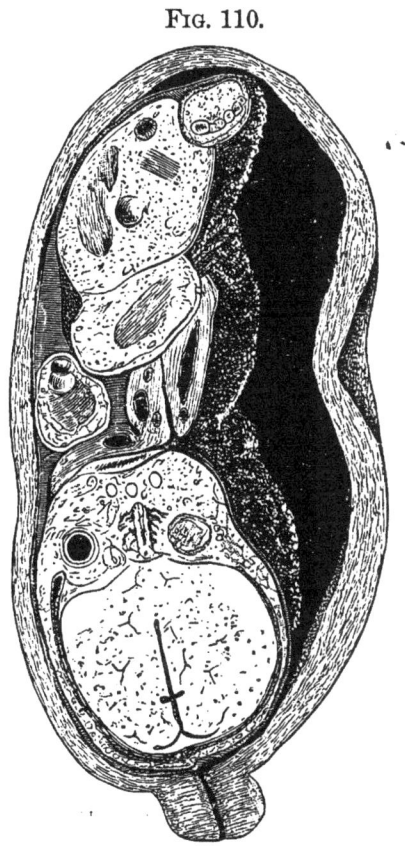

Frozen section of the uterus of a woman who died of accidental hemorrhage at the Maternité de Beaujon. (Pinard and Varnier.)

Symptoms and Diagnosis of Accidental Hemorrhage.

The symptoms resemble those of rupture of the uterus, but are not so severe.

In the **apparent variety** the fact of hemorrhage is obvious. It usually takes place early in labor or during the later months of pregnancy. Severe localized pain at the placental site is not infrequent. The uterus may bulge at this point.

Placenta prævia is readily distinguished by a careful vaginal examination.

Concealed hemorrhage is generally revealed by the systemic effects. Rapid pulse, pallor, cold extremities, restlessness, sighing respiration, and collapse may be present. If labor has begun, the uterine contractions cease or become weak, though the patient may complain of more or less continual pain at the placental site. On abdominal examination the uterine wall may be found bulging at the seat of the hemorrhage and the fœtal heart-sounds are feeble and irregular. Rupture of the uterus may be distinguished from concealed accidental hemorrhage by the fact that the former occurs late in labor, usually after rupture of the membranes, and that the presenting part of the fœtus recedes.

Prognosis.

In apparent hemorrhage the prognosis is good for the mother, but not favorable for the child. If labor does not come on at once, there is danger of infection of the blood-tract between the edge of the placenta and the os, resulting in sepsis.

In the concealed hemorrhage the percentage of mortality for both mother and child is high. Death results from hemorrhage, shock, extreme anæmia, or sepsis. The fœtal mortality is due to interference with the uteroplacental circulation.

Treatment.

External variety : If the external hemorrhage is moderate in amount, a full dose of opium (liq. opii sed., $\mathfrak{m}$xxv) and rest in bed for a few days will be the only treatment required. The patient's temperature should be taken twice daily for a week or ten days, and if evidences of infection of the blood-tract occurs the uterus should be emptied. When the blood-loss is alarming it may be necessary to induce labor. The os should be dilated digitally to permit rupture of the membranes. A Barnes or Champetier de Ribes bag may then be introduced into the cervix and left there till it is expelled, when forceps may be applied, should the forces of Nature fail in promptly effecting delivery. When it is required to empty the uterus immediately, the cervix should be dilated rapidly ; if necessary, it should be incised and version performed.

Concealed variety : If the patient's condition is such as to forbid active obstetric interference, the treatment should be directed to combating the effects of the shock and hemorrhage (see Treatment of Post-partum Hemorrhage).

The fundus should be compressed by means of a snugly fitting binder and pad. The foot of the bed should be elevated.

When the patient's condition permits, the uterus should be emptied by means of manual dilatation of the cervix and version. The placenta in these cases should be removed manually, and a hot intra-uterine injection should be given after the uterus has been emptied.

The after-treatment should be directed to controlling the effects of severe hemorrhage, and to securing good uterine contraction.

Retained Placenta.

This condition is of frequent occurrence. The placenta is usually completely detached, and lies in the dilated lower uterine segment or in the upper part of the vagina.

Causes: Feeble uterine contractions, or, more frequently, improper methods of placental expression, generally give rise to the condition. A full bladder or rectum may lead to retention of the placenta.

Treatment : The proper application of Credé's method of expression is usually all that is required in the way of treatment. The uterus may be steadied and held in position by laying one hand across the suprapubic region of the abdomen, while the other firmly squeezes the fundus and at the same time exerts pressure in the axis of the pelvic inlet *during a uterine contraction.* This method will rarely fail to secure expulsion of the placenta. Very occasionally it may be necessary to introduce a couple of fingers into the vagina, so as to reach the lower edge of the placenta and hook it forward.

Adherent Placenta.

In this condition, which is rare, the placenta is not only retained, but is also **adherent** to the uterine wall. The adhe-

sion is rarely complete; a part of the placenta is usually
detached. The torn sinuses bleed profusely, as the uterus

FIG. 111.

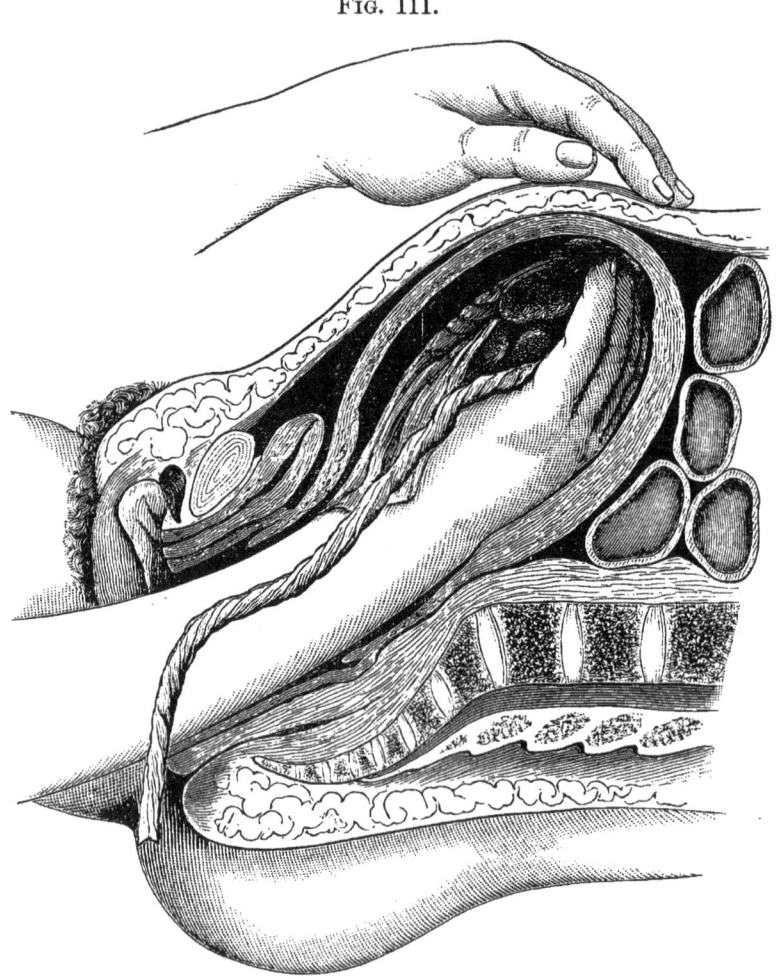

Artificial removal of adherent placenta. (Modified from Ribement-Dessaignes and
Lepage.)

cannot contract properly on account of the portion of the
placenta which remains adherent.

Causes: The most frequent cause is a placentitis (or decidual inflammation) of specific origin. Chronic endometritis

and placental degenerations, due to chronic nephritis in the mother, may give rise to adherent placenta.

Treatment: If Credé's method of expression fails and the hemorrhage is profuse, the cavity of the uterus must be entered and the placenta gently separated and removed.

To perform this operation one hand grasps the fundus securely, while the other is inserted into the vagina and follows up the cord as a guide till the placenta is reached. A detached edge is then felt for, the finger-tips inserted between the placenta and the uterine wall, and by gentle lateral movements of the hand the separation is completed and the placenta gently grasped. The outer hand then makes friction over the fundus until a contraction has been stimulated, when the internal hand and placenta are slowly withdrawn (Fig. 111).

The internal hand and the placenta should never be withdrawn until uterine contraction has occurred, on account of the danger of producing inversion of the uterus. The hand should then be re-introduced and the whole uterine cavity explored to make sure that no fragments of placental tissue have been retained. A hot intra-uterine douche should then be given. It is advisable to administer a full dose of ergot as soon as the uterus has been emptied.

MATERNAL DYSTOCIA.

The subject of **maternal dystocia** may be divided into three headings :

1. Anomalies in the forces of labor ;
2. Anomalies in the pelvis ;
3. Anomalies in the maternal soft structures.

1. ANOMALIES IN THE FORCES OF LABOR.

Precipitate Labor.

Excessive power in the expulsive forces of labor may result in the very speedy completion of the act.

Etiology: The condition is usually due to *undue excitability of the sympathetic nervous system,* rather than to excessive muscular development. It may therefore be met with in

18—Obst.

young primiparæ, as well as in women of more advanced age and of greater muscular development. The rule is that the precipitancy occurs in the *second stage* of labor, the first stage being quite normal.

Conditions causing relaxation of the pelvic floor, as debilitating diseases, previous laceration, etc., favor the occurrence of precipitate labor.

Powerful emotions, such as fear or anxiety, may act by increasing the force of the uterine contractions.

Sudden and powerful uterine contraction with the patient in the erect posture may result in the rapid expulsion of the fœtus, which may fall to the floor and receive serious injury. Thus it not infrequently happens that women are suddenly delivered while sitting in a privy or water-closet, and the child may fall into the cesspit or bowl of the closet and perish before aid is secured.

Prognosis : Lacerations of the vagina and perineum, hemorrhage from partial or complete separation of the placenta, inversion of the uterus, and occasionally retention of the placenta, associated with hour-glass contraction of the uterus, may be mentioned as sequelæ of precipitate labor.

The sudden evacuation of the uterine contents may lead to severe or even fatal syncope on the part of the mother. The fœtal mortality is somewhat greater than normal.

Treatment : When the uterine action is powerful and the fœtus descends rapidly, it may be *held back* by inserting the fingers in the vagina and resisting the advance of the presenting part, while at the same time chloroform is administered to the mother. The patient should be instructed to keep the mouth open, and to pant or cry out during each pain.

If a previous labor has been precipitate, the woman should be kept constantly in bed after the onset of labor. If the pains tend to become too powerful, chloral should be freely administered. Fifteen or twenty grains may be given at a dose, and repeated at intervals of twenty minutes until a drachm has been given or the action of the drug has been obtained. It is advisable to administer chloroform while waiting for the chloral to be absorbed into the system.

The management of the *third stage* of labor demands special care, for in these cases there is often a complete absence of contraction after delivery of the child ; hence the uterus becomes extremely relaxed in the intervals between the pains. The fundus should be kept well under control, firm friction made between each pain to stimulate contraction, and plenty of time should be given before attempting to expel the placenta.

If, after the expulsion of the placenta the uterus does not remain contracted, a hot (120° F.) intra-uterine douche should be given, followed by a hypodermic injection of ergot (aseptic) ℔ xx. The fundus should be controlled until the uterus remains firmly contracted.

Delayed Labor; Uterine Inertia.

When the expulsive action of the uterus is **unable to overcome the normal resistance** of the maternal passages, labor is delayed and the pains are said to be " weak."

Causes: The commonest causes of uterine inertia are premature rupture of the membranes, rigid os, a distended bladder or rectum, and general debility of the patient. Obliquity of the uterus; overdistention, as in multiple pregnancy or hydramnios; degeneration of the uterine muscle-fibres from inflammation or too frequent childbearing; malpresentation; uterine tumors or tumors of neighboring structures; and low attachments of the placenta, may all be mentioned as causes of uterine inertia.

Diagnosis: Before making a diagnosis of uterine inertia care should be taken to ascertain if the bladder and rectum have been emptied. By external examination the contraction of the uterus may be felt to be weak, for the organ will not assume the intense hardness associated with good uterine action. By vaginal examination in the first stage the bag of waters does not become tense during a pain, or if the membranes have ruptured the presenting part does not descend.

Examination should then be made to ascertain that the labor is not delayed by some obstruction.

The **prognosis** depends on the stage of labor and the cause of the inertia. In the first stage there is little danger to either mother or child unless the membranes have been long ruptured. In the second stage of labor there is danger to both mother and child from prolongation of the labor.

No hard-and-fast rule as to how long delay might be without danger can be laid down. When the head is low in the pelvis prolonged delay may cause serious injury to the maternal parts from pressure of the head. The condition of the mother and child should be carefully watched. Danger to the child is manifested by a slowing of the fœtal heart's action, while danger to the mother is indicated by local œdema and a rising pulse and temperature. It may be said that a delay of over six hours in the second stage warrants the artificial termination of the labor.

Treatment: This depends on the stage of labor and the cause of the inertia. The first duty is to ascertain the cause of the delay, and, if possible, remove it. The bladder and rectum should be emptied. The prolongation of the first stage of labor may have exhausted the patient, and when this is the case no effort should be made to stimulate uterine contractions until the patient has been restored by a good rest, and, if possible, sleep. This may be accomplished by giving her a hypodermic injection of morphine ($\frac{1}{4}$ gr.), and repeating it in half an hour if necessary. At the same time she may be given some hot broth or milk, or some sherry and a biscuit, to maintain her strength.

Chloral is to be preferred to morphine, as it seldom arrests the progress of labor. Two drachms of the syrup of chloral may be given in a cupful of warm milk, and repeated in half an hour if required. On waking, the patient may be given some hot broth or egg-nog. If the contractions do not then set in with increased power, efforts may be made to stimulate the uterus to action.

Strychnine (gr. $\frac{1}{30}$), administered hypodermically, is probably the most valuable uterine stimulant. Quinine in large doses (gr. xv), repeated in half an hour, acts well in some cases; but the author has failed to find it completely satisfactory.

Ergot is only mentioned to be condemned, for it tends to induce tetanic uterine action, and thus interferes with the placental circulation. *It should never be used until the uterus has been emptied.* Hot vaginal douches (120° F.), given at intervals of half an hour, often prove of great value.

Alcohol has proved a very satisfactory uterine stimulant in the author's experience; it is best given in the form of sherry, as recommended by Hirst, and should be slowly sipped, the patient being informed that it will surely bring back the pains and hasten the delivery.

In very obstinate cases a *sterilized bougie* may be inserted into the uterus, and the vagina packed lightly with sterile gauze, as for the induction of premature labor. The introduction into the cervix of a Champetier de Ribes bag or of a Barnes bag is a very useful but troublesome method of treatment. These not only stimulate the uterus to action, but dilate the cervix, and thus assist in overcoming the resistance offered by the os.

The *bag of waters* should not be ruptured until the os is dilated, unless it is evident that there is an excess of liquor amnii present, and that this is the probable cause of inefficient uterine action.

When inertia is present in the *second stage* of labor the patient may be allowed to walk about, in the hope that the descent of the head under the influence of gravity will set up uterine action by reflex stimulation of the pelvic floor.

Pressure on the fundus with the patient in the dorsal position may prove of value when employed during uterine contractions. When other measures fail resource must be had to the forceps to terminate labor.

2. ANOMALIES OF THE PELVIS.

The great majority of anomalies of the pelvis are of the nature of **contraction**. Contractions in the diameters of the pelvic brim give rise to the most serious consequences both to mother and to child, in proportion to the degree of obstruction offered to the passage of the fœtus.

Frequency: Until recently it was commonly believed that abnormal pelves were much more rarely met with in America than in Europe; but the more general practice of pelvimetry which has prevailed in obstetric clinics during the past decade has revealed the fact that in America deformity of the pelvis is met with in about the same proportion of women as in Europe.

The records of European clinics show a wide variation in the percentages reported, the difference extending from 1.2 per cent. in Russia to 24.3 per cent. in Saxony. Von Winckel considers that from 10 to 15 per cent. of German women have deformed pelves; but that in only 5 per cent. is the obstruction serious enough to be noticed.

Among American observers,[1] Flint, in New York, found

[1] Davis, E. P., American Journal of Obstetrics, Jan., 1900.

1.42 per cent. of pelvic contraction; Reynolds, in Boston, 1.13 per cent.; Crossen, in St. Louis, 7 per cent.; Dobbin, in Baltimore, 11.45 per cent.; and Williams, in Baltimore, 13.1 per cent. Davis, from the records of 1224 patients, concludes that 25 per cent. of the women in the United States have pelves smaller than the average, while 7 per cent. have pelves larger than the average.

Hirst states that deformed pelves are by no means rare among native-born women in the Eastern States.

Classification: Various classifications of pelvic anomalies have been employed in different countries, but the following, taken from Jewett's *Practice of Obstetrics*, will be found sufficiently comprehensive to meet all requirements:

I. Pelves normally proportioned but abnormal in size:
    1. Uniformly enlarged (justomajor).
    2. Uniformly contracted (justominor).

II. Pelves with anomalies of size, shape, inclination, or combinations of these:
    1. Those with minor developmental peculiarities:
        (*a*) Masculine;
        (*b*) Shallow;
        (*c*) Deep;
        (*d*) Funnel-shaped.
    2. Anteroposteriorly contracted:
        (*a*) Flat non-rachitic;
        (*b*) Flat rachitic.
    3. Obliquely contracted:
        (*a*) By imperfect development of one sacral ala (Naegele pelvis);
        (*b*) By imperfect or abolished use of one limb;
        (*c*) By spinal curvature.
    4. Transversely contracted:
        (*a*) By imperfect development of both sacral alæ (Robert pelvis);
        (*b*) By kyphosis of the spine.
    5. Compressed pelvis:
        (*a*) Malacosteon;
        (*b*) Pseudomalacosteon rachitic.
    6. Spondylolisthetic.

7. Pelves distorted by injury, tumors, anchylosis of joints.
8. Deformity due to spinal curvature:
   (*a*) Kyphotic;
   (*b*) Scoliotic;
   (*c*) Kyphoscoliotic;
   (*d*) Lordosis.

Diagnosis: *Theoretically* it is the duty of the physician to take careful measurement of the pelvis of every woman he is called upon to attend in labor; practically, this is rarely done until delay in the progress of labor calls attention to the fact that possibly some obstruction exists in the pelvis.

Deformity of the pelvis is *most frequently* met with in those women who in childhood have suffered from malnutrition, rickets, or tuberculosis of the vertebræ or joints of the lower limbs, or who early in life have suffered from accident to a limb which has resulted in shortening, dislocation, etc.

Malnutrition and *hard work* early in life not infrequently result in flattening of the pelvic brim. *Rickets* may lead to various serious pelvic deformities. A *history* of late dentition, prolonged indigestion, of not walking after the second year, would suggest this disease. An examination of such a patient might reveal the square head, pigeon-breast, beading of the ribs, or bending or twisting of the long bones common to this disease. Usually these patients are of short stature.

Diseases or *accidents* resulting in deformity of the spine or lower limbs when they have occurred *early in life* result in abnormal development of the pelvis.

Failure of the head to descend into the pelvis at or before the onset of labor, associated with undue prominence of the abdomen, should always suggest obstruction at the pelvic brim when these conditions are found present in a primipara with a vertex presentation.

Pelvimetry.

Deformities of the pelvis may be detected by *external* and *internal palpation;* and by *measurements*, both external and internal, of those diameters of the pelvis which are accessible.

For *taking pelvic measurements* the examiner's fingers, a

tape-measure, and a pair of modified calipers, known as a pelvimeter, are usually employed. The pelvimeter devised by
Baudelocque in 1775 (Fig. 112) is probably the best, though
many others have since been invented.

FIG. 112.

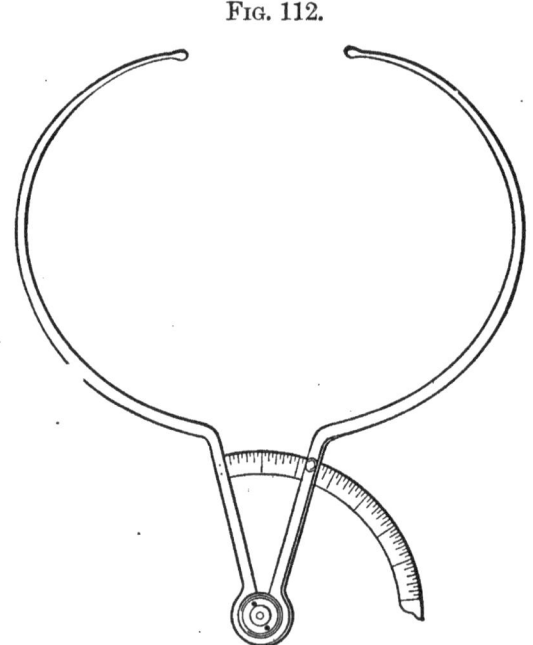

Baudelocque's pelvimeter.

Methods of Taking Pelvic Measurements.

External measurements : The clothing of the patient having
been rolled well out of the way and the lower part of the body
covered with a sheet, she lies on her back close to the edge of
the bed, while the physician stands beside her looking toward
her head. He then takes the pelvimeter and holds a rod in
each hand, the tip of an index-finger being on each knob, and
the reading surface of the scale held so as to be easily read.

The knobs of the pelvimeter are then placed on the *anterior
superior spines of the ilia* or on the tense fascia lata just below
them, as suggested by Winckel. In the normal pelvis this
measurement should be about 10¼ inches (26 cm.) ; the knobs
of the pelvimeter are then moved along the *external edges of
the iliac crests* until the greatest distance is found, the measure-

ment of which should be about 11 inches (28 cm.). The length of these measurements, as well as any important difference between them, enables us to draw our conclusions as to the development of the innominate bones, and the *width of the transverse diameter at the inlet.*

The patient is then made to turn on her side, with the thighs slightly flexed. The knob of one rod is then placed in the depression *just below the spine of the last lumbar vertebra* and firmly held in this position, while the other knob is placed on the symphysis pubis at a point about one-eighth of an inch below its upper border, and pressed firmly into position. The measurement thus obtained should be about $7\frac{1}{2}$ inches (19 cm.), and is known as the *external conjugate*, or the *diameter of Baudelocque.* To obtain an idea of the true conjugate $3\frac{1}{2}$ inches (9 cm.) should be deducted from the measurement of the external conjugate, to allow for the thickness of bone and soft tissues ; this would give the normal true conjugate, 4 inches (10 cm.).

The *oblique diameters of the brim* may be measured by placing one knob of the pelvimeter in the depression marking the posterior superior spine of one side, and the other knob on the anterior superior spine of the opposite side. In symmetrical pelves these measurements are usually equal, and should be about 9 inches (22.5 cm.).

The *circumference* of the pelvis may be measured by placing a tape-line around the body, so that it will pass just over the symphysis, under the iliac crests, and over the middle of the sacrum behind. In a woman of average development and with a normal pelvis this measurement should be about $35\frac{1}{2}$ inches (90 cm.).

The other external measurements of importance are those of the *outlet of the pelvis.* The *transverse diameter* of the outlet is measured by placing the knobs of the pelvimeter on the inner sides of the ischial tuberosities. Contraction of the outlet of the pelvis is one of the commonest varieties of pelvic deformity encountered in America, Williams stating that anomalies of the outlet are to be met with in every twelfth patient, hence the importance of ascertaining the measurement of this diameter. The *anteroposterior diameter* may be measured by placing one knob of the pelvimeter on the under border of the symphysis pubis and the other knob on the skin over the lower border of the tip of the sacrum. From this 1.3 cm. must be deducted to allow for thickness of the bone, etc. This measurement can be better obtained by placing the tip of the middle finger of the left hand, inserted into the vagina, against the end of the sacrum and pressing the edge of the hand against the lower border of the symphysis, the point of contact being marked by the index-finger of the right hand and the distance measured after the left hand has been withdrawn.

Internal measurements : A good general idea of the capacity of the pelvic canal may be obtained from a careful vaginal

FIG. 113.

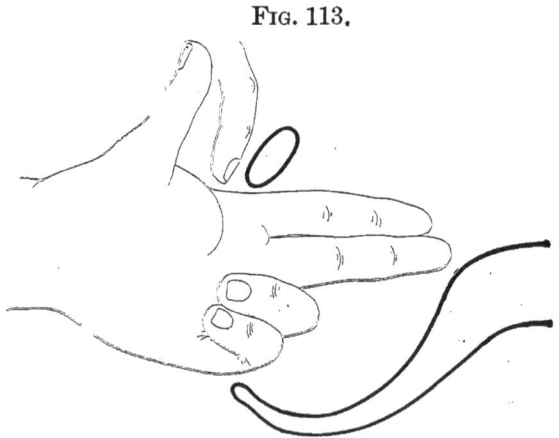

Internal pelvimetry. Measuring the diagonal conjugate with the hands. (Jewett.)

examination. The points of importance in this examination are the thickness, height, and inclination of the pubis ; the condition of the lateral walls as regards projections, etc.; the condition of the sacrococcygeal joint ; the curve of the sacrum ; and the condition of the promontory, if this can be reached.

The *diagonal conjugate*—i. e., the measurement from the promontory to the subpubic ligament—can usually be obtained without much difficulty provided the examination is made carefully and methodically.

The patient is put in the lithotomy position with the buttocks projecting over the edge of the bed or table. The examiner then introduces the first two fingers of the left hand into the vagina and extends them inward and upward until the tip of the second finger rests upon the promontory of the sacrum (Fig. 113). Care must be taken not to mistake the last lumbar vertebra for the first sacral, or *vice versâ*. The radial side of the hand is then raised until the impress of the subpubic ligament is felt upon it. With a finger-nail of the other hand the point of contact is marked, and both hands then withdrawn. With a pelvimeter the distance between the mark and the tip of the second finger is then measured. This is the length of the diagonal conjugate. From this measurement $\frac{2}{3}$ inch (1.75 cm.) should be deducted to obtain the true conjugate diameter. This average difference between these two diameters depends upon the height of the symphysis ($1\frac{1}{2}$ inches, 4 cm.), a normal angle between the axis of the pubis and the true conjugate (105 degrees), a normal thickness of the symphysis, and a normal height of the promontory.

When the height of the symphysis is greater than $1\frac{1}{2}$ inches (4 cm.), about $\frac{3}{4}$ inch (2 cm.) should be deducted from the diagonal conjugate.

Pelves Normally Proportioned but Abnormal in Size.

Uniformly Enlarged Pelvis (Justomajor).

Definition: This form of pelvis preserves all the characters of the normal, but all its measurements are increased. It is generally to be found in women of great stature, though it is met with occasionally in women below the medium height.

Diagnosis: All the measurements are found to be in excess of the normal while preserving their relative proportion.

Influence on pregnancy and labor: During pregnancy the uterus tends to remain longer in the pelvis than in the normal condition, thus giving rise to disturbances of the bladder and of the rectum. For the same reason the pressure-symptoms in the latter part of pregnancy are often severe, and may render locomotion difficult.

The condition predisposes to precipitate delivery. The imperfect resistance offered to the head in its descent may lead to loss of flexion, and thus retard rotation.

Uniformly Contracted Pelvis (Justominor).

Definition: In this type of pelvis the form is preserved, but its size is diminished.

Three **varieties** of the justominor pelvis are usually described: of these, the most common is the *juvenile*, in which the bones are small and slender; the *masculine*, in which the bones are heavy and thick; and the *dwarf*, or pelvis nana, in which the bones are thin and fragile, and the cartilaginous junctions between the constituents of the ossa innominata are retained.

Occurrence: The uniformly contracted pelvis is usually to be found in under-sized women, though it may be met with

FIG. 114.

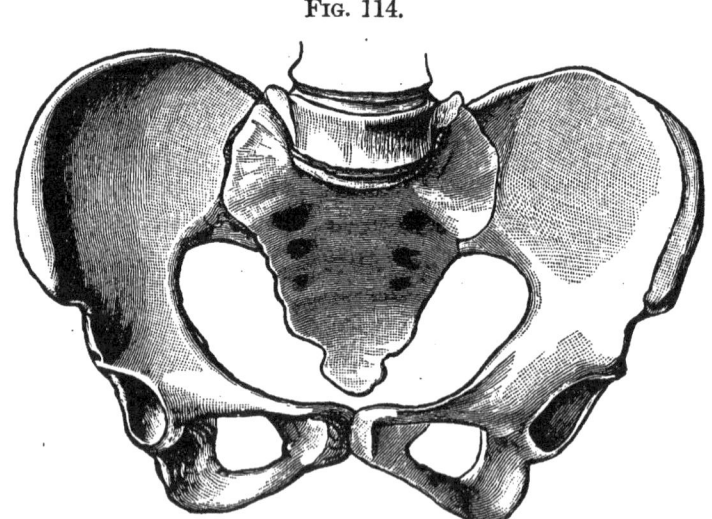

Generally contracted dwarf pelvis. (After Winckel.)

in women of average height, or even in tall women. It is most commonly met with in America in shop- and factory-girls.

Etiology: The causation of the justominor pelvis has not been satisfactorily explained. It is generally the result of arrested development due to unfavorable hygienic surroundings and bad nutrition in early life.

Characteristics: The generally contracted pelvis approaches the infantile in type (Fig. 114). The alæ of the sacrum are narrow, while the sacrum itself is short and has lessened forward inclination as compared with the normal. The promontory is high but not prominent. The pubic bones and symphysis have a lessened inclination outward. Thus when the patient stands erect the inclination of the pelvic entrance to the abdominal axis makes a more obtuse angle than would be the case in a normal pelvis (Fig. 115).

Usually the contraction is not very great. The conjugate diameter is seldom below 9 cm. (3½ inches).

Diagnosis: Careful pelvimetry will show that all the measurements are below normal, with the exception possibly of the external conjugate diameter, which is longer than would be expected, on account of the posterior position and lessened inclination forward of the sacrum. In this form of contracted pelvis the measurement of the pelvic circumference is generally far below the normal, 90 cm. (35½ inches).

Influence of labor: The increased resistance offered to the descent of the head results in flexion being more marked than it is in the normal pelvis. The head generally enters the brim in the oblique diameter.

Fig. 115.

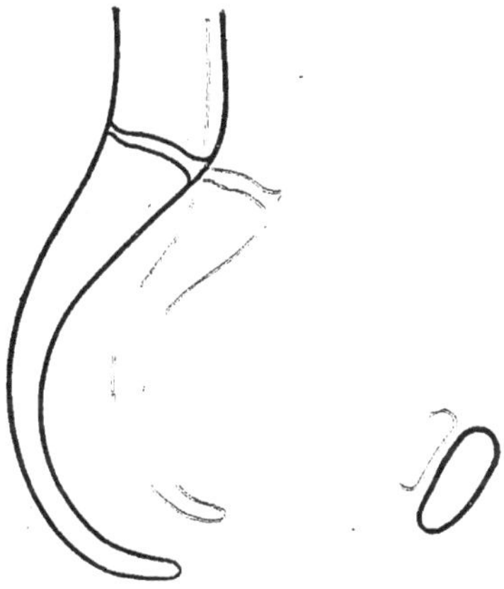

Diagram showing difference between normal and justominor pelvis on vertical mesial section.
Black, normal. Red, justominor.

In *breech cases* the child's head must be well flexed, by the operator putting his finger in its mouth and drawing down the chin before an attempt is made to secure engagement in the brim

Labor is usually prolonged, and the head undergoes much moulding, the caput succedaneum being unusually large. The suboccipitobregmatic diameter of the head is compressed and the occipitomental elongated (Fig. 116).

Treatment: If the head is advancing under the influence of uterine action, no interference is called for. The patient's strength must be sustained by appropriate nourishment, and opium may be used hypodermically to relieve her sufferings. Plenty of time must be allowed to secure good moulding of the head.

When labor *is delayed* and advance of the head ceases, then forceps should be tried. The axis-traction forceps should be employed. As a rule, when the contraction is not over one centimetre the head can be extracted if it be fairly soft and has been allowed to become well moulded.

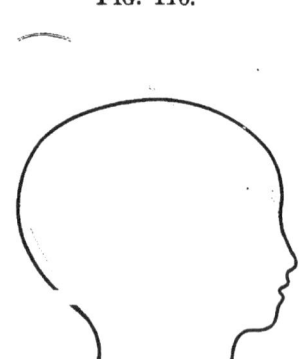

FIG. 116.

Diagram showing head unmoulded and moulded by labor in a justominor case.
Black, unmoulded.
Red, moulded.

If moderate efforts at extraction with the forceps fail to bring about advance of the head and the child is still living, *pubiotomy* should be performed.

Version is not to be recommended on account of the difficulty in securing the proper amount of flexion necessary to permit the engagement of the after-coming head in the pelvic brim.

Pelves with Anomalies of Size, Shape, Inclination; or Combinations of These.

Minor Developmental Peculiarities.

Masculine pelvis: In this pelvis the bones are heavy and strong, and the whole pelvis is masculine in character.

Labor may be prolonged and difficult on account of delay either in the brim or the outlet. Forceps are frequently required to accomplish delivery.

Shallow pelvis: The distance between the brim and the outlet is relatively less in this form of pelvis than in the normal. As a rule, labor is easy, though occasionally forceps are required.

Deep pelvis: There is an abnormal increase in the distance between the inlet and the outlet in this form of pelvis. Provided the diameters are normal, labor is not interfered with.

Funnel-shaped pelvis: In this form of pelvis the sacrum is narrow and has little perpendicular curve, and thus the depth of the canal is increased (Fig. 117). In this form of pelvis the contraction is most marked at the outlet, and may be in the anteroposterior diameter, or in the lateral, or in both. The pelvis thus approaches the masculine in type.

Influence on Labor: The mechanism of labor is interfered with and the head tends to become extended in the cavity of the pelvis; thus backward rotation of the occiput is likely to occur. Labor is usually prolonged, the delay occurring when the head is at the outlet. There is greater risk of extensive rupture of the perineum. The soft parts at the pelvic outlet are likely to be injured by undue pressure of the head.

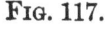

FIG. 117.

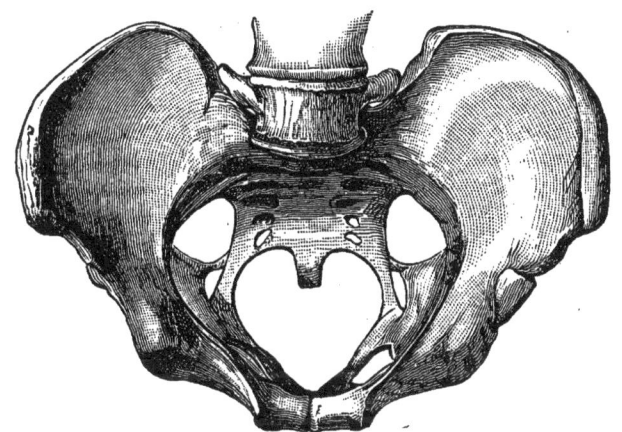

Funnel-shaped pelvis. (After Winckel.)

Treatment: In the lesser grades of contraction the woman may be delivered spontaneously or by forceps. In the higher grades the Cæsarean operation may be required. Pubiotomy may be employed when the contraction in the outlet is not marked and efforts at extraction by means of the forceps fail.

Flat Pelves.

Shortening of the conjugate diameter of the brim is the main characteristic of flat pelves.

Simple Flat Pelves; Non-rachitic.

Schröder states that this variety of deformed pelvis is more frequently seen in Europe than all the other forms put

together.   In America the simple flat, and the generally contracted, are the two varieties of pelvic deformity most frequently met with.

Hirst, in a series of 316 pelves in women of American
birth, found flattening to exist in 5.6 per cent.   Davis, in a
series of 1224 pelves, found the simple flat in 5.7 per cent.

Characteristics: The sacrum is small, and pressed downward and forward between the iliac bones; as it is not rotated

Fig. 118.

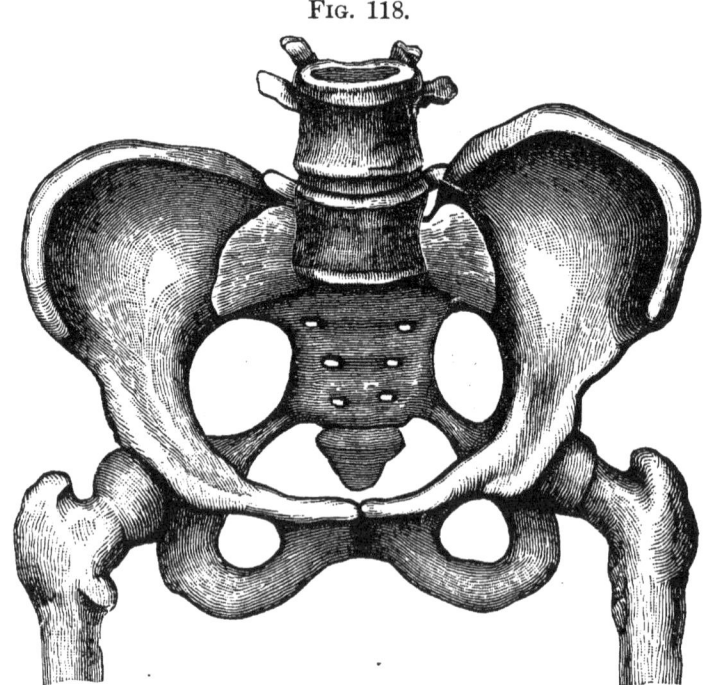

Flat non-rachitic pelvis.   (After Kleinwächter.)

forward on its transverse diameter, the anteroposterior diameter of the pelvis is therefore contracted throughout its whole
extent.   The transverse diameter remains as great as in the
normal pelvis (Fig. 118).

Frequently in flat pelves there is a *double promontory*, so
that a line drawn between the second sacral vertebra and the
symphysis is often as short as, or shorter than, the true conjugate.

The *degree of contraction* is usually not great, as it is rarely below 8 cm. (3⅛ inches), and usually not under 9.5 cm. (3¾ inches).

Etiology: The condition is usually congenital, though hard work in youth, too early walking, and excessive standing on the feet may be mentioned as causative factors.

Diagnosis: This pelvis may be found in small or in large women. There is usually nothing in the patient's history or appearance to suggest the deformity, unless she has had difficulty in previous labors. By pelvimetry the transverse measurements will be found to be normal, while the anteroposterior diameter will be diminished.

The Flat Rachitic Pelvis.

Characteristics: Rachitis leads to increased condensation in the bones; hence in the flat rachitic pelvis they are heavier, thicker, and somewhat smaller than in the normal. The sacrum is wider than in the normal pelvis.

The *iliac crests* are more or less everted at their anterior ends, so that the interspinal diameter is equal to or greater than the intercristal. The ilia are flattened, so that the fossæ are not so distinctly hollowed out nor are the iliac wings as expanded as in the normal pelvis. The *pelvic brim* is kidney-shaped, not heart-shaped, as in the normal pelvis. The *conjugate* is diminished; and the *transverse diameter* relatively or absolutely increased. At the *outlet* the transverse diameter may be widened and the anteroposterior be either normal or increased (Fig. 119).

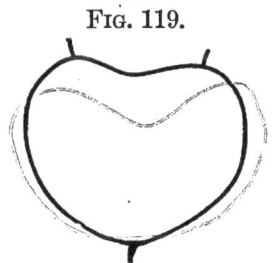

Fig. 119.

Diagram showing outline of brim of normal and of flat rachitic pelvis. Black, normal. Red, flat.

The *pubic arch* is wider than normal, and the symphysis is deeper and is rotated on its transverse diameter, so that its upper border converges toward the promontory. Thus the relation of the true conjugate to the diagonal conjugate is not the same as in the normal pelvis (Fig. 120).

19—Obst.

In the rachitic pelvis the *conjugata vera* may be diminished to any extent, depending on the degree of deformity present.

FIG. 120.

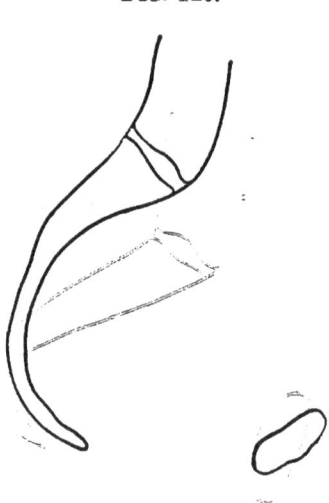

Diagram showing difference between normal and rachitic pelvis on vertical mesial section
Black, normal.   Red, rachitic.

Etiology : Rachitis in its early stages causes a softening of the bones and ligaments. The weight of the body tends to push the promontory of the sacrum downward and forward ; this causes a rotation of the sacrum on its transverse diameter, and tends to elevate the lower part of this bone and the coccyx upward and backward. The strong ligaments attached to the lower part of the sacrum prevent its movement upward and backward, and the result is a sharp bending of the bone produced in the neighborhood of the fourth sacral vertebra.

Besides the weight of the body, the *action of the muscles* attached to the pelvis helps to bring about the deformity. The increased separation of the ischial tuberosities is due to the action of the abductor and rotator muscles of the thighs. The degree of deformity produced by rachitis depends on the date of its appearance, its severity, its duration, and the habits of the child.

Diagnosis : The history of the woman, her appearance, and the examination and measurements of her pelvis will permit the establishment of a diagnosis.

The rachitic woman is usually under-sized. She may have a square-shaped head or deformed thorax (pigeon-breast), beading of the ribs, and curved long bones, which may be enlarged at the ends. When she lies on a flat surface with the limbs well extended lordosis is generally present.

Pelvic measurement will show that the relation of the spines and crests of the ilia is altered. The external conjugate and the diagonal conjugate diameters will be found diminished. On account of the increased depth of the symphysis and the divergence of its lower margin, $\frac{3}{4}$ inch (2 cm.) must be deducted from the diagonal conjugate, instead of the average $\frac{2}{3}$ inch (1.75 cm.).

Care must be taken to ascertain if a *double promontory* is present; and if so, the conjugate should be measured from the projection of the sacrum which is nearer the symphysis.

Mechanism of Labor in Flat Pelves.

The contracted condition of the conjugate prevents the entrance into the pelvic inlet of the presenting part; hence the abdomen is usually more or less pendulous.

The presenting part, if it is the **head**, is usually found at the onset of labor to be resting in one or other iliac fossa; or it may be firmly pressed down upon the brim in a transverse position, so that its longest diameter is accommodated to the longest diameter of the pelvic inlet.

Malpresentations are common, and prolapse of the cord and of the extremities is not infrequent.

The **first stage** of labor is usually prolonged, because of the non-descent of the head. The membranes protrude from the os in a cylindrical pouch. **U**nfortunately the bag of waters usually ruptures early; and in this case dilatation can only be effected by a retraction of the cervix over the head.

In the **second stage** of labor the descent of the head is resisted by the projection of the sacral promontory. Thus the occiput is pushed to one side till it comes into contact with the lateral brim of the pelvis, the iliopectineal line, where it is arrested. The sinciput not being resisted, then descends, and thus extension of the head occurs; this brings the small bi-temporal, instead of the larger biparietal, diameter of the head into relation with the contracted conjugate.

The movement " **rounding the promontory** " then takes place. The posterior parietal bone becomes arrested on the promontory, so that the head becomes obliquely displaced by turning on its anteroposterior diameter. Thus the sagittal suture, instead of remaining in the middle of the pelvic inlet, approaches the promontory, as the anterior parietal bone slips past the upper border of the symphysis and enters the cavity of the pelvis. Then the posterior parietal bone slips past the promontory, and the head enters the pelvic cavity in an extended position (Fig. 121).

Once the **obstruction at the superior strait is passed,** the head usually descends with ease and rapidity, the rest of the mechanism going on normally. Occasionally rotation of the head fails, and owing to the width of the transverse diameter of the pelvis it is expelled from the vulva in its original transverse or in an oblique position.

Head-moulding : The caput succedaneum is generally not exaggerated. Usually the child's head shows what is known as the " promontory mark." This may be only a red mark on the parietal region, between the anterior fontanelle and the parietal eminence which was in contact with the promontory. Occasionally there may be an actual depression of the parietal bone in this region. Sometimes a gutter-like groove may be noted in a line running outward and forward on the child's skull. Usually the posterior parietal bone is depressed below the anterior, which overlaps it at the sagittal suture.

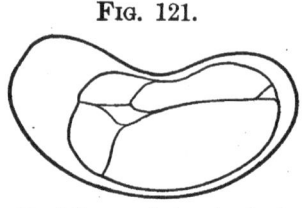

FIG. 121.

Moulding of head during passage through flat rachitic pelvis.

Treatment of Labor in Flat Pelves.

Care should be taken to **keep the membranes intact** as long as possible, by keeping the patient in bed during the first stage of labor, and by warning her against " bearing down " during the pains.

If the conjugate is not greatly diminished, the **head will usually engage,** provided it be given plenty of time to mould. *To this end* the uterine contractions should be controlled by means of hypodermic injections of morphine or of Battley's solution. The patient's strength should be maintained by the administration of nourishing broths, egg-noggs, etc. If the child's head be not unduly ossified, this treatment in the large proportion of cases will prove successful.

Should the head not descend, interference should not be delayed too long, for there is danger that the pressure of the head may result in necrosis of the cervical tissue over the promontory and of the anterior vaginal wall behind the symphysis.

Delivery by the employment of axis-traction forceps must then be attempted; for this operation the patient should be placed in Walcher's position. Should the forceps operation fail, delivery of a living child can only be effected by recourse to pubiotomy or to Cæsarean section.

Obliquely Contracted Pelves.

Obliquely contracted pelves **result** from:
(*a*) Imperfect development of one sacral **ala**;

FIG. 122.

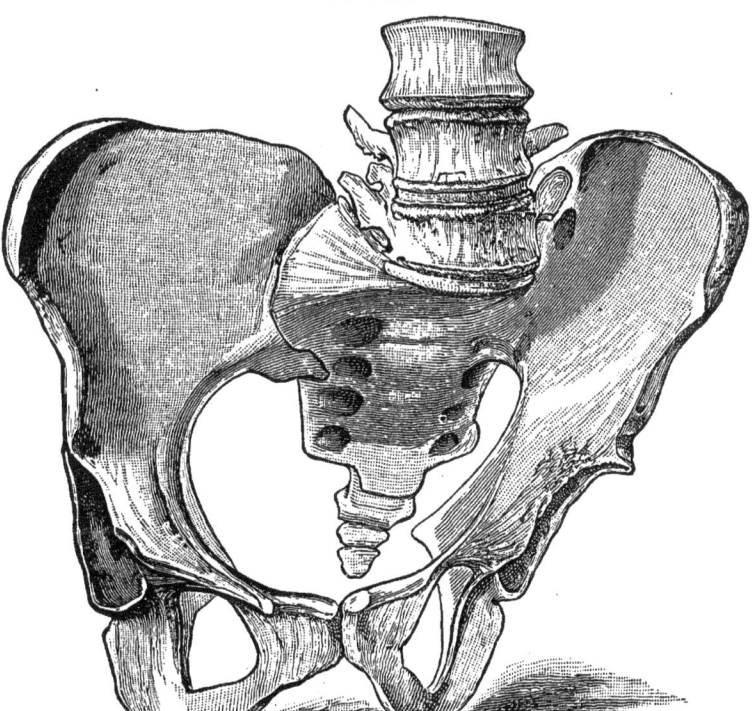

Singly obliquely contracted pelvis. (After Winckel.)

(*b*) Imperfect or abolished use of one limb; or
(*c*) Lateral curvature of the spine.

In these pelves the pelvic inlet has an oval shape, with the small point directed to the atrophied side of the pelvis (Fig. 122).

The **diagnosis** is based upon the history of the woman, and a careful examination and measurement of her pelvis.

Influence on labor: The mechanism of the head in passing through an obliquely contracted pelvis is the same as in the case of a justominor pelvis. The head usually enters the brim

FIG. 123.

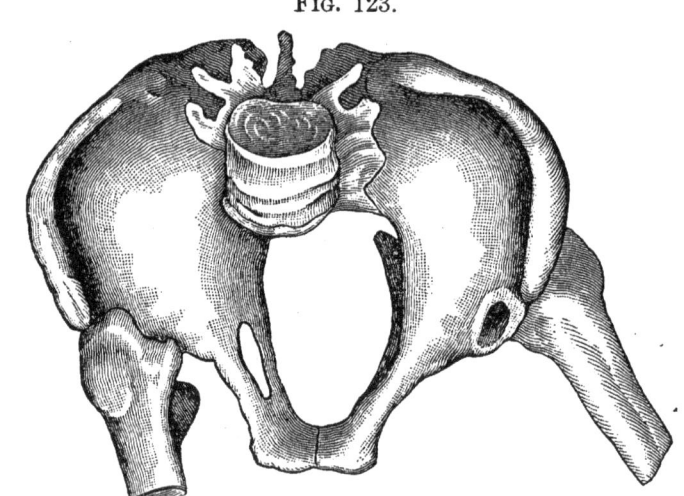

Transversely contracted pelvis. (After E. Martin.)

in extreme flexion, with its long diameter in relation to the long, oblique diameter of the pelvis. The long, oblique diameter is usually that of the diseased side. As the head descends rotation may fail and the occiput may turn toward the sacrum.

Treatment: The long diameter of the head should always be brought into relationship with the long oblique diameter of the pelvis by manual rotation, should Nature have failed to accomplish this before the onset of labor.

Should descent of the head be delayed, the axis-traction forceps should be tried. Should these fail, Cæsarean section is the only operation available.

Should the condition be diagnosed early in pregnancy, premature labor may be induced, provided the deformity of the pelvis is not extreme.

Transversely Contracted Pelves (Fig. 123).

Transverse contraction of the pelvis **results** from :
(*a*) *Imperfect development of both sacral alœ* (Robert pelvis) ;
(*b*) *Kyphosis of the spine.*
This is a very **rare** deformity.
As delivery " per vias naturales " is impossible, **Cæsarean section** must be employed.

Compressed Pelves.

Two **varieties** of compressed pelves have been described, the *malacosteon* and the *pseudomalacosteon.*

Malacosteon.

Characteristics : The whole pelvis is greatly altered in shape. There is a marked bending of the iliac wings, the anterior superior spines turning inward. The pelvic brim is triradiate,

Fig. 124.　　　　　　Fig. 125.

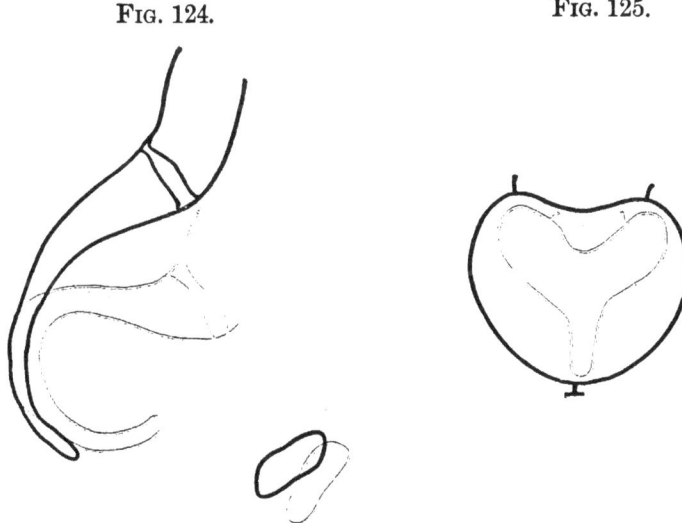

Diagram showing difference between normal and malacosteon pelvis on vertical mesial section.

　　Black, normal.
　　Red, malacosteon.

Diagram showing outline of brim of normal
and of malacosteon pelvis.

Black, normal.
Red, malacosteon.

owing to the promontory and the acetabula being approximated. The pubic bones are close together and project as a
beak. The curve of the sacrum is greatly exaggerated and
the coccyx points upward into the pelvic canal (Figs. 124,
125, and 126).

Etiology: The condition is brought about by great softening
of the bones resulting from osteomalacia (mollities ossium).
This disease is met with chiefly in Europe, and is characterized

FIG. 126.

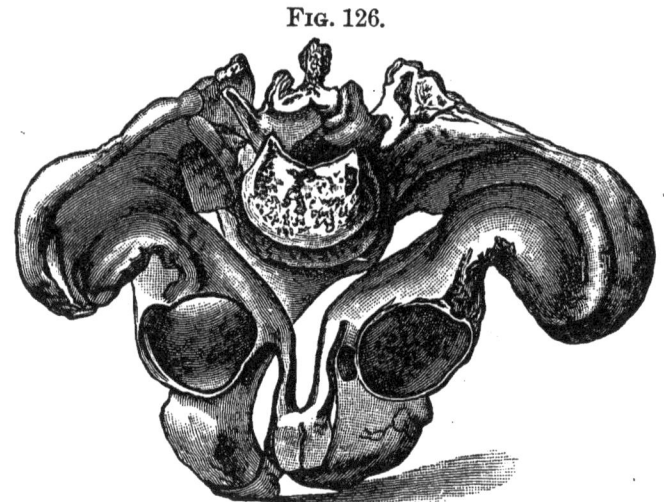

Malacosteon pelvis, seen from above.   (After Winckel.)

by a removal of the lime salts from the bones. It usually
develops during the puerperium, but also occurs in pregnancy.
The deformity results from transmission of the weight of the
body through the pelvis to the lower limbs.

Diagnosis: This is based upon the history of the woman
and an examination of the pelvis.

Treatment: When the bones are soft delivery may be effected
by means of forceps; when the bones are hard and the deformity permanent, Cæsarean section must be performed should the
pelvic contraction be extreme.

Pseudomalacosteon (Rachitic).

This deformity of the pelvis, produced by severe **rachitis**,
may closely approximate that produced by osteomalacia.

While the deformity of the true pelvis is very much as in the malacosteon, the iliac wings are widely separated as in the typical rachitic condition.

Spondylolisthetic Pelves.

Definition: The name applied to this variety of pelvic deformity indicates the condition—"spondylolisthesis," a slipping down of the vertebra, being derived from σπόνδυλος, "vertebra," and ὀλισθησις, "a slipping down."

FIG. 127.

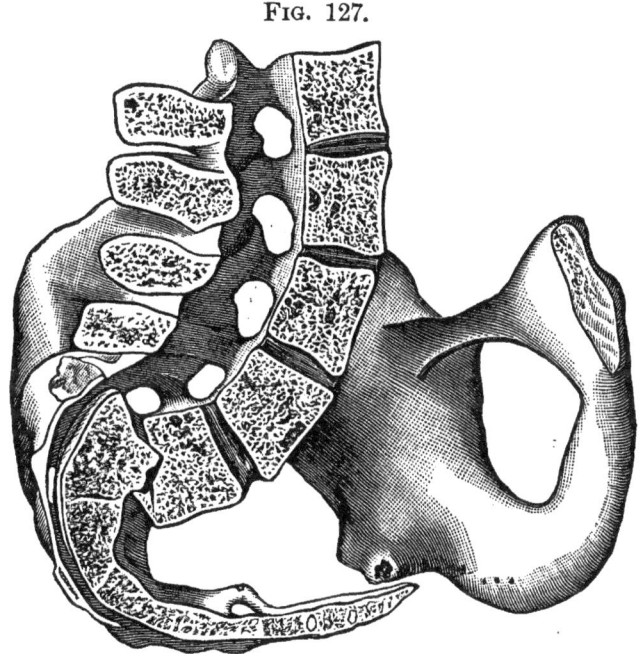

Spondylolisthetic pelvis. (After E. Martin.)

The deformity is **due to** a dislocation of the last lumbar vertebra in front of the sacrum. The body of the former is usually found to have slipped down in front of the first sacral vertebra, to which it has become attached by bony union. An exaggerated lordosis is produced, so that two or more of the lumbar vertebræ descend into the pelvic inlet and obstruct its anteroposterior diameter. The sacrum is pushed downward and backward, and to compensate this the anterior half of the pelvis is raised, so that the height of the symphysis is increased (Fig. 127).

The pelvic inlet is thus diminished both laterally and antero-posteriorly.

Etiology: Injury, disease, and developmental defects are usually mentioned as predisposing causes.

The **diagnosis** is somewhat difficult unless the condition is well marked. The stature of the woman is diminished, and the ribs may come into actual contact with the iliac crests. Lordosis is extreme and the shoulders are carried well back when the patient is erect. The posterior superior iliac spines are widely separated. The pelvic inclination is altered, so that the vulvar region is carried somewhat forward.

Internal examination reveals the projection of the lumbar vertebræ. It may be possible to feel the lower end of the aorta pulsating.

Treatment: The deformity is of the nature of a flattening of the pelvis, so that the mechanism of labor resembles that which occurs in the flat rachitic pelvis. The obstruction to labor depends entirely upon the projection of the lumbar vertebræ. The treatment is conducted on the same lines as in flat pelvis.

Pelves Distorted by Injuries, Tumors, or Disease.

Luxation of the femur: This condition, which is usually congenital, rarely produces such deformity of the pelvis as seriously to obstruct labor.

Tumors: The commonest tumors which occur in connection with the pelvis are *exostoses* of the joints. Fibroma, sarcoma, carcinoma, and enchondroma of the pelvic bones may distort the pelvis and so lead to obstruction (Fig. 128).

Treatment: When the growth is not excessive, delivery by the natural passages may be possible. When such is not the case, Cæsarean section must be performed. Pubiotomy may be employed in suitable cases, when the sacro-iliac joints are not involved in the tumor.

Fractures of the pelves: Deformity the result of fracture of the pelvic bones is rare.

Separation of the symphysis pubis: This accident may *occur* as a result of great force being exerted in the extraction of the head by means of forceps, or after version has been performed. Osteomalacia, rachitis, syphilis, and tuberculosis, or any profound cachexia, may predispose to the occurrence of this accident.

Diagnosis: The patient generally complains of sharp pain at the moment of separation of the joint. The condition may be recognized by introducing the index-finger into the vagina behind the joint and grasping it between the finger and thumb.

Fig. 128.

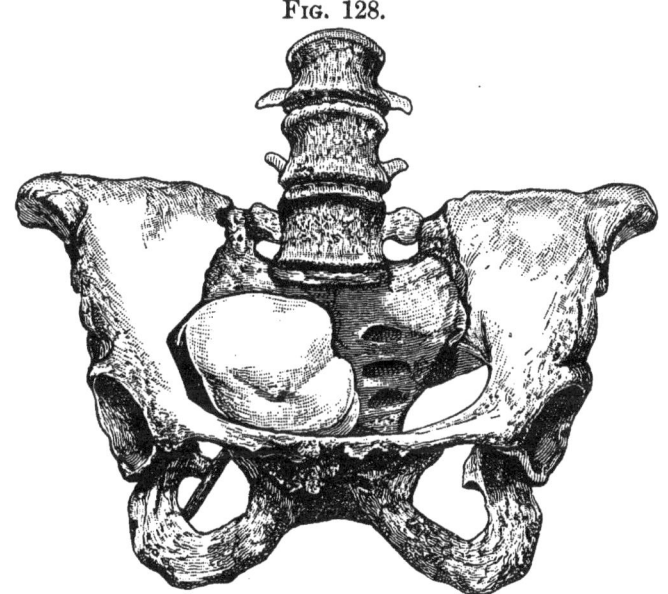

Malignant growth of posterior wall of pelvis which necessitated Cæsarean section in a case of Dr. Cameron.

Treatment: This consists in the application of a firm pelvic girdle as recommended for use after the operation of symphysiotomy.

Anchylosis of pelvic joints: This condition may affect any of the pelvic joints. When the symphysis is affected it has but little influence on labor. Anchylosis of the sacro-iliac joints may result in serious pelvic deformity. Not uncommonly the sacrococcygeal joint is affected, in which case obstruction may occur at the outlet. Fracture of the coccyx is the usual result.

Split pelvis: Want of complete development of the anterior wall of the pelvis results in this condition. It does not cause any obstruction to labor, but is likely to be associated with precipitate delivery.

Pelvic Deformities Due to Spinal Curvature.

Kyphosis: The degree of pelvic deformity resulting from kyphosis depends on the situation of the hump; the nearer this is to the sacrum the greater is the deformity of the pelvis. Generally the kyphosis occurs about the junction of the dorsal and lumbar vertebræ.

Treatment: If the degree of contraction is slight, labor is usually easy. There exists an old saying that "hunchbacks

Fig. 129.

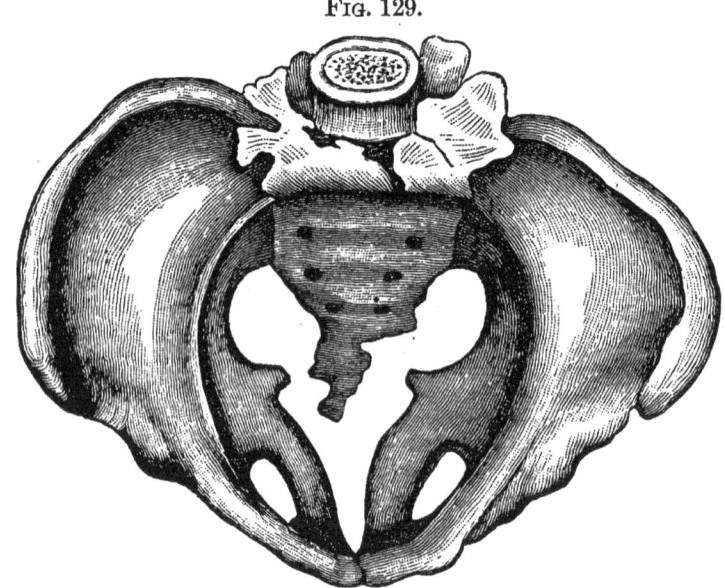

Lordotic pelvis. (After Kleinwächter.)

have easy labors." When delay takes place forceps may be required to effect delivery. In extreme contraction the Cæsarean operation is demanded.

Lordosis is a rare condition, and is usually secondary to spinal disease or pelvic deformity. To a certain degree it affords compensation; but, as a rule, it is not sufficient, and a rotation of the sacrum occurs, so that the upper end is thrown backward and downward (Fig. 129). The pelvic canal tends to become funnel shaped on account of the projection forward of the lower part of the sacrum and the partial obliteration of the promontory.

At the *inlet* the conjugate is increased; the diameters at the *outlet* are usually more or less diminished.

Scoliosis: The effect of scoliosis on the pelvis depends on the situation and extent of the spinal curvature. The lower it is and the earlier it occurs, the more serious are the effects produced in the pelvis. There is usually some degree of oblique contraction present in the pelvis of a patient the subject of scoliosis. The condition is frequently associated with rachitis.

The *innominate bone*, toward which the lumbar vertebræ are curved, receives the greater part of the body-weight, and is therefore pushed upward, inward, and backward by the extra pressure exerted on it by the head of the femur. The *acetabulum* on this side is displaced upward and inward toward the sacrum. The *symphysis* is thus pushed toward the opposite side. Thus the greatest degree of pelvic contraction is *on the side of the spinal convexity.*

In *labor* the largest part of the head generally descends on the roomier side of the pelvis, through which it may pass when in a state of good flexion.

In cases in which the pelvic deformity is extreme the Cæsarean operation must be resorted to.

Kyphoscoliosis: Rachitis may produce both kyphosis and scoliosis in the same woman. If the kyphosis is situated high up, but little effect may be produced on the pelvis.

3. ANOMALIES OF THE MATERNAL SOFT STRUCTURES.

Anomalies of Uterine Development.

Varieties: Labor may be complicated in many ways in a patient who has a double or septate uterus. Malpositions of the fœtus are common. The unimpregnated half may cause obstruction by its bulk, as it usually undergoes considerable increase in size in sympathy with the impregnated half. If the placenta is attached to the septum, severe hemorrhage may take place owing to imperfect contraction. Rupture of the septum or of the uterus may occur.

The decidual membrane which has formed in the impregnated half of the uterus may be retained, and, undergoing proliferation after delivery, may give rise to septic infection.

In all cases of anomalous development of the uterus **labor-pains** are usually short and inefficient.

Pregnancy in a **rudimentary horn** is a most dangerous condition, and when diagnosed it should be treated as a case of ectopic gestation.

Treatment : Forceps or version must be resorted to in most of these cases in order to effect delivery. The former should be chosen in preference to the latter when possible. Cæsarean section may be necessary.

Abnormal Conditions of the Cervix.

Varieties : Atresia, cicatricial conditions, contraction, and rigidity of the cervix, may all give rise to more or less obstruction in the first stage of labor.

Atresia is a very rare condition, and it is very seldom complete. The situation of the external os may be recognized as a dimple. Pressure upon this with a blunt instrument, such as the tip of a uterine sound, is usually all that is required to perforate it, after which dilatation usually proceeds rapidly.

Cicatricial contraction of the cervix is usually due to old laceration, or it may arise from a repair operation, from cauterization, or from syphilis or cancer.

Rigidity of the Cervix.

Etiology : When not due to *organic changes*, it is said to be *functional.* Functional rigidity is common in highly sensitive young women and in elderly primiparæ. It is usually due to some imperfection in the nerve-supply of the uterus, and is frequently associated with inefficient uterine contractions.

Treatment : When the rigidity of the cervix is functional in origin it may usually be overcome by the employment of nerve sedatives and hot douches. Syr. chloral. hydrat., ℥iss, should be administered in warm milk. Ten minutes later a hot vaginal douche (115° F.) should be given, at least two quarts of water being used. Every succeeding ten minutes a dose of chloral and a hot douche should be given in alternation, till the patient has received three doses of chloral and three hot douches, should the cervix not yield before. In the author's experience this plan of treatment has rarely failed.

In some cases a hypodermic injection of morphine, gr. ¼, is all that is required. Painting the cervix with a 2 per cent. solution of cocaine has been highly recommended. Occasionally a few whiffs of chloroform with each pain act like a charm in relieving this condition when it occurs in a highly nervous patient.

When these methods fail, artificial dilatation by means of the fingers or by the introduction of a hydrostatic bag may be necessary.

In extreme cases it may be necessary to make several small incisions, one-quarter to one-half inch deep, in the cervix before proceeding to artificial delivery.

Impaction of the Anterior Lip of the Cervix.

Occurrence: This condition may occasionally obstruct the advance of the head at the outlet. The anterior lip in these cases is caught between the head and pubes, and, becoming swollen and œdematous, may actually protrude at the vulva. After labor it may slough.

The proper **treatment** is to attempt to push it up in the intervals between the pains. If it be very œdematous, it may be necessary first to make a number of small incisions into it to permit the escape of serum, when its reduction may be accomplished without difficulty.

Displacements of the Uterus.

Anterior displacement of the uterus at the time of labor is not infrequent. It is generally due to a lax condition of the abdominal walls.

Treatment consists in the application of a tight abdominal binder, and in keeping the patient on her back in a half-reclining posture during labor.

Lateral displacement to one or other side may take place. The pregnant uterus is usually tilted slightly to the right side. When the lateral inclination is excessive part of the propulsive force of the uterus is lost, on account of the pressure of the presenting part against the lateral wall of the pelvis.

Treatment: Lateral displacement of the uterus may be corrected by making the patient lie on the side opposite to that to which the fundus is directed.

Retrodisplacement of the gravid uterus has already been referred to. Should the case go on to full term the distention of the uterus to accommodate the fœtus is accomplished by the stretching of the anterior wall, while the fundus and the posterior wall remain within the pelvis. The condition is known as " posterior sacculation " of the uterus.

In these cases the cervix is always displaced anteriorly and is pressed close to the abdominal wall.

Treatment: Cæsarean section is seldom necessary in these cases, as delivery can usually be effected by artificial dilatation of the cervical canal and subsequent internal version.

Prolapse of the pregnant uterus is possible, but these cases never go to full term. The prolapse of the uterus at term is usually partial, and only the elongated cervix escapes from the vulva, the fundus being in its usual position (Fig. 130). In labor the cervix may be retracted within the vagina ; or if it be rigid it may become œdematous, and by its bulk prevent delivery of the child.

Treatment: When possible the cervix should be pushed into the vagina, and retained there till dilatation occurs, when forceps may be applied and the child delivered. When the cervix is rigid and œdematous it should be freely incised and dilated, to permit the application of forceps to the child's head. An assistant may counteract the traction of the forceps, by pushing up the cervical tissues during the extraction of the child.

Ventrofixation or **suspensio uteri** may lead to obstruction in labor if the fundus has been attached too low down on the anterior wall. If the fundus is so firmly attached to the abdominal wall that it is prevented from rising, the anterior wall of the uterus remains crowded down over the pelvic inlet, while the posterior is distended and greatly thinned.

FIG. 130.

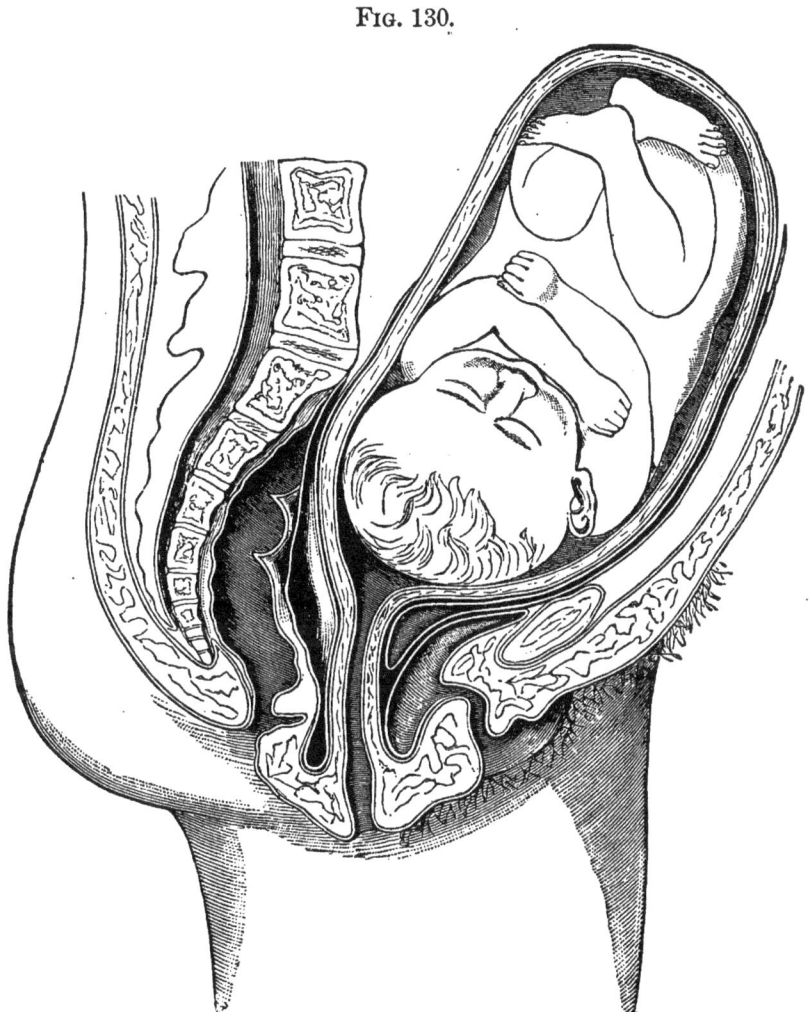

Elongated cervix with procidentia during labor.   (Barnes.)

The *complications* of labor which have been recorded in such cases are: inertia uteri, transverse position of the child, displacements of the head, cervical rigidity, rupture of the uterus, and severe hemorrhage during the third stage of labor.

20—Obst.

Treatment: If the obstruction offered by the folded and thickened anterior uterine wall be so great as completely to cut off the pelvic inlet, Cæsarean section must be performed. In some cases it may be possible to deliver the child by means of version, the danger of this operation being rupture of the thinned-out posterior wall of the uterus. The writer in one case was able to push the anterior wall out of the way sufficiently to permit the application of the forceps to the head, which was then drawn down.

Abnormal Conditions of the Vagina and Vulva.

Longitudinal and **transverse septa** may be present in the vagina and obstruct the advance of the presenting part of the foetus. They are seldom very dense in structure and are easily ruptured. If they do not yield, they may be divided between ligatures.

Unruptured hymen: This condition may be found present in labor; it causes but slight obstruction; occasionally it may be necessary to incise it.

Atresia of the vagina: Narrowing of the vagina may be due to maldevelopment or to cicatricial contractions after previous injury.

Treatment: Hot douches followed by injections of sterilized sweet oil may be employed to soften the part. Dilatation may be effected by the use of a hydrostatic bag.

Rigidity of perineum: The perineum may be so rigid as to prevent advance of the foetus. This condition is common in muscular women and in elderly primiparæ.

Treatment: In these cases the forceps may be required to draw down the foetus. During delivery the perineum may be softened by the free use of hot fomentations, care being taken to smear the parts with vaseline, to prevent burning. When laceration is certain, episiotomy may be performed.

Hæmatoma: This condition is, when present, found at the vaginal orifice.

Treatment: If large enough to obstruct labor, the tumor should be excised and the contents cleared out; after delivery, if hemorrhage from the cavity takes place, it should be packed with iodoform gauze.

Varicose veins when present seldom obstruct labor. They may rupture or be so bruised as to slough afterward.

Œdema of the vulva due to heart or kidney disease may obstruct labor. Multiple punctures should only be resorted to in extreme cases, as there is great risk of sepsis or gangrene following delivery.

Abnormal Conditions of the Bladder.

Distended bladder: This is a not uncommon cause of delay in labor, and should always be borne in mind. The urine should be removed with a sterile, long, soft catheter, the presenting part being pushed up so as to permit access to the bladder. In cases in which it is impossible to pass the catheter perforation through the abdominal wall may be required.

Cystocele: In this condition the bladder may protrude through the vulva.

Treatment: The urine must be drawn by means of a soft catheter, and the prolapsed part afterward pushed gently up above the presenting part of the fœtus. If reduction prove impossible, the part must be held up while the child is extracted by means of the forceps.

Vesical calculus: If small, the calculus may not obstruct labor. If possible, it should be pushed up above the symphysis.

When large, it may be extracted after dilating the urethra; or it may be necessary to incise the bladder through the anterior vaginal wall. After labor the incision may be sutured.

Tumors of the Genital Canal and Neighboring Organs.

Carcinoma of the cervix: It may be said that, as a rule, when this condition is present at full term serious obstruction to labor results. Spontaneous delivery may occur if the disease is limited to the anterior lip and is not surrounded by a large area of cicatricial infiltration.

Hemorrhage and sepsis are likely to arise during the puerperium.

Cæsarean section is the proper *treatment,* if the disease is fairly extensive.

Fibromyomata.

The obstructions to labor resulting from the presence of fibro-myomata depend on the **situation** of the new growth.   If it springs from the lower uterine segmen or cervix, it may become incarcerated in the pelvis and absolutely prevent the descent of the child (Fig. 131).

Fig. 131.

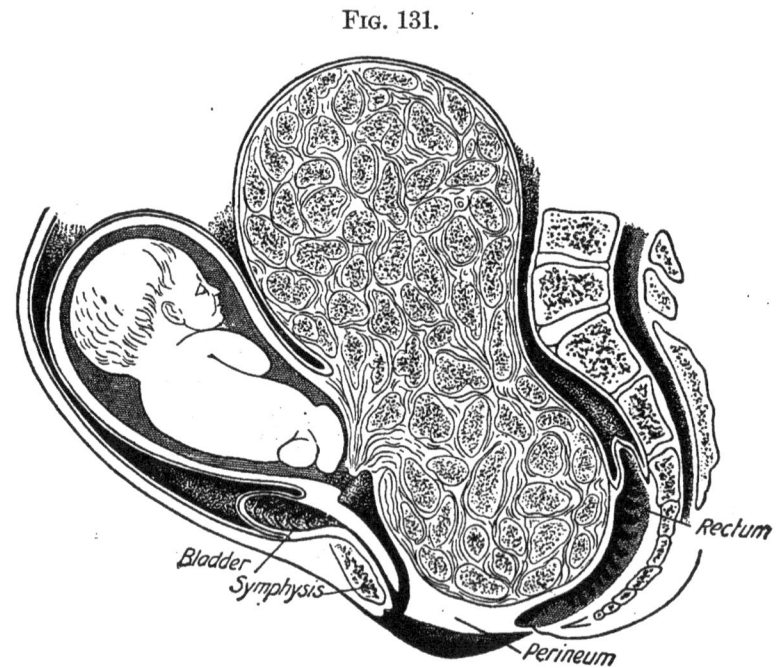

Myoma uteri complicating pregnancy.   (After Spiegelberg.)

Effects : They lead to malpresentations and malpositions of the fœtus, to prolapse of the cord, to adherent placenta, and to hemorrhage.   The labor-pains are likely to be inefficient.   A tetanic condition of the uterus is not infrequently met with in these cases.

The pressure of the tumor may produce severe contusions or fractures of the fœtal skull.   The tumor may be so injured during labor that sloughing and gangrene may follow and give rise to septic infection.

When the tumor is situated on the anterior wall it may be displaced upward by uterine contraction, and thus cease to obstruct the advance of the child.

Diagnosis: When situated low down in the uterus a fibroid tumor may be mistaken for the fœtal head. A careful examination should prevent this mistake.

Prognosis: This depends upon the early recognition of the condition and the treatment adopted. The experience of the writer leads him to consider the presence of myoma a grave complication of labor. In a series of 300 of these cases collected by Lafleur the mortality for the mothers, of delivery by the natural passage, was 25 to 55 per cent. and 77 per cent. for the children.

Treatment: When the tumor or tumors are *situated high up* labor may terminate naturally. In some cases labor is prolonged on account of uterine inertia, and must be terminated by version or forceps.

When the *tumor is small* and situated *low down*, it may be possible to push it up out of harm's way by placing the patient in the knee-chest position. If this fails, it may be possible to extract the child by means of the forceps with the woman in Walcher's position. If this be impossible, Cæsarean section must be performed, or else Porro's operation.

If the tumor is *submucous* and attached to the cervix, it may be possible to remove it by enucleation even after labor has begun. After labor the tumor cavity should be packed with iodoform gauze.

In *all cases* in which delivery takes place through the natural passages there is great *danger of hemorrhage* from imperfect contraction of the placental site. Should hot intra-uterine douches and hypodermics of ergot fail to control the hemorrhage, the cavity of the uterus must be packed with sterilized gauze. The gauze may be left in the cavity for one or two days, and, if necessary, it may then be renewed.

Polypi.

Mucous polyps usually spring from the cervical canal or anterior lip of the cervix, and when present may obstruct labor.

Even if small, these polypi should be **removed** at the time of labor, by transfixing and tying the pedicle, and cutting them away.

Ovarian Cysts.

These **rarely** complicate labor. If discovered during pregnancy, they should be removed. Small ovarian tumors may prolapse and cause obstruction in the pelvis.

Treatment: If the tumor be found below the brim at the time of labor, efforts should be made to push it up into the abdominal cavity. To do this it may be necessary to anæsthetize the patient and to place her in the knee-chest position. If it be impossible to reduce the tumor, it may be tapped from the vagina. This operation cannot be recommended, as it exposes the patient to the danger of peritonitis, from escape of the contents into the peritoneal cavity. It is better to perform Cæsarean section, and at the same time remove the tumor. If the cyst only partially occludes the pelvic inlet, it may be possible to effect delivery by version or forceps.

Vaginal cysts, dermoid cysts, swellings of the tubes and broad ligaments, prolapse of a floating kidney to the pelvic inlet, hydatid cysts of the pelvis, and tumors of the liver or spleen may be found to cause obstruction in labor.

Rupture of the Uterus.

Occurrence: Rupture of the uterus may take place during pregnancy, labor, or the puerperal period. In the vast majority of these cases the rupture takes place during the second stage of labor, and consists of a laceration of some portion of the uterine wall.

Frequency: This accident is said to occur about once in 4000 cases, but the writer is of the opinion that it occurs much more frequently than is generally thought, as practitioners are not prone to report these cases when they occur in private practice.

Etiology: The most frequent cause of rupture of the uterus is overdistention of the lower uterine segment, the result of *some obstruction* which prevents the descent of the presenting part of the child.

Thus pelvic deformity, overgrowth of the child, hydro-cephalus, a tumor blocking the pelvis, rigidity of the soft parts, or malpresentations, result in contractions of the uterus forcing the child's body into the lower uterine segment, which becomes enormously distended, while the upper segment, with its walls greatly thickened, is drawn up until it forms a dis-tinct tumor, which can be felt through the abdominal wall above the child.

There is usually a *well-defined line* between the thickened upper segment and the distended lower segment. This line is generally visible, as well as palpable, running obliquely across the abdomen somewhat below the umbilicus. This is the retraction-ring, or so-called " contraction-ring of Bandl." When the limit of the capacity of the lower uterine wall in stretching and thinning is reached rupture takes place.

When the *uterine wall is weakened* from any cause, such as a blow or fall during pregnancy, fatty or other degeneration, or from malignant or other disease, it may give way, even with-out much distention of the lower segment and before the membranes have ruptured.

Finally, rupture may occur during *unskilful attempts* at version, the high application of forceps, or separation of an adherent placenta.

Rupture of the uterus has been recorded as following the *administration of ergot* to hasten the expulsion of the child.

Site of the rupture : The tear usually begins in the wall of the lower uterine segment and runs transversely. When the rupture is spontaneous it usually occurs in the lateral wall. When due to traumatism the anterior wall is usually the site of the laceration.

The *extent of the tear* varies from a small rent limited to the muscular coat to complete penetration into the abdominal cavity. Usually the edges of the wound are jagged and irregular, and infiltrated with blood.

INCOMPLETE RUPTURE : When *only the muscular coat is torn*, the peritoneal covering of the uterus may be stripped off for a considerable distance beyond the tear, the sac thus formed becoming filled with blood-clot.

COMPLETE RUPTURE : The fœtus and placenta may escape

into the peritoneal cavity when the *rent is extensive,* and the intestines may prolapse into the vagina.

Symptoms: Rupture of the uterus when extensive is usually accompanied with alarming symptoms. The uterine contractions have probably been vigorous for some time, and the woman's suffering becomes extreme. Complaint is usually made of continuous and severe cramp-like pain in the lower part of the abdomen.

On *abdominal examination* the uterus will be found in a state of almost tetanic contraction with the lower segment greatly distended. The retraction-ring may be palpable, or even visible. Suddenly there is a peculiar sharp, lancinating pain, the woman gives a loud cry, and asserts that something has torn. The sound of the tear may be audible. Then follows absolute cessation of uterine action. Blood flows from the vagina, and symptoms of profound shock rapidly develop.

On making a *vaginal examination,* the presenting part will be found to have receded ; a loop of intestine may be encountered, or the hand may pass through the rent into the abdominal cavity.

When the rupture is only partial, there may be no symptoms until after the birth of the child. There may be a moderately severe hemorrhage before the placenta comes away. Uterine action is usually poor, and there may be some difficulty in expelling the placenta. The uterus tends to remain flaccid, and there may be some post-partum hemorrhage. None of these symptoms may suggest the condition actually present. The rapid development of septic peritonitis may lead to an intra-uterine examination being made within twenty-four or forty-eight hours, when a partial laceration will be discovered if the uterine cavity be carefully explored.

The author has had experience of one case in which there were *no symptoms* to indicate that rupture had taken place, beyond a somewhat severe hemorrhage with the expulsion of the placenta. On the second day of the puerperal period the patient developed a slight temperature, and on the third a severe hemorrhage took place. On making an intra-uterine examination a rent, sufficiently large to admit two fingers was found in the posterolateral wall just above the external os.

The **prognosis** depends on the site and extent of the laceration as well as upon the treatment. The maternal mortality under the best treatment runs as high as 60 per cent., while the mortality of the infants is as high as 90 per cent.

Complete rupture is much more likely to prove fatal than is partial rupture, on account of the involvement of the peritoneal cavity. More than one-half of the cases perish within twenty-four hours of the accident. The causes of death are sepsis, hemorrhage, and shock.

Treatment: When vigorous uterine contractions fail to cause advance of the presenting part, the condition of the lower uterine segment should be ascertained. When the retraction-ring of Bandl is to be felt half-way between the pubes and the umbilicus labor should be terminated as rapidly as possible, in order to guard against the occurrence of rupture. The procedure to be adopted will depend on the conditions present. Before operating the patient should be anæsthetized to the surgical degree, and if this fails to relax the uterus completely a hypodermic injection of morphine may be given.

When rupture has taken place the physician's first duty is to empty the uterus and to control hemorrhage. If the child has not escaped into the peritoneal cavity, it should be delivered rapidly by the application of forceps or by craniotomy. The placenta should then be removed manually, and the site and extent of the laceration examined.

In *incomplete laceration* it is sufficient to irrigate the cavity of the rent with a hot antiseptic solution, such as formalin (1 : 500) and to pack it gently with sterile gauze. This treatment should be repeated at intervals of from twenty-four to forty-eight hours until the rent has healed.

When the rupture is found to be *complete* the treatment depends on its site and extent. When it is small and situated low down, and but little if any foreign matter has escaped into the peritoneal cavity, the rent may be irrigated and packed with iodoform gauze. In such a case a close watch should be kept for symptoms of peritonitis ; and if such develop the abdomen should be promptly opened, the peritoneal cavity cleansed, and thorough vaginal and abdominal drainage provided.

When the rupture *is extensive* the abdomen should be promptly opened and the peritoneum cleansed of all clots and other foreign matter. If the edges of the wound are ragged and infiltrated with blood, no sutures will hold; in this case some authors recommend that the uterus be removed, while others claim excellent results from merely providing for good vaginal and abdominal drainage.

The condition of *shock*, if present, should be treated by saline injection, strychnine, digitalis, and brandy, and the application of heat to the surface of the body.

In the author's experience, limited to four cases in which treatment was possible, most excellent results followed careful irrigation and gauze packing. In two of these cases the perforations, though small, extended completely through the uterus. The hemorrhage was severe in all four cases, but could be fairly well controlled by pressing the uterus firmly down into the pelvis from above.

After the hot douche the blood ceases to flow for a short period; this time must be utilized by quickly packing the cavity of the rent with gauze, which may be guided into place along the fingers of the left hand placed in the cervix.

Great care must be exercised in removing the gauze packing, when this is necessary; it must be drawn out bit by bit, slowly and gently, in order to avoid starting a hemorrhage. The most rigid asepsis is required in the performance of each dressing of the laceration. The gauze packing should not be too firm, though sufficient should be inserted to prevent bleeding, but not so tightly packed as to prevent free drainage.

Inversion of the Uterus.

Occurrence: This accident is fortunately extremely rare. It is met with more frequently in private than in hospital practice. Inversion of the uterus may be acute or chronic. It is with the acute form the obstetrician has to deal. The inversion may be *partial* or *complete*.

In **partial inversion** the fundus may be the site of a cup-shaped depression, or it may actually prolapse sufficiently to protrude from the os.

In **complete inversion** the uterus is turned inside out, and may protrude from the vulva, appearing as a rounded mass between the patient's thighs.

Etiology: Complete inertia uteri, or uterine paralysis, at the close of the second stage of labor, is the most important predisposing cause. It may occur spontaneously, and immediately follow the birth of the child.

It has been produced by unskilful attempts at placental expulsion. *Traction on the cord,* to aid the expulsion of the placenta, has brought about inversion. When there is an actual or relative shortening of the cord it is possible that the traction on the placental site may drag down the fundus so as ultimately to produce inversion.

Symptoms: The inversion usually takes place suddenly, and is associated with severe shock, pain, and hemorrhage. Vesical and rectal tenesmus may be present. The pain is usually severe, while the hemorrhage is rarely profuse. By abdominal examination the absence of the uterine tumor will be noticed. On making an internal examination the inverted fundus will be found either protruding from the os or possibly completely filling the vagina.

Diagnosis: Inversion of the uterus can usually be diagnosed by a careful external and internal examination. The only condition from which it must be differentiated is prolapse of a uterine polypus. The most important point in distinguishing between these conditions is the presence or absence of a uterine cavity. This can usually be demonstrated or excluded satisfactorily by the introduction of a uterine sound.

Prognosis: In the acute form the mortality-rate is extremely high. Death may take place in a few hours from shock, hemorrhage, or exhaustion, or later from septicæmia.

Recovery has followed spontaneous reposition, and after separation of the inverted organ by sloughing.

Spontaneous reposition is more likely to occur when the inversion is partial than when it is complete.

Treatment: Reposition by *taxis* is the only treatment usually available. If the placenta is still attached to the uterus, it should be separated before reposition is attempted. The uterus should be douched with a hot antiseptic solution. The patient should then be anæsthetized and placed in the lithotomy position. The body of the uterus should be gently pushed back within the vulva, and the operator's hand inserted into the vagina and well back toward the sacrum, having the palm directed upward. The finger-tips then grasp the lower uterine segment and exert pressure upon it, in a direction *upward* and *forward*, toward the anterior abdominal wall, and in the axis of the pelvic inlet.

After the reposition has been completed the hand should be kept within the cavity until a contraction occurs, when it may be gently withdrawn. A hot intravaginal douche should then be given, and strychnine (gr. $\frac{1}{20}$) combined with ergotine (gr. $\frac{1}{50}$) administered hypodermically.

If efforts at immediate reposition fail, it should be attempted again within a few hours.

If it be impossible to reduce the inversion, measures should be taken to prevent the occurrence of septic infection, and the case left for operative treatment at a later date. If infection occur, the best method is vaginal hysterectomy.

PATHOLOGY OF THE PUERPERAL PERIOD.

HEMORRHAGES DURING THE PUERPERIUM.

Post-partum Hemorrhage.

Definition: Excessive loss of blood from the genital canal immediately following the birth of the placenta, or taking place within twenty-four hours of labor, is usually termed post-partum hemorrhage.

Etiology: The commonest cause of this grave accident is mismanagement of the third stage of labor. Spiegelberg has stated that severe post-partum hemorrhage is almost without exception the fault of the medical attendant. It is certain that this accident is met with much more frequently in private practice than in well-organized maternities, the reason being that in these institutions the attendants are individuals of special skill.

Uterine inertia is a frequent cause of post-partum hemorrhage. The uterus fails to retract properly after the expulsion of the placenta; hence the placental sinuses remain patent, and blood is poured out into the uterine cavity, where clots form, which acting as a foreign body may stimulate contractions. These contractions are usually weak and inefficient, while the intra-uterine clots are more or less firmly attached to the walls, and hence difficult to dislodge. In the intervals between the contractions more blood is poured out, until finally by this process the uterus may become distended to its full capacity. The external hemorrhage may be insignificant in amount, though it is usually greatly in excess of the normal.

Other conditions which predispose to hemorrhage are: precipitate labor; overdistention of the uterus, as in hydramnios, twin pregnancy, etc.; a distended bladder or rectum; the retention of small portions of the placenta or membranes; tumors and other new growths in the uterus; and exhaustion following a prolonged and difficult labor.

Certain *constitutional conditions* predispose to this accident, as nephritis, extreme anæmia, and hæmophilia.

Severe post-partum hemorrhage may result from *lacerations* in the lower part of the birth-canal. Lacerations of the cervix involving the circular artery, or of the vulva involving one of the bulbs of the vestibule, may occasion severe hemorrhage.

Symptoms: The hemorrhage may occur with or after the expulsion of the placenta. It may be an abrupt, sharp hemorrhage, or simply steady dribbling which by its persistence results in an extensive loss of blood. The bleeding may be external, internal, or both.

The *pulse* is the most certain indicator of the severity of the hemorrhage. If after delivery the pulse-rate shows a tendency to become more rapid, the possibility of hemorrhage must be borne in mind. It is a good rule not to leave a patient whose pulse-rate is 100 or more to the minute till all possibility of the occurrence of hemorrhage has passed.

In a *severe case* symptoms indicative of extensive blood-loss rapidly develop. The pulse becomes rapid and thready; respiration is shallow, rapid, and sighing; the patient becomes restless in her movements, tossing herself about and calling for air. She may complain of thirst. Her skin becomes cold and covered with a clammy sweat. If the hemorrhage continues, syncope, convulsions, and death bring the painful scene to a close.

The **diagnosis** is seldom difficult, though in conditions of severe shock occurring immediately after labor all the symptoms of severe hemorrhage may be present, except evident loss of blood and a relaxed uterus.

The blanched face, clammy skin, rapid, thready pulse, and sighing respiration, all indicate hemorrhage; though the external loss of blood may have been out of all proportion to the symptoms present. On palpation of the abdomen the hard globular uterus will be missed from its usual location half-way between the umbilicus and symphysis, and the soft, boggy fundus may be found reaching almost up to the ensiform cartilage.

In cases in which the hemorrhage arises from lacerations of the lower part of the birth-canal the fundus will be found in its usual position, firmly contracted, in spite of the fact that blood is escaping from the vulva. An internal examination by means of a speculum, if necessary, will reveal the bleeding point.

Prognosis: These cases rarely terminate fatally when skilled assistance is at hand. The greater the loss of blood the graver is the prognosis. The most unfavorable cases are those in which the blood lost is thin and watery, and fails to clot properly, as this is indicative of a blood dyscrasia.

Treatment of Post-partum Hemorrhage.

This accident can usually be **prevented** by the proper management of the third stage of labor. The directions given for the management of the third stage of labor constitute an outline of the preventive treatment of post-partum hemorrhage.

The **prompt, energetic treatment** of a case of post-partum hemorrhage calls for self-control, readiness in resource, and presence of mind on the part of the physician. His object is to secure good, firm contraction of the uterus. It is well to have clearly in mind a routine treatment to secure this object.

The first thing to be done is to **stimulate the uterus** to action by making vigorous friction over the fundus, through the abdominal wall. As the organ becomes outlined on contracting, pressure may be exerted in the manner recommended for the expulsion of the placenta. Such compression may lead to the expulsion of clots from the genital canal, and further hemorrhage may cease. If this fortunate result does not follow, the free hand should be inserted into the vagina and passed into the uterus, and adherent clots may be loosened and broken up by scraping the walls with the finger-tips. The uterus should then be rubbed and kneaded between the external and internal hands, so as to stimulate contractions. As soon as contraction has been secured the internal hand should be withdrawn and an intra-uterine douche of hot sterilized water should be given. To be effectual, the water should be between 115° and 125° F., and at least a gallon should be employed. A fountain-douche should be used, and the nozzle, either of glass or metal, should be carried to the fundus. While the douche is being given the fundus should be kneaded through the abdominal wall.

If the hemorrhage is not checked by this means, then the uterine cavity must be **tamponed with strips of sterile gauze** fastened end to end.

The **technique** of this procedure is very simple. The anterior lip of the cervix is seized with a tenaculum-forceps and drawn down to the vulva. The end of a strip of gauze is then seized by means of a pair of uterine dressing-forceps and guided to the fundus; then the whole cavity is firmly packed. It is not necessary to pack the vagina as well, but after removing the tenaculum from the cervix a strip of gauze may be placed in the upper part of the vagina to keep the cervix in place. The gauze may be left in place from twenty-four to forty-eight hours and then gently removed. It is seldom necessary to repeat the intra-uterine packing.

As soon as the uterus has been **emptied of clots** a hypodermic of ergot (aseptic, Parke, Davis & Co.), ʒss, should be given, and repeated in half an hour if required.

Having checked the hemorrhage, the physician's duty is then to combat the evil effects of severe loss of blood.

Treatment of Acute Anæmia.

The pillows should be removed from beneath the patient's head and the **foot of the bed raised** on some books or bricks.

Hot-water bottles should be applied to the extremities of the patient, and she should be covered with warm blankets. If there is a tendency to syncope, a hypodermic injection of strychnine nitrate (gr. $\frac{1}{30}$) and nitroglycerin (gr. $\frac{1}{100}$) should be given.

As soon as possible a quart of water at 110° F., containing two teaspoonfuls of common salt, should be **injected into** the rectum. For this purpose a soft-rubber catheter should be attached to the nozzle of a fountain-syringe, so that the injection may be carried as far up as possible.

If the heart's action fails to improve, **hypodermic injections** of ether, strychnin, and nitroglycerin may be employed.

Nausea and **vomiting** are frequent in these cases, and there is but little absorption from the stomach until these cease. As soon as the stomach will retain anything, small quantities of hot coffee, hot brandy and water, or warm milk may be given and frequently repeated. When reaction has been established a hypodermic of morphine (gr. $\frac{1}{8}$) should be given to quiet the patient.

In **desperate cases** the saline solution may be sterilized, and injected beneath the breasts or directly into the median basilic vein :

To **insert the salt solution** beneath the breasts a large exploring-needle may be used. A glass funnel and a piece of rubber tubing complete the apparatus. These should be sterilized after being fitted together for use. The breasts are then washed with soap and hot water, and rubbed with alcohol. Having filled the funnel, the physician grasps the breast firmly with one hand, lifts it from the chest-wall, and with the other hand the needle (with the solution flowing from it) is plunged boldly into the loose tissue beneath the breast. Care should be taken to prevent the entrance of air.

Intravenous injection is seldom used on account of the time required to perform the operation, and because the methods before given answer the purpose just as well. For the method of operation the reader is referred to works on surgery.

Convalescence in these cases is slow and tedious. The patient should not be allowed to sit upright for two or three weeks. The diet should consist largely of fluids, and iron in some form should be administered.

Puerperal or Secondary Hemorrhage.

Definition: This term is used to denote hemorrhage from the genital canal of a woman occurring at any time after the first twenty-four hours to the end of the puerperium.

Etiology: The most frequent cause of secondary hemorrhage during the puerperium is the retention of portions of placenta and membranes. Clots in the uterine cavity or the dislodgement of clots in the placental site, displacements of the uterus, relaxation of the uterus, fibroids, polypi, partial rupture, the separation of a slough, and overdistention of the bladder or rectum may be mentioned as giving rise to puerperal hemorrhage. Sudden emotion or constitutional causes may result in hemorrhage during the puerperium.

Diagnosis: Having the causes in mind, it is the duty of the physician to make a careful external and internal examination in all cases of secondary hemorrhage. The diagnosis should rarely prove difficult.

The **treatment** depends on the cause of the hemorrhage. After emptying the bladder the cavity of the uterus should be explored. Fragments of placenta and membranes or clots should be removed and a hot intra-uterine douche given. If the cause is found to be other than those just mentioned, appropriate treatment should be inaugurated.

Hæmatoma.

Definition: In this form of hemorrhage the effusion of blood is interstitial. The result of this accident is the formation of a tumor varying in size with the degree of the hemorrhage. The most frequent situation of hæmatoma is in one or other labium, rarely in both. It may occur in any portion of the genital canal outside of the uterus.

Etiology: A varicose and congested condition of the pelvic veins predispose to the occurrence of this accident. The determining cause is usually direct injury of the tissues from pressure of the fœtal head or from forceps. Forcing or straining on the part of the woman may lead to the rupture of an engorged vein, and so give rise to the condition. It may occur before or after the completion of labor.

21—Obst.

Treatment: If possible, the absorption of the effused blood should be encouraged. Care should be taken to avoid its manipulation in performing the toilet of the vulva. Frequent gentle irrigation with warm, mild antiseptic solutions may be employed. If absorption is delayed, the tumor should be incised, the contents turned out, and the cavity packed with iodoform gauze. If on incising the tumor a bleeding vessel is found, it should be tied before packing the cavity. Frequent dressing and rigid asepsis are necessary to prevent the occurrence of infection.

SUBINVOLUTION.

Definition: When the process of involution of the puerperal uterus is arrested or retarded the organ is said to be in a condition of subinvolution.

Etiology.

Any condition which prevents a rapid *diminution in the blood-supply* of the puerperal uterus may be said to be a cause of subinvolution. Any condition which *interferes with contractions* of the muscular tissues of the puerperal uterus tends to give rise to subinvolution.

The following conditions which tend to **interfere with the diminution of the blood-supply** of the puerperal uterus may be mentioned as giving rise to subinvolution: hyperplasia of the endometrium, the result of local congestion or of mild septic infection; laceration of the cervix; small fibroids; metritis, generally septic in origin; retention of secundines or clots; uterine displacements; chronic constipation; and the resumption of the ordinary duties of life too soon after abortion or labor.

Conditions giving rise to subinvolution by **interfering with uterine contractions** are: the retention of large clots or fragments of the placenta, or placentæ succenturiatæ; displacement of the uterus from overdistention of the bladder; large intramural fibroids; and peritoneal adhesions from old or recent inflammatory attacks.

Subinvolution is practically always the **result** of some *local disorder*. *Constitutional disturbances* very exceptionally give rise to the condition, though in women with general lack of tone, with flabby muscles and diminished eliminative powers, subinvolution may occur without any evidence of a distinct local cause.

Diagnosis of Subinvolution.

The diagnosis is usually easy.

By the **tenth day** of the puerperal period the fundus uteri should be on a level with or a little below the brim of the pelvis. Later, if the condition is suspected, the depth of the uterus may be measured by means of the intra-uterine sound.

The **lochia**, instead of becoming pale and puriform, remains bloody and its discharge is prolonged. The condition is usually associated with constipation and a coated tongue.

Ahlfeld has drawn attention to the fact that free perspiration during the puerperium is usually associated with firm uterine contractions; when **perspiration fails** to appear he always looks for uterine relaxation.

Treatment of Subinvolution.

In the **earlier period** of the puerperium the uterus may be stimulated to contraction by gentle friction of the fundus through the abdominal wall for ten minutes or so, three or four times daily. A pill containing ergotin, gr. j; quinine, gr. j; and strychnine, gr. $\frac{1}{30}$, may be given three times daily.

Should this treatment fail to improve matters and there is no diminution in the loss of blood, the **cavity of the uterus should be explored** with the finger. If necessary, the curette and placental forceps may be used, being followed by a douche of hot formalin solution (1 : 500), and the introduction of a wick of gauze to the fundus. The latter acts by stimulating the uterus to contraction and by favoring drainage. The gauze should be removed at the end of forty-eight hours and a hot vaginal douche once or twice daily may be ordered. Daily free evacuation of the bowels should be secured.

If the uterus be **displaced**, it should be put in proper position and retained there by means of a pessary.

Occasionally the condition of subinvolution is not discovered until **late in the puerperal period**, after the woman has been walking about for some time. In such cases the cavity of the uterus should be painted with Churchill's solution of iodine, and a vaginal tampon of wool saturated with boroglycerin should be inserted two or three times a week.

ANOMALIES AND DISEASES OF THE NIPPLES AND BREASTS.

Anomalies of the Nipples.

Supernumerary nipples are of frequent occurrence.

Defects of the nipples are chiefly important as they may interfere with nursing.

Inversion of the nipple is a very common condition, which may be congenital or acquired. This defect may constitute an absolute impediment to lactation.

During the last month of pregnancy attempts should be made to draw out the nipples by means of a breast-pump. When the nipples are small or imperfectly developed daily gentle traction upon them by the nurse or physician may result in improvement. If this fails, a nipple-shield must be employed to enable the child to nurse.

Anomalies of the Breasts.

Absence of mammæ: While imperfect development of the mammæ is common, their complete absence is a very rare condition. It is usually associated with deformities of the pelvic sexual organs.

Hypertrophy of the mammæ: This condition is also rare. When present it does not of necessity contraindicate nursing.

Supernumerary mammæ: Supernumerary breasts are to be met with comparatively frequently. They occur with no regularity of situation; the most frequent position is below the true mammæ; they have been found over the pubes, on the buttocks, shoulders, and in the axillæ. In most cases no hereditary influence can be traced.

Anomalies in Milk Secretion.

Deficient Secretion.

Complete absence of milk-secretion is a rare condition; but *deficient milk-secretion* is only too frequently encountered.

Etiology: *Lack of development* of the glandular tissue of the breasts is the most common cause of deficient secretion of milk. This lack of development may be due to hereditary causes, or to continuous pressure from tight clothing; or it may be associated with maldevelopment of the other sexual organs of the body.

The *size of the breasts* is no indication of their ability to furnish milk. This function depends entirely upon the amount of glandular tissue present in the breasts. Some women with well-developed breasts have but little glandular tissue, and therefore make poor nurses; while others with apparently but poor development of these organs have a rich and abundant supply of milk for their offspring.

The secretion of milk may be diminished by the occurrence of fever, hemorrhages, chronic diarrhœa, and insufficient nourishment; serious organic diseases also result in diminished milk-secretion. Emotions profoundly affect the secretion of milk; prolonged grief is a well-known cause of deficient secretion.

The *return of menstruation,* while it may affect the quantity and quality of the milk secreted, cannot be said invariably to produce this result. It may be stated that, as a rule, the return of this function has but little influence on milk-secretion.

Treatment: But little can be suggested in the way of treatment; good, plain food and plenty of it; moderate exercise in the open air; three or four glasses of milk daily between meals, and a wineglassful of extract of malt thrice daily, constitute about all the treatment possible. There is no medicinal galactagogue of any value in the experience of the writer.

Excessive Secretion—Polygalactia.

In this condition, which is not infrequently met with, the secretion of milk is **in excess** of the demands of the child.

Treatment: The bowels should be kept relaxed and the quantity of fluids imbibed reduced. The breasts may be compressed by means of a tightly fitting breast-binder. The woman should take plenty of hard exercise daily in the open air. If this treatment fails, the excess of milk must be pumped out at regular intervals.

Galactorrhœa.

This term is applied to an **excessive secretion** of milk which persists after weaning. The flow of milk is not necessarily excited by suckling the child. The milk is thin and watery, the *quantity* being excessive. One or more breasts may be affected, and the condition seriously impair the general health. The condition may last for years.

Etiology : Nothing definite is known as to the causation of this condition. It has been attributed to a relaxation or paralysis of the circular muscular fibres surrounding the milk-ducts.

Treatment : These cases frequently offer very stubborn resistance to all treatment. Firm compression of the breasts by means of a breast-binder and the administration of potassium iodide (gr. x t. i. d.) and of fl. ext. ergot (℞ x). for a considerable period constitute the usual treatment. General tonics and iron should be administered.

Engorgement of the Breasts.

Etiology : Reference has already been made to the fact that occasionally with the establishment of lactation the breasts may become congested and engorged. This condition of engorgement may occur at any time throughout the period of lactation. Exposure of the breasts to cold air and hypersecretion of milk are the most common causes of this condition.

Symptoms : The breasts quite suddenly become engorged with milk, to such an extent as to occasion very considerable distress to the patient. The pain and tenderness may be the occasion of more or less elevation of temperature.

Treatment.

To relieve the patient it is necessary to remove the excessive amount of milk and to prevent further engorgement of the breasts. The breasts may be emptied by permitting the infant *to nurse;* by the *breast-pump;* and by *massage.*

If the child fails to empty the breasts, the milk remaining

may be drawn off by means of the **breast-pump.** Probably the most satisfactory breast-pump is that known as the " English " pump. That part of the pump which is applied to the breasts should be free from jagged, rough edges, otherwise these may produce some abrasions.

Massage of the breasts: When properly performed this is a very efficient aid in relieving congestion and engorgement. It should never be employed if there is evidence of interstitial inflammation of the breasts.

The patient, being in the dorsal position, is directed to support her breast by placing her forearm under it and drawing it up. The breast is then anointed, with warm oil, after which the operator begins the manipulations by placing his finger-tips, separated as widely as possible, at the periphery of the breast. A rapid though gentle stroking movement is then made toward the nipple, the finger-tips being brought gradually together so as to meet at the termination of the stroke. Each segment of the gland is thus rapidly stroked in succession, each movement terminating at the nipple. The pressure exerted by the finger-tips should be gradually increased, short of producing severe pain. This stroking movement in about five minutes usually ceases to cause pain. Then the operator supporting the breast in the palm of one hand, with the finger-tips of the other hand selects a *nodule* of induration, which he strokes toward the nipple, gradually employing deeper and firmer pressure. Each nodule of induration is thus treated in succession.

Nodules which this manipulation fails to soften may then be compressed by placing the hand flat upon them and exerting steady gentle pressure downward against the chest-wall. The pressure thus exerted should be greatest at the periphery of the gland. After a few moments of steady pressure, gentle rotary movements of the hand may be made over the lumps. If pain is complained of, the stroking movements should be resumed.

The breast should then be grasped with both hands so as to encircle it completely ; and the whole gland gently raised and compressed, while the two index-fingers are quickly stroked toward the nipple to favor the escape of milk. These various manipulations should be repeated at short intervals until the

328 PATHOLOGY OF THE PUERPERAL PERIOD.

glands have been softened and emptied of their contents, when a pressure-bandage should be applied.

The most satisfactory **breast-bandage**, in the opinion of the writer, is the Y-bandage, which was first employed in the Boston Lying-in Hospital. This may be made of two pieces of soft, unbleached cotton or bird's eye towelling, about thirty-six inches long and ten or twelve inches wide. I have used ordinary hand towels for this purpose, and find they answer admirably. These are folded into strips about three or four inches wide; one of these is folded end to end, and the doubled end turned over so as to convert the strip into an L-shape, when the free ends are separated. The apex of this strip is then pinned with three or four safety-pins to one end of the other strip, so as to form the Y-bandage.

The breasts are then *dusted* with powdered starch or other dusting-powder, and the longer arm of the bandage slipped under the patient's back at the lower part of the scapular region until the apex of the fork is just external to the outer edge of the left breast. The patient then lifts her breasts upward and toward each other, while the lower arm of the fork is drawn tightly across the chest beneath the breasts; the inferior border of this arm should extend at least an inch below the lower margins of the breasts.

The upper arm of the fork is then drawn across the chest above the breasts in such a way that its upper border extends an inch beyond the upper margins of the breasts. The free ends of the two arms of the fork should thus meet at the outer margin of the right breast, where they should then be drawn tight and securely pinned with safety-pins to the strip which has been passed beneath the back. The free end of the back strip may then lie over the apices of both breasts. The strip passing underneath the breasts is then pinned to the binder to keep it from slipping up; shoulder-straps may then be pinned to the upper arm of the fork and fastened behind to the back strips, thus keeping the upper arm of the fork from slipping down. The hollow between the breasts may then be filled with cotton, and this held in place by two safety-pins joined together and pinned to the upper and lower arms of the fork.

In place of this the **Murphy binder** may be employed. It is made of a strip of thick gray cotton, forty inches long and ten inches wide. In the upper border of this strip a narrow notch is cut for the neck and two deep notches for the arms. The binder is applied tightly over the breasts and pinned in front. When it is desired to make applications to the nipples, two circular holes the size of a silver half dollar can be cut in the Murphy binder; the margins of these holes should be button-hole stitched.

In cases in which the engorgement is intense and the breasts so sensitive that manipulation is impossible much relief can be given by the application of **hot compresses**. Flannel soaked in hot water and carbonate of ammonium (ℨj to the pint), wrung dry, and then applied to the breasts, and repeated at intervals of five minutes, soon gives relief and permits the application of the breast-binder.

In these cases a *free action of the bowels* should be obtained by the administration of teaspoonful doses of Rochelle salt in warm water, at intervals of fifteen minutes till purgation is induced.

Sore Nipples.

Etiology and symptoms: The child in nursing may macer-ate the superficial epithelium of the nipples. Small superficial ulcers may thus be formed at the apices or at the bases of the nipples, which are difficult to heal because the child in nursing separates their edges. The pain caused by this condition varies between simple tenderness at the moment the child seizes the nipple, and the acutest agony during the whole act of suckling. Erosion of the nipples occurs most frequently in primiparæ.

Treatment.

Prophylactic treatment should be begun toward the end of pregnancy, as has been mentioned. Close attention to cleans-ing of the nipples and of the child's mouth is of supreme im-portance. After nursing, the nipples should be washed with boric-acid lotion and carefully dried. At least once a day the child's mouth should be swabbed with pledgets of cotton soaked in glycerinum boracis.

Painting the nipples, by means of a camel's-hair brush, with the compound tincture of benzoin, or a 10 grain to the ounce solution of silver nitrate, will be found very satisfactory treatment in more severe cases. Deep fissures are best treated by daily touching them carefully with the solid stick of nitrate of silver.

In some cases extreme tenderness of the nipples may be complained of, and yet the most careful examination fail to reveal any trace of either erosion or fissure. In these cases extract of witch-hazel (ext. hamamelidis) will be found very useful; it may be employed pure or diluted with two or three parts of boiled water.

A very satisfactory ointment for eroded nipples is the following:

R̥. Argyrol,   gr. l;
　　Bals. Peru.,   ʒj;
　　Lanolini,   ʒiij;
　　Vaselin,   ad ʒj.
Sig. Apply after nursing and cover with waxed paper.

In all cases in which the nipples are tender a glass and rubber **nipple-shield** should be employed while nursing. The shield should be kept surgically clean.

In some cases it may be necessary for the mother not even to attempt to nurse the child for twenty-four hours, or even longer. In these cases the breasts may be emptied by means of **massage,** the breast-pump not being used unless it prove absolutely necessary.

In very exceptional cases nothing but **weaning** will result in permanently relieving the condition.

Inflammation of the Breasts—Mastitis.

Varieties: Three forms of mastitis are usually described: the most frequent variety is the *parenchymatous,* or *glandular,* in which the acini of the gland are primarily the site of the inflammation. In the *subcutaneous* variety the connective tissue immediately beneath the skin is attacked. In the *subglandular* or *post-mammary* form the connective tissue between the gland and the chest-wall is the site of the inflammation.

The inflammation is but rarely confined to one of these localities, so that clinically two or all three may be combined, especially in cases which do not receive prompt treatment. Usually mastitis begins in the acini of the gland, whence it spreads to the connective tissue and approaches the skin surface.

Frequency: Mastitis occurs in about 6 per cent. of all nursing women, though it is most frequently met with in primiparæ. It may terminate by resolution or by suppuration.

Etiology: All forms of mastitis are of *microbic origin.* The infection is usually due to the entrance of staphylococci, either the aureus or albus, though streptococci or other pus-producing organisms may give rise to the condition.

The infection usually *arises* in a fissure or abrasion of the nipple, and spreads either by means of the *lymph-channels* into the connective tissue; or directly along the *epithelium of a duct* to an acinus, possibly to several. The inflammation may at first be confined to the epithelium, but soon spreads to the surrounding connective tissue. Impaired general health and local mechanical injuries are important predisposing causes.

Milk stasis was at one time thought to be the cause of mastitis, but pathologists have proved that stasis alone will not produce the condition. It is possible that stasis of milk results in impairment of the epithelium of the ducts and thus renders infection more liable to occur.

A possible source of infection is the *blood*. Escherich states that staphylococci which have gained access to the blood through infection of the genital canal are excreted in the milk.

Symptoms of Mastitis.

All forms of mastitis are accompanied by the signs of inflammation.

The **onset** of the inflammation is generally characterized by a distinct chill or by a sense of chilliness. The temperature begins to rise and the patient complains of pain and tenderness in the affected breast.

In the **parenchymatous** form one or more tender nodules will be found in the affected breast. The skin overlying these nodules may or may not be reddened. Pressure on these nodules usually produces a sharp, cutting pain.   The temperature may rise to 104° F., or even higher.

In the low **interstitial** form the pain is not so distinctly localized and no nodule can be felt in the breast.   The temperature rises more gradually and chilly sensations are more frequent than a distinct rigor.   The skin over the affected area quickly becomes reddened, and it will be frequently noticed that the site of the inflammation corresponds to a fissure in the nipple. This form of inflammation is very difficult to abort and usually results in abscess formation, though if the breast be opened early but very little pus may be found.

Treatment of Mastitis.

Abortive : The indications are to secure complete rest for the affected gland by (*a*) absolutely prohibiting nursing from either breast; (*b*) removing by means of massage and the breast-pump the contents of the glands, and (*c*) reducing the local blood-supply.

It is important to decide if possible whether the **inflammation** is of the parenchymatous or of the interstitial form.   The mode of onset, condition of the nipple, appearance and feel of the breast, and the fact that the parenchymatous form occurs most frequently, will afford assistance in making a diagnosis.

If the type of inflammation present is **parenchymatous,** the routine of treatment may be given as follows : the breasts are emptied by means of *massage* and the breast-pump, all manipulations being as gently carried out as possible.   The nipples are then cleansed and an antiseptic dressing applied, as previously recommended.   A tightly fitting Murphy binder is then applied so as to secure as firm compression of both breasts as is possible, without increasing the pain in the affected parts. Then an ice-bag may be placed outside the binder over the affected portion of the gland.   The ice-bag should be kept constantly applied for from twelve to twenty-four hours, the length of time being determined by the relief of pain and subsidence of temperature.

The lessening of the local blood-supply of the gland may be obtained by the derivative action of saline cathartics, which should be freely administered as previously recommended.

If **after twenty-four hours** the temperature has dropped and the pain disappeared, the pressure on the breasts may be reduced by loosening the binder somewhat. The ice-bag may then be removed for an hour or two, but should be used intermittently till all tenderness of the breast disappears and the flow of milk has been re-established. In rare instances the ice-bag is not well borne by the patient, in which case a compress wrung out of a solution of lead and opium (1 : 40) should be applied over the affected portion of the gland and covered with oiled silk or a layer of non-absorbent cotton, over which the Murphy binder may be lightly applied.

The treatment of the **interstitial form** of mastitis differs somewhat from the preceding. In this form massage should be avoided, as only tending to aggravate the condition. The Murphy binder should be applied so as merely to support the breasts, but not to compress them ; otherwise the treatment of the two forms is the same. In spite of all treatment a large proportion of these cases terminate in abscess formation.

Mammary Abscess.

The pus may be **located** in the gland-substance or in the submammary connective tissue.

Symptoms: It is not always possible to be certain that suppuration has taken place from the symptoms given. Fluctuation, the most certain sign of abscess formation, is rarely to be found until late.

Severe throbbing or stabbing pain suggests abscess formation, especially when accompanied with chilly sensations, a higher grade of temperature, and greater rapidity of pulse. Usually a bluish discoloration and some œdema of the skin mark the locality where the abscess will " point," especially in the more common parenchymatous form.

In the *interstitial form* the pus tends to burrow extensively, and no actual abscess may be discernible though the whole gland is found to be riddled with pus-tracts. If such a case be left too long, the pus will be found " pointing " in several places.

Surgical Treatment.

Preliminary: The patient should always be anæsthetized before attempting to open or treat a mammary abscess, unless it be superficial and about to point.   The whole breast should be well scrubbed with soap and hot water, followed by solutions of permanganate of potassium and oxalic acid.

Incision: By careful palpation the pus collection is located, and an incision is then made in the skin over its most dependent portion in a line radiating from the nipple.   Through this opening a grooved director is then inserted and passed in all directions until pus is encountered, when a pair of artery-forceps is introduced and opened so as to dilate the tissues sufficiently to permit the introduction of a finger into the abscess-cavity.   All, adjacent cavities should then be searched for and freely opened, and all friable tissue broken down.   Additional openings should be made to secure free drainage.   The walls of the abscess-cavity should be gently scraped with a Volkmann spoon.   All the openings should then be irrigated freely with an antiseptic solution, such as formalin, 1 : 500.

Drainage: Instead of employing rubber tubes for drainage, gutta-percha tissue which has been sterilized by soaking in formalin solution, and then folded in strips about half an inch wide and six or eight inches long, will be found much more serviceable.   Several of these strips should be drawn through the openings, so as to secure drainage in all directions.   An antiseptic surgical dressing is then applied, and the breast firmly bandaged with a broad roller bandage, so as to secure even compression throughout, or a Murphy bandage may be applied.

After twenty-four or thirty-six hours the dressings should be removed and the abscess-cavity thoroughly irrigated with boric-acid or formalin solution.   The gutta-percha tissue drains should be reinserted and a fresh dressing applied.   As soon as the discharge has almost ceased, the gutta-percha tissue drainage may be dispensed with and firm compression of the walls of the cavity secured by means of antiseptic compresses placed under the bandage or binder.   The most equable pressure is secured by means of a large bath-sponge which has been boiled and then wrung out of 1 : 5000 bichloride solution.   This should be slightly hollowed out so as to fit over the breast, to which it is directly applied and covered with oiled silk and the bandage or binder.   This dressing should be removed daily and the sponge cleansed in a solution of 1 : 5000 bichloride. The breast should also be washed with the same solution before the dressing is reapplied.

Nursing: The child may be applied to the sound breast to keep up the flow of milk, provided the mother's general health is such that it is not desirable to discontinue nursing.

In the **interstitial form** of abscess but very little pus may be found on incising the breast. All nodules should be opened, as the pus tends to burrow very extensively in this form, and special care should therefore be given to providing for free drainage.

Abscesses of the areola: The glands of Montgomery may become infected and result in the formation of small superficial abscesses in the areola.

Treatment: Each suppurating gland should be opened, and its walls curetted and then swabbed with strong bichloride or formalin solution.

Galactocele: This is a milk tumor which may form as the result of occlusion of one of the lactiferous ducts. Beyond causing a little pain these milk tumors are of no importance.

Treatment: Massage may result in causing the milk to flow and thus relieve the condition. Rarely these tumors persist for a long time, and may become so large as to necessitate their being tapped and drained.

Arrest of Lactation.

Indications: When the child has perished at birth or when the constitutional condition of the mother is such as to preclude the possibility of nursing, it is necessary to prevent the activity of the mammary glands.

Method: Before the first appearance of breast engorgement a tightly fitting *Murphy binder* should be applied. *Free purgation* should be induced by means of salines when the patient's strength will permit. The amount of fluids ingested should be restricted, the patient's thirst being relieved by rinsing the mouth frequently with weak tea.

If the engorgement of the breasts tends to *become excessive,* the binder may be removed once or twice daily to permit of *massage* or the use of the *breast-pump.* The breasts may then be covered with glycerite of belladonna and the binder or bandage reapplied. Usually under this treatment the breasts become inactive in less than a week.

To arrest lactation when the woman *has been nursing* for some time, firm compression of the breasts by means of the Y-binder combined with the use of salines will be sufficient. The milk usually flows away readily under the compression exerted by the Y-binder, and there is no disposition of the breasts to become engorged and caked.

Massage and the use of the pump should be omitted as long as the milk flows away freely. In a few days the breasts will cease flowing, when a Murphy binder may be applied and worn till the breasts become soft.

After prolonged lactation there is but little difficulty in drawing away the milk when the child is weaned gradually. Should secretion persist it may be necessary to employ compression and to give atropine internally.

INTERCURRENT DISEASES IN THE PUERPERIUM.

Miscellaneous Diseases.

Scarlet fever : This is a rare complication of the puerperium. It almost always appears within three days of labor; the throat complications are slight, the rash appears quickly, is rapidly diffused, and is usually of an intense dark-red color. Convalescence is usually tedious. Occasionally the pelvic organs are profoundly affected by this disease, and when this is the case the prognosis is very grave.

When the attack is a frank one and the genitalia are not much involved the *prognosis* is not unfavorable, though the condition is a grave one.

Measles : The puerperium is rarely complicated by this disease unless the attack has occurred during pregnancy and has led to premature expulsion of the ovum. The condition predisposes to hemorrhage and also to pneumonia.

Variola: This is a very grave complication of the puerperium.

Rotheln: This disease does not markedly affect the puerperium. In two or three cases which have come under my notice the disease was very mild in character, though in one the rash was very marked.

Erysipelas: This disease usually affects the genitals when it occurs during the puerperal period. It is seldom manifested by a cutaneous eruption. When the genitals only are affected the prognosis is very grave, and it is impossible to distinguish the case from one of ordinary streptococcus infection.

Erythematous rashes: Puerperal erythema is not an infrequent condition.

In *simple cases* there is apt to be a moderate elevation of temperature, and the lochia may become offensive. There may be some uterine or pelvic tenderness. The condition is therefore looked upon as a mild septic infection.

Erythema may be mistaken for scarlet fever, and it is not infrequently associated with grave septicæmia.

Diphtheria: This disease may affect the throat or the genitals, in the latter case a variety of general sepsis ensues.

Pneumonia: This disease constitutes a very grave complication of the puerperium. It not infrequently occurs secondary to septic infection. Its treatment will be discussed in the section on puerperal infection.

Rheumatism; arthritis: The diagnosis between septic arthritis and simple acute rheumatism is a matter of great difficulty during the puerperium. Simple rheumatism tends to affect several joints, while the arthritis is septic in origin and usually only one large joint is affected. In the latter case there may be little evidence of general septic infection. Simple rheumatism usually runs its ordinary course and does not affect the puerperium, nor is it affected greatly by it.

The *treatment* of acute rheumatism is the same as when it occurs at any other time. In *septic arthritis* recovery is the rule, but with a greatly damaged joint. Local treatment only is of service, general medication being of little use.

Malaria.

The puerperal state, it is generally admitted, **predisposes** to malarial attacks. Women who are subject to malaria usually manifest the disease after delivery, probably as a result of the traumatism of labor.

The **malarial attack** is usually of a mild type, but occasionally it may be extremely severe. The disease, which usually manifests itself about the third day after delivery, predisposes to puerperal hemorrhage; it also modifies milk secretion, especially during the exacerbation of fever. It is not generally admitted that the germs of disease can be transmitted in the milk to the nursing infant.

Diagnosis: Malaria occurring during the puerperium must be differentiated from septic infection or typhoid fever. The diagnosis is occasionally a matter of considerable difficulty. The fever in malaria is frequently continuous at first, but soon becomes remittent in type.

In doubtful cases the *blood should be examined* for malarial organisms, and Widal's test for typhoid reaction should be applied. A bacteriological examination of the uterine lochia should also be made, for it is quite possible that malarial poisoning may be associated with septic infection in some cases. With these tests at one's disposal we should not remain long in doubt as to the origin of the fever in any given case.

Treatment: Usually it is necessary to give large doses of quinine to control the fever during the puerperium. When the daily dose of quinine is 20 grains or under, it is seldom necessary to remove the child from the breast; but when this dose is exceeded the infant is likely to suffer from the effects.

Puerperal Anæmia.

After delivery the blood begins to undergo a change in constitution by which it is converted from the hydræmia of pregnancy to the normal proportion of its constituent parts in the non-gravid condition.

This change is usually completed by the end of the second week of the puerperal period.

Many causes may interfere with this process of involution

of the blood, such as sepsis, severe blood-loss at the time of labor, or any wasting or depressing disease. In such cases the anæmia tends to assume a pernicious form if treatment is neglected.

Careful **blood examinations** should be made from time to time in these cases in order to judge of the effect of treatment.

The **treatment** consists in the administration of tonic drugs and careful feeding. Iron and arsenic, in the form of the compound Blaud pill, usually give satisfactory results. In some cases in which iron is not well borne arsenic alone will succeed.

Hemorrhoids.

Great discomfort is frequently caused by an attack of hemorrhoids during the earlier days of the puerperal period.

Treatment: The bowels should be freely opened, and great relief may be obtained by the application of hot compresses wrung out of hot lead-and-opium solution (1:40). In some cases the application of ice is more comforting to the patient. An ointment composed of equal parts of ung. gallæ cum opio, ung. stramon. and ung. bellad. will further relieve pain.

Diseases of the Urinary Organs.

Retention of urine: Patients not infrequently complain of inability to urinate after delivery. The condition may be the result of injury to the urethra or the anterior vaginal wall during labor. Many women are unable to empty the bladder while lying in bed. In others the flow of the urine over small abrasions of the vulva sets up irritation, which they seek to avoid by holding the urine as long as possible. The relaxed condition of the abdominal walls and the consequent diminution of intra-abdominal pressure to some extent interfere with the function of micturition during this period.

Treatment: The nurse should be instructed to see that the patient empties the bladder at least twice daily. For this purpose, if unable to pass water otherwise, the patient may assume a kneeling posture, or may be raised carefully so as to be able to sit on the bed-pan. Hot applications may prove of assistance, as may also the stimulus caused by the sound of running water.   If these means fail, the nurse should be instructed to pass the catheter into the bladder, and to observe the strictest antiseptic precautions in so doing.

Incontinence of urine: This condition may result from over-distention of the bladder from retention of urine.   This is the commonest cause.   Other causes of the condition are paresis of the sphincter muscle and vesicovaginal or vesico-uterine fistula.

A *careful examination* will reveal the cause of the condition. The *treatment* must vary with the cause of the incontinence.

Cystitis: This is unfortunately a common complication of the puerperal state.   It is usually due either to injury from overdistention of the bladder or to careless catheterization.

Symptoms: Frequent micturition, associated with burning and tenesmus, is the most usual symptom ; the temperature may rise to 102°–103° F., and the pulse become rapid.   The urine is usually found to contain mucus and pus in varying quantities.

Treatment: Prompt and energetic treatment is usually de-manded to prevent the infection spreading to the ureters and kidneys.   The bladder should be irrigated daily with a warm solution of boric acid (gr. xv–ʒj).   The diet should consist of milk only, and the following mixture should be ordered :

> ℞. Sod. bihor.,
>   Ac. benzoic.,   āā ʒss ;
>   Inf. buchu,   ʒvj.—M.

Sig. A tablespoonful in a wineglassful of water three times daily.

Or, urotropin, gr. vj, g. 6. h., in a tumblerful of Vichy Celestin.

If the condition persist after irrigating with boric solution, the bladder should be distended with a solution of silver nitrate (gr. ss–ʒj), all of which should be allowed to drain away with the exception of about an ounce, which may be left in the bladder.

Pyelonephritis: This condition may follow an infection of the bladder by extension of the disease along the ureters, or it may result from a general septic infection.

Diagnosis can usually be made by an examination of the urine.

Treatment: Stimulation, support, the administration of

urotropin, and daily irrigation of the bladder constitute the treatment of this condition.

Hæmaturia: Bloody urine is sometimes seen after labor, and may follow severe contusion of the bladder either by the child's head or the forceps. Not infrequently the condition is due to the persistence of vesical hemorrhoids which developed during pregnancy. Usually the blood disappears from the urine in a few days without treatment.

Diseases of the Nervous System.

Neuritis and Myelitis.

Neuritis following labor is due either to (*a*) nerve injury the result of pressure by the child's head or by forceps; or to (*b*) nerve disease the result of septic infection.

Neuritis due to injury: The injury to the lumbosacral plexus may be so slight as to produce nothing but a partial loss of power associated with but slight pain or tenderness on movement, which subsides without special treatment in a few days. In more severe cases the pain may be intense and constant, while paralysis and atrophy of the affected muscles may follow, being associated with anæsthesia. Pressure on the sacral plexus by means of the finger introduced into the rectum gives rise to intense pain.

Neuritis due to septic infection may assume almost any type, being multiple, diffused, or isolated, while either motor or sensory nerves may be affected. Occasionally in this form the median or ulnar nerves may be affected.

Myelitis is generally the result of septic infection, though Hirst mentions having met with a case which proved fatal, and in which no septic focus or apoplexy could be discovered at the post-mortem.

Treatment: In the acute stage fixation and extension of the part affected will give the greatest relief. Alternate hot and cold applications, and the administration of phenacetin or, if necessary, opium, will secure further relief from pain. When this stage has subsided massage, electricity, and passive movement, combined with the administration of pot. iod. (gr. x–xv t. i. d.), will hasten the restoration of the part to usefulness.

Cerebral Hemorrhage and Embolism.

A woman the condition of whose arteries predisposes her to **cerebral hemorrhage** is much more likely to be stricken with this accident during labor than at any other time. Hemiplegia is not infrequently found to follow an attack of eclampsia.

Cerebral embolism when it is not within the puerperium generally follows an endocarditis or phlebitis of septic origin.

Puerperal Insanity.

Occurrence : Mental derangement manifests itself in connection with childbearing most frequently during the puerperal period, rarely during lactation, and but exceptionally during pregnancy.

The term puerperal insanity is here used to designate the occurrence of mental derangement at any time between the birth of the child and the termination of lactation. The condition is most likely to occur in connection with the first confinement, though in a small number of cases mental derangement may first manifest itself with the second or third parturition.

Etiology : *Predisposing causes :* In many cases there is present a hereditary disposition to mental derangement. A woman with an unstable nervous system is manifestly unsuited to bear the nervous strain incident to pregnancy, parturition, or lactation. Chorea, epilepsy, and hysteria previously existing predispose to the development of insanity in connection with the puerperal period. Alcoholism and the narcotic habit should be mentioned as predisposing causes.

Exciting causes : Marked anæmia, sepsis, albuminuria, eclampsia, great physical or mental exhaustion, and profound emotion have been cited as exciting causes of this condition. *Mental anxiety* in connection with domestic worry, desertion, and illegitimate pregnancy may be mentioned as an exciting cause.

Forms : Two forms of insanity are ordinarily met with, the *maniacal* and the *melancholic :* the former occurs much more frequently during the puerperal period ; while the latter is generally associated with lactation.

Puerperal insanity—symptoms : In both forms *prodromal*

symptoms usually manifest themselves. These are irritability, restlessness, complaints of petty annoyances, and periods of depression, alternating with conditions of nervous tension. A condition of general ill-health is usually manifested by loss of appetite, indigestion, constipation, and flatulence. The patient is usually pale, the pulse is irritable and quick, and she is inclined to sudden outbreaks of tearfulness.

The condition may deepen rapidly, and fever develop, and delusions and hallucinations become manifest. The language becomes obscene, and frequently erotic manifestations become evident. The patient becomes uncontrollable, and is violent in her actions; she may attempt to destroy her infant or attack her attendants.

In the *melancholic form* the patient becomes morose, depressed, and listless; delusions of persecution are of frequent occurrence. She accuses her husband of infidelity, or of even worse crimes. She hears voices telling her to kill herself, which she may attempt to do unless closely watched.

In some cases the *prodromal symptoms* may be *so slight* as to escape observation; or the condition may be regarded as one of ordinary neurasthenia, when suddenly the patient may attack and destroy her infant or attendant, or may accomplish suicide.

When a woman during the puerperal period manifests excessive irritability or unusual loquacity or taciturnity, associated with sleeplessness and constipation, a close watch should be kept on all her actions, and she should on no account be left alone with her infant.

Diagnosis: Usually this can be made without difficulty. The delirium of mania must be distinguished from that of fever and that of delirium tremens.

Prognosis: About two-thirds of all cases recover their reason in from two to six months. Of the other third, 10 per cent. die of sepsis or exhaustion, and the balance remain permanently insane.

Mania is less likely to result in permanent insanity than is melancholia; but it may be said that the patient's life is in greater danger from mania than from melancholia. The older the patient, the more rapid the pulse, and the more persistent the elevation of temperature, the more grave is the prognosis.

When eclampsia bears a causal relation to the condition the prognosis is distinctly more favorable, for these patients recover much quicker than in any other variety.

Treatment of Puerperal Insanity.

When possible, patients suffering from this affliction should be removed to **special institutions** for treatment, and the earlier this is done the better. When this is impossible the patient should be isolated with two or three attendants who are strangers to her. She should never be left for one minute alone, the windows should be securely fastened, and all unnecessary furniture removed from the room.

When **in mania** it is necessary to keep the patient in bed, this may be done by covering her with a strong sheet fastened at the sides and foot of the bed; otherwise instruments of restraint should never be employed, but a sufficient number of attendants should always be at hand to control the patient if this be necessary.

The treatment otherwise should be largely **symptomatic**. Nutrition should be promoted by every means possible, but sedation should be avoided.

It is always well to begin by securing a free action of the **bowels**. This may be accomplished by the administration of a mercurial with a subsequent saline. The regular administration of intestinal antiseptics, as salicylate of sodium or naphthalin (gr. v t. i. d.), is advisable.

Sleep may be promoted by giving paraldehyde ($\mathrecsp{3}j$–ij) at night. Instead of this, sulfonal or trional in 20 grain doses may be employed.

Hydrotherapy is of advantage both as controlling the temperature and in securing sleep.

The **diet** should consist of milk in generous quantities at first; later, eggs and meat may be added as digestion improves. Stimulants should be employed when necessary. Malt extracts are valuable adjuvants to the diet.

Forced feeding by means of the œsophageal tube may be required in rare instances, and it may be replaced at intervals by nutrient enemata.

Iron and **arsenic** should be given regularly in full doses, as soon as the condition of the digestive tract permits of their employment.

As soon as possible the patient should be kept constantly in the **open air** during the daytime; and exercise short of fatigue should be encouraged.

The fact that **pelvic conditions** have much to do with the development of this condition renders it necessary to make a careful examination of the state of these organs in all cases. All abnormal conditions should be corrected as far as possible. In many cases operative treatment has been followed by brilliant results; but to accomplish this, such procedure should be adopted early in the history of the case.

Sudden Death in the Puerperium.

The most **common causes** of sudden death in the puerperal period are *pulmonary embolism, entrance of air into the uterine sinuses,* and *heart-failure.*

Pulmonary Embolism and Thrombosis.

Etiology: Some authorities claim that primary and spontaneous coagulation of blood may take place in the pulmonary artery.

The most generally accepted view is that pulmonary embolism results from the separation of a portion of a thrombus which has formed in some peripheral vein. Thrombosis most commonly takes place either in an iliac, femoral, or uterine vein.

Symptoms and diagnosis: This accident may occur at any time during the earlier weeks of the puerperal period. The symptoms usually develop with *great suddenness,* and their severity depends on the size of the embolus. When the obstruction of the pulmonary artery is complete, death may be practically instantaneous; or it may be preceded by precordial oppression, great dyspnœa, and cyanosis. Usually the patient utters a sharp cry; the respirations become shallow, gasping, and irregular, and in a few seconds cease altogether. In cases in which the embolus is small the onset of symptoms is not so sudden; but they are similar, though not so severe. Death may not take place for several days, and very rarely recovery may follow. The symptoms usually follow some sudden movement, such as sitting up, laughing, straining at stool, etc.

The following may be cited as **an illustrative case** : the patient, a multipara, had made a perfect convalescence after an uneventful labor, when on the morning of the thirteenth day, after being gently moved to a sofa placed alongside of her bed, she suddenly gave a gasp, fell back on the pillows, and in a moment lost consciousness. Cyanosis rapidly developed, and the respirations became labored and ceased inside of five minutes. The pulse at first was rapid and strong, but quickly became thready, and ceased shortly after the failure of respiration.

At the *autopsy* there were found in certain of the larger veins in connection with the uterovaginal plexus large, well-formed thrombi; a thrombus was found to extend into the right internal iliac vein, where it ended abruptly with a truncated and apparently broken-off end. Both right and left pulmonary arteries were found absolutely occluded with firm red clot at their very origin. Nothing abnormal was found elsewhere in the body.

Treatment : Usually death takes place before any treatment can be inaugurated. In all cases in which there is evidence of venous thrombosis *prolonged* and *complete rest* should be enjoined. From an examination of the records of four of these cases which came under the observation of the writer, in none of which there existed any evidence of thrombosis before the onset of the fatal symptoms, the only abnormal condition common to all was a somewhat increased pulse-rate. In all four the pulse-rate is never recorded as being below 80, though death took place in each between the tenth and the fifteenth days of the puerperal period. In view of this fact the writer is in the habit of keeping all cases having an unusually high pulse-rate as quiet as possible for at least four weeks after the birth of the child, or until the pulse-rate becomes normal.

In *mild cases* in which treatment is possible the indications are to keep up the body-temperature by the application of heat externally, to stimulate the cardiac and respiratory organs by the administration of appropriate remedies, and to secure the most absolute physical and mental rest for the patient.

Entrance of Air into the Uterine Sinuses.

Causation : This is a very rare accident. Air may find entrance into the uterine sinuses in the course of intra-uterine manipulations, such as the introduction of the hand, the giving of an intra-uterine douche, or by aspiration following a change in posture of the patient.

Symptoms : These are practically the same as in pulmonary embolism.

Treatment : This consists in the hypodermic administration of stimulants and the employment of artificial respiration. Inhalation of oxygen gas, in order to inflate the lungs and to expel the air emboli, has been suggested.

Fever during the Puerperium due to Other than Septic Causes.

Elevation of temperature may occur in the course of the puerperal period quite independently of *septic infection,* from such causes as exposure to cold, constipation, emotion, or reflex irritation of any kind.

Emotional fever : Profound psychical impressions, such as grief, anger, fear, or even excessive joy, may give rise to some elevation of temperature, especially when experienced during the early puerperium. The mechanism of this elevation of temperature is not susceptible of explanation in the present state of our knowledge.

In maternity hospitals emotional fever is frequently met with in cases of *illegitimate pregnancy* about the tenth day of the puerperium, as a result of anxiety on the part of such patients in regard to their ability to provide for themselves and their children in the immediate future. In emotional fever the temperature may rise to 104°–105° F.; but the cause being usually transient the temperature quickly falls to normal.

Exposure to cold : Elevation of temperature may follow exposure of the breasts or abdomen to cold ; too low a temperature in the lying-in room or insufficient bed-clothing may expose the patient to a chill, which is usually followed by some elevation of temperature.

The administration of some warm drink and the application of external heat usually cause the fever to disappear promptly.

Constipation: This is a not infrequent cause of elevation of temperature during the earlier part of the puerperium. The fever is probably due to the irritation of retained animal alkaloids.

The administration of a dose of castor oil will probably result in a drop of the temperature to normal as soon as the bowels have been evacuated.

Fever from reflex irritation: The effect of constipation when it occurs in the puerperium is an example of reflex irritation of the nervous system producing fever which at other times would have no such result.

Irritation from *engorgement of the breasts* frequently results in elevation of temperature, as has been mentioned elsewhere.

Several times we have met with cases of fever in which no cause could be found to explain the condition until segments of a *tapeworm* or a round worm appeared in the stools. Following the administration of appropriate remedies the worms were expelled and the temperature promptly returned to normal.

Tympanites: Tympanites, or overdistention of the intestines with gas, is not infrequently met with in the earlier part of the puerperal period. This condition may or may not be attended with fever. When this condition is associated with elevation of the temperature care must be taken to distinguish it from peritonitis.

Treatment: Turpentine enemata at short intervals, combined with the internal administration of small doses of calomel, usually relieve the patient.

Usually it is necessary to start the treatment with an enema of hot soap-water and turpentine (ʒij to Oj). Then calomel (gr. $\frac{1}{10}$) should be given every hour. At the end of six hours a dose of Epsom salt (ʒss, in two ounces of hot water) may be given; and if this is not effectual in an hour an enema containing glycerin (ʒj), turpentine (ʒij), Epsom salt (ʒss), and water (ʒiij) should be given.

The calomel should be kept up for two days, and then reduced to two or three doses daily. As these cases are due to paralysis of the muscular coats of the intestine, a hypodermic of strychnine (gr. $\frac{1}{30}$) should be given every four or six hours until the condition improves.

Puerperal Septic Infection.

The general term **puerperal septic infection** is here employed to designate the many and varied diseased conditions resulting from infection of the female genital tract during labor and the puerperium, by microörganisms.

Frequency: Previous to the introduction of the antiseptic method of conducting labor the mortality-rate from septic infection varied between 10 and 15 per cent. in the large maternity institutions. As the result of the application of rigid antisepsis and asepsis to hospital practice the mortality from septic disease has been reduced to a low fraction of 1 per cent.

In private practice the beneficial results of the antiseptic method are much less marked than in hospital practice. Epidemics of puerperal infection are now but rarely heard of, but the mortality-returns still show a large proportion of deaths following parturition.

That septic conditions frequently complicate the puerperium is evidenced by the overcrowded condition of the gynæcological clinics in all parts of the country. A very large proportion of these gynæcological cases present conditions which owe their origin to febrile affections arising during the puerperal period.

Bacteriology.

The **streptococcus** is the microörganism most frequently associated with the occurrence of puerperal sepsis. It is to be found in nearly all fatal cases.

The **staphylococcus aureus** is the next most frequent cause of puerperal septic infection. Not infrequently mixed infections with streptococci and staphylococci are encountered.

The **gonococcus, bacillus coli communis, bacillus diphtheriæ, bacillus aerogenes capsulatus, pneumococcus,** and **bacillus typhosus** may be mentioned as rare causes of puerperal septic infection. These may be found pure or mixed with streptococci; when the latter is the case the infection is generally exceptionally virulent.

The *gonococcus* plays an important part in the production of puerperal sepsis. Krönig has found it to be present in 50 out of 179 cases presenting febrile puerperia. It appears usually to cause a mild infection, unless associated with a streptococcus, in which case the infection is usually very virulent.

Sapræmia: There is a considerable class of cases in which the symptoms are due to the absorption of toxic products produced by organisms within the genital tract which do not make their way into the blood-current. These are mostly of an anaërobic nature, belonging to the *putrefactive* class of microörganisms, of which little is known. They usually produce gas, and hence give rise to frothy, foul-smelling discharges.

Recently a great deal of bacteriological work has been carried out in the study of **the vaginal secretion**. It has been practically proved that the normal vagina in pregnancy is free from pathogenic microörganisms, at least in its upper third. The vaginal secretions are commonly strongly acid in their reaction, due to the presence of a so-called vaginal bacillus, which in its life-processes produces lactic acid. It is probably this acid condition of the vaginal secretions, associated with a certain leukocytosis due to chemotaxic action, which results in the rapid destruction of the pathogenic bacteria should they find entrance to the vagina.

It has been proved that pathogenic bacteria introduced into a normal vagina perish in from eleven to twenty hours through the germicidal action of the normal secretions. Preliminary antiseptic vaginal douches have been proved to inhibit the germicidal action of normal vaginal secretions. Pathogenic bacteria have been found to flourish from eight to sixteen hours longer in the healthy vagina after antiseptic douching than when no douching was employed.

The **cervix** has been usually found to contain in its lower part a few pathogenic bacteria of greatly diminished virulence. Its upper part is invariably sterile in the normal condition. The uterine cavity normally is entirely free from microörganisms, both in the pregnant and in the non-pregnant condition.

The microörganisms to be found in the lower part of the **vagina** are usually non-infectious; but should pathogenic bacteria be present, their virulence is invariably greatly diminished as a result of the germicidal action of the normal secretions.

Pathology of Puerperal Septic Infection.

The **consequences** of infection of the genital tract of the puerperal woman by microörganisms are extremely variable. The infection may be limited to lesions of the vulva or vaginal outlet, or may rapidly spread from this locality to the uterine cavity. In the most virulent cases no lesion may mark the locality in which the germs have effected an entrance, and yet the patient may succumb with extreme rapidity.

It is the *endometrium* which is affected in the majority of cases of puerperal septic infection. This *endometritis* may be *septic* or *putrid*, according as it is the result of infection by pyogenic or putrefactive microörganisms.

The mildest form of puerperal septic infection is the **puerperal ulcer.** These puerperal ulcers are simply infected lacerations of the vaginal outlet and vulva. They usually present a dirty, greenish-yellow appearance and are bathed in a purulent secretion. Formerly these were termed diphtheritic ulcers, but it is very rare that they result from infection with the Klebs-Löffler bacillus.

Usually they cause but little symptomatic disturbance, and therefore their presence may pass unnoticed.

True puerperal vaginitis may occur, but is rare; it is characterized by an inflammation of the vaginal mucosa, which swells and softens, becoming bathed in a purulent secretion. Lacerations in the vagina when infection occurs usually become covered with a pseudodiphtheritic membrane. Rarely, true diphtheritic vaginitis may occur.

Endometritis: After labor the more or less lacerated condition of the endometrium, and the uneven placental site with its thrombosed sinuses, render the uterine cavity specially susceptible to the reception and propagation of infective organisms. Hence the most common lesion associated with puerperal septic infection is endometritis.

The infection may be limited to the placental site; or may extend over the whole of the endometrium.

When the infection is *limited to the placental site* the organisms develop in the thrombi in the placental sinuses, setting up a phlebitis which may be limited to the uterine wall, or may extend to the surrounding veins, and thus give rise to secondary infection elsewhere.

When the *whole endometrium* is involved the mucosa is converted into a stinking, necrotic layer, which is bathed in a bloody discharge. The quantity of necrotic material formed is often considerable, and it recurs with great rapidity after its removal by the curette. It consists of necrotic decidual débris

FIG. 132.

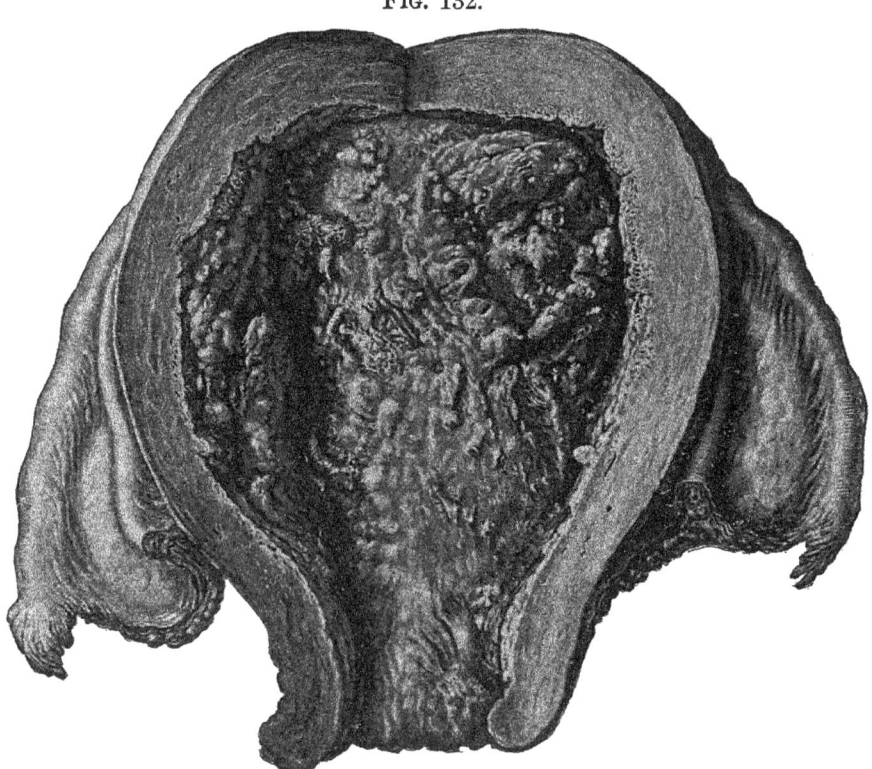

Uterus from patient dying on the tenth day from a pure streptococcus infection.

and fibrin-exudate loaded with microörganisms (Figs. 132 and 133).

When the infection is due to the *streptococcus* or to the *staphylococcus*, the odor of the lochia may not be affected. Thus in the most virulent cases the lochia may remain sweet throughout; but when the *colon bacillus* or any of the *putre-*

fective germs are present the discharges become foul in the extreme.

In a large number of cases Nature succeeds in limiting the infective process to the endometrium, which it does by forming

FIG. 133.

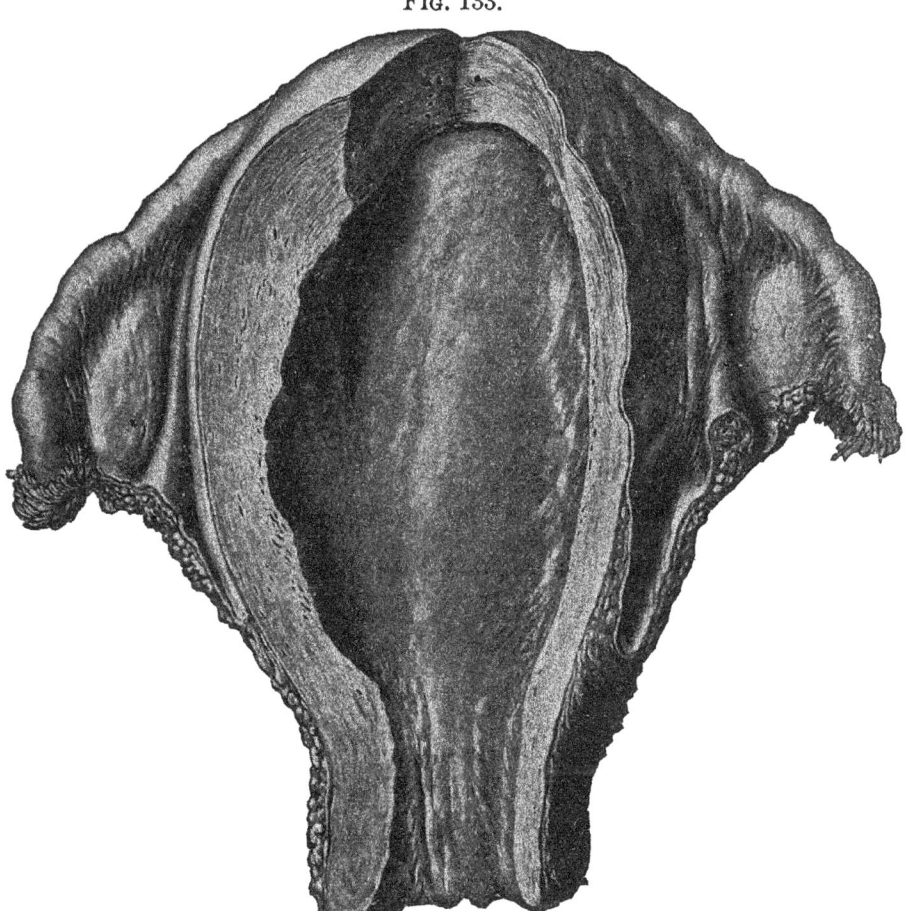

Uterus from patient dying on the tenth day from a mixed infection—streptococcus and colon bacilli.

a barrier or obstruction immediately below the necrotic layer. This barrier consists of a layer of small-cell infiltration, designated the *zone of reaction.* Beneath this zone the tissues are usually quite normal.

23—Obst.

Thus *on section* we find an internal layer consisting of necrotic decidua and fibrin-exudate swarming with microorganisms; below this is a layer of small-cell infiltration, the " zone of reaction," containing few if any bacteria, while under this is the normal uterine tissue.

Such is the condition found when the infection is due to putrefactive microörganisms, as in *putrid endometritis*, so-called by Bumm and Döderlein; or when, if due to pyogenic bacteria, these are possessed of but little virulence.

In the so-called **septic endometritis** (Bumm and Döderlein), when the infective organisms are virulent streptococci or staphylococci, the zone of small-cell infiltration may be but imperfectly formed, or even entirely absent; while the superficial necrotic layer may be lacking, or if present be very thin. In this case the extension of the infective process occurs by means of the lymphatics, and soon spreads through the uterine wall to the peritoneal layer, thus setting up a metritis, lymphangitis, and finally a septic peritonitis. This *lymphangitis* usually results in the formation of numerous small abscesses throughout the uterine wall, though usually most marked just beneath the peritoneum.

Parametritis: This inflammation of the connective tissue contiguous to the uterus frequently follows intra-uterine infection during the puerperium. The extension of the microörganisms usually proceeds along the lymphatics from the endometrium to the peri-uterine connective tissue. Occasionally the infection may originate in laceration of the cervix.

The infective inflammation of the peri-uterine connective tissue produces extensive *œdema*. This may result in resolution, or in suppuration and abscess-formation. When extension of the infection occurs along the lymphatics in the anterior portion of the pelvis, the inflammatory œdema surrounds the greater vessels of the thigh in the neighborhood of the inguinal region, giving rise to one form of *phlegmasia alba dolens.*

Salpingitis: The Fallopian tubes in a certain number of cases become infected by direct extension of the inflammation from the uterine cavity. Occasionally the infection may be carried to the tubes as well as ovaries, by means of the lymphatics.

Peritonitis : This condition usually arises as the result of the rapid extension of infection from the uterine cavity by means of the lymphatics as already described.

Peritonitis may rarely occur in consequence of the rupture of a pus-tube, or of an ovarian or parametritic abscess. Septic peritonitis is usually the direct cause of death in the vast majority of fatal cases.

Pyæmia : As already mentioned, the infective microörganisms may penetrate the thrombi at the placental site. This results in a condition of septic phlebitis, which may be limited to the veins in the uterine wall or may extend to the veins in the neighborhood. The thrombosis may extend as far as the inferior vena cava. These infected thrombi may break down, and small portions may be swept by the blood-current to distant parts of the body, thus setting up a condition of pyæmia.

These *infected emboli* may be deposited in the abdominal viscera, the lungs, the brain, spinal cord, the joints, or in the subcutaneous tissue at any portion of the body surface, where they give rise to abscesses. In these cases there is very little involvement of the uterus, infection then being limited usually to the placental site. Death in these cases is usually due to exhaustion following a long suppurative process.

Phlegmasia alba dolens: This condition is known to the laity as " milk leg," as· it was popularly supposed at one time to be due to a metastasis of milk. It occurs as the result either of the extension of a thrombosis from the uterine veins to those of the lower extremities, or of a septic parametritis spreading to the connective tissue of the thigh.

In *thrombotic phlegmasia* the swelling of the affected limb usually begins about the foot, and rapidly extends to the thigh.

In *cellulitic phlegmasia* the swelling begins in the thigh and spreads down the limb.

In *both)forms* the affected limb becomes enormously swollen. In the first form there is usually more or less tenderness along the course of the femoral vein, which is usually marked by a line of inflammatory redness.

Modes of infection: The most common mode of infection is the introduction of septic material into the genital canal, on the *hands* or *instruments* of the physician or midwife ; *con-*

tact with secretion from *wounds* of any kind, such as infected abrasions on the hands of a nurse or physician.   *Air-infection* may account for a very small proportion of cases.

The *water* used to douche the patient after labor may carry pathogenic germs into the genital canal.   *Contact* of the vulva with dirty bed-clothes or personal linen, or with infected vulvar pads, may account for some cases.

In one case in the author's experience infection was probably due to the *dirty hand of the patient,* who could not be restrained from scratching the vulva.

As has been shown, the normal vagina is practically sterile, so that when infection occurs it is generally the result of the *introduction of pathogenic material from without.*   Epidemics of septic infection have been stamped out in maternities by avoiding all internal examinations.   The best morbidity and mortality records have been obtained in institutions where vaginal examinations have been eliminated as far as possible.

Auto-infection may he held to account for a very small proportion of cases of puerperal sepsis.   In these cases the pathogenic germs are held to be resident in the body, and not to have been introduced from without, during or after labor. The microörganisms may be lodged in the vagina, cervix, or urethra, as in cases of gonorrhœa.   Endometritis antedating conception may account for the lodgement of germs in the uterine mucous membrane, which in the favorable conditions existing after delivery may become virulent and set up septic infection.   In the same way an old pus-sac in one of the tubes may rupture during labor and cause a septic peritonitis.

Symptomatology.

The symptoms of septic infection may **develop** within the first twenty-four hours after delivery ; but, as a rule, nothing out of the ordinary is to be noted until the third or fourth day.

The **onset** of infection may be attended with a sense of malaise and possibly a slight headache.   As the temperature begins to rise the patient develops a more or less severe chill, which may amount to an actual rigor.   The temperature quickly rises to 103° F. or higher, and the pulse becomes very rapid. Usually there is only one chill, but the temperature remains persistently elevated.

The *lochia* may become scant, but as a rule the discharge increases in amount. It may remain bloody or may rapidly become purulent. In the most virulent cases and in those due to pure streptococcus infection, very little, if any, odor is to be noticed.

Profuse foul-smelling lochial discharge indicates a putrid endometritis; or a mixed infection due to pyogenic as well as putrefactive organisms.

With the onset of endometritis either of the septic or the putrid form, **involution** of the uterus at once ceases, thus favoring the spread of the infection, in that the lymph-channels, being free from compression, remain patent and thus offer less resistance to the passage of microörganisms.

If the infective process **extends beyond the uterus,** the symptoms which then develop depend upon the tissues involved. Symptoms indicative of peritonitis, parametritis, or pyæmia may thus ensue.

Peritonitis: The onset of this complication is indicated by the occurrence of intense pain, which is at first limited to the lower zone of the abdomen, but gradually extends as the whole peritoneum becomes affected. As paralysis of the intestines takes place marked tympanites occurs. In fatal cases death usually takes place within the first ten days of the puerperium.

Parametritis: This complication, as a rule, develops when the endometritis is apparently subsiding. Its onset is frequently attended with a chill; the temperature, which has probably fallen, again becomes elevated and pursues a more or less irregular course. The extension of the inflammatory process to the parametrium may usually be detected by a vaginal examination. The infiltrated tissues surrounding the uterus become hard and tense to the feel. This inflammation may end in resolution or in *abscess-formation*—one large or several small abscesses may form. The pus may burrow about and make its way into the bladder, rectum, vagina, or peritoneal cavity. Occasionally such an abscess may point at Poupart's ligament, or even above the crest of the ilium.

Pyæmia : In cases of pyæmia the initial symptoms of infection are not so marked as in the other forms. The temperature does not remain constantly elevated, but assumes the hectic type. Chills are usually of frequent occurrence.

The subsequent symptoms depend upon the organs invaded by the infected thrombi. Most commonly with pyæmia we have symptoms of an infectious bronchopneumonia developing. This generally proves rapidly fatal.

In **true septicæmia,** which is the most virulent form of septic infection, the organisms make their way so rapidly into the general blood-current that they fail to become localized in any one organ. This is the most rapidly fatal form of infection; death may occur on the third or fourth day of the puerperium, the poison being so virulent as to induce a condition of profound shock.

Diagnosis of Puerperal Septic Infection.

If on the third or fourth day of the puerperal period a woman develops **a temperature** of 101° F., or more, which persists for twenty-four hours, the condition present is almost certainly one of septic infection provided there is no other apparent cause to account satisfactorily for the symptoms.

The most common **causes** of an elevation of temperature early in the puerperium, *not associated with* septic infection, are : constipation, irritation from the breasts, and emotional excitement, fright, or grief. Malaria and typhoid fever may complicate the puerperium, and may be confounded with septic infection.

A diagnosis of **malaria** is only possible when the presence of the plasmodium has been demonstrated in the blood.

A diagnosis of **typhoid fever** is not permissible in the absence of Widal's blood-serum test.

Before making a diagnosis of septic infection, careful, systematic **physical examination** of the patient should be made.

A careful examination of the characters of the **lochial discharge** may render possible a diagnosis of which variety of endometritis is present in a given case of puerperal septic infection.

In all cases the physician should make an **ocular** examination of the *vulva, vagina,* and *cervix* in a good light, employing for this purpose a large speculum.

As it is desirable to know what **organisms** are concerned in the production of the infection, a *culture* may be taken from the interior of the uterus. This may be accomplished with but little difficulty by the method recommended by Professor Williams, of Baltimore.

The **apparatus** necessary consists of a glass tube, 20 to 25 cm. in length and 3 to 4 mm. in diameter, with a slight bend at one end so as to facilitate its introduction into the uterus. This may be sterilized after placing it in a long test-tube of thick glass, which contains in its lower extremity a pledget of cotton-wool, while its upper end may be closed 'by a cotton plug (Figs. 134–136).

Williams thus describes the **method** to be followed in obtaining a culture from the uterine cavity : " When we wish to make cultures from the uterus, our hands and the external genitalia should be thoroughly disinfected, the patient placed in the Sims position, and a sterilized Sims or Simons speculum introduced so as to retract the posterior vaginal wall ; then the cervix is caught with a volsellum forceps and brought down to the vulva ; the vaginal portion of the cervix is then carefully cleansed with a bit of sterilized cotton, and the sterile lochial tube is removed from its tube and introduced into the uterus as high up as it will go, care being taken to avoid touching the external genitals in the operation. To the end of the lochial tube which protrudes from the vulva a syringe, which draws well, is attached by means of a rubber tube. Suction is made whereby a certain amount of the uterine contents is drawn up in the tube. The tube is then withdrawn and its ends sealed with sealing-wax, when it can be carried to the laboratory without fear of contamination. On reaching the laboratory it is broken in its middle portion and cultures are taken from its contents, which we know represent the uncontaminated lochia from the upper part of the uterus."

When there is *undoubted evidence* of endometritis the **interior** of the uterus should be **explored** by means of the **sterile finger.** This procedure can be carried out when the culture has been

Fig. 135.

Fig. 134.

Fig. 136.

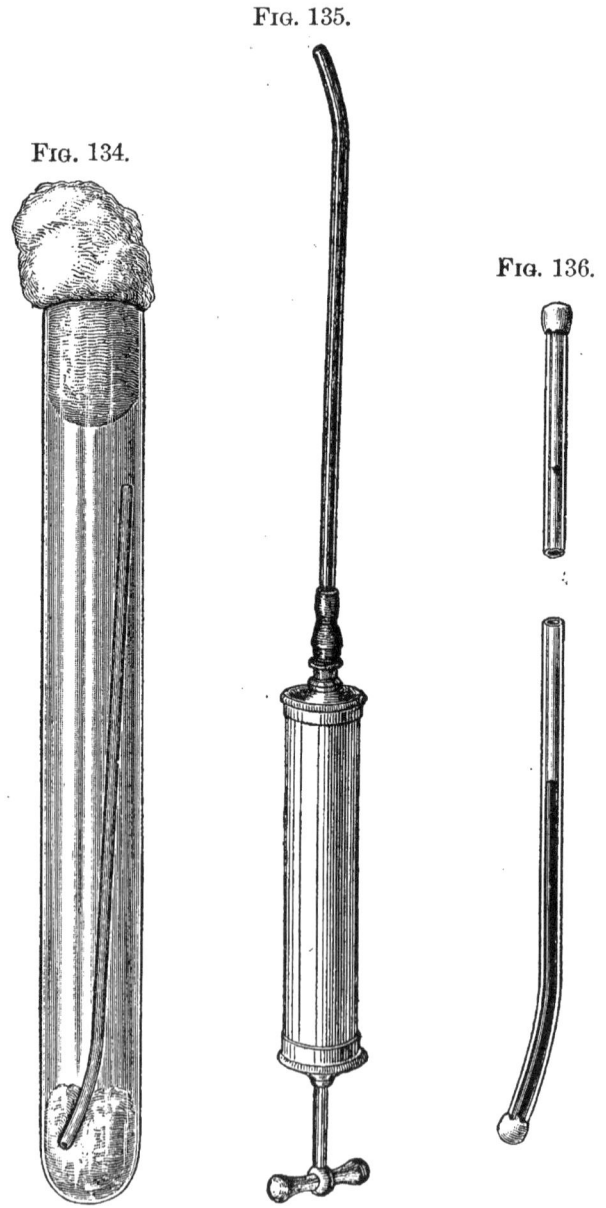

obtained.   By this means important information may be obtained which will indicate the line of treatment to be pursued.

When the *walls* of the uterine cavity are *rough*, the probability is that we have to deal with a *putrefactive endometritis;* or one due to a pyogenic organism of a low degree of virulency. When the cavity is perfectly *smooth* the infection is probably due to virulent *streptococci* or *staphylococci.*

Treatment of Puerperal Septic Infection.

Prophylaxis: The occurrence of puerperal septic infection is to be prevented by the observance of the most scrupulous *asepsis* in the method of conducting labor. This subject has been fully dealt with in the section on the management of labor, to which the reader is again referred.

Prophylactic *douches* should not be employed except when the vaginal secretion presents marked evidences of abnormality. *Vaginal examinations* should be made as infrequently as possible during labor; in normal cases more than one or two are seldom necessary.

All vaginal and vulvar *lacerations* which extend deeper than the mucosa should be *sutured* immediately after the conclusion of labor.

During the first *two weeks* of the puerperal period the most rigid asepsis should be observed in the care of the external genitals. The subject has been discussed in this work on the section in the management of the puerperium.

Local Treatment.

If on examination of the vulva **sloughing** surfaces are discovered, these should be painted daily with tincture of iodine.

When **sutured wounds** of the vaginal outlet present evidences of **infection**, the stitches should be removed in order to secure free drainage.

Endometritis is the condition most frequently present in puerperal septic infection.

As previously mentioned, the cavity of the uterus should be explored and a portion of the lochia removed for examination.

The method of treatment to be followed will depend in a large measure on the conditions present in the uterine cavity.

The indications are to remove all débris and shreds of broken-down tissue and to cleanse thoroughly the interior of the uterus. The *routine* use of the curette in all cases of puerperal endometritis is mentioned only to be condemned, as in certain conditions this treatment may result in the production of far more harm than good.

When the **walls** of the uterine cavity are found to be **perfectly smooth** there is absolutely no indication for the employment of the curette, as there is nothing present that can be removed by it. The cavity should be douched thoroughly with a gallon or two of hot sterile formalin solution (1 : 500).

If the **bacteriological examination** of the lochia reveals that the infection is due to *streptococci,* further local treatment is to be avoided.

If the **interior** of the uterus be found **rough and jagged,** and covered with more or less false membrane, the walls of the cavity should be systematically scraped with a blunt curette (Mundé's), though many prefer the fingers for this purpose. *After curetting,* the walls should be explored by the finger-tips to make sure that all débris has been removed by the curette. A *douche* of hot formalin solution (1 : 500) may then be employed to cleanse the cavity thoroughly.

This treatment usually results in a marked improvement of the symptoms, the temperature falls within a few hours, and the lochia becomes more normal in type. Should the temperature not yield to the first injection, the treatment may be repeated daily, provided there is no evidence that the infection has extended beyond the uterus, in which case local treatment should be abandoned.

Bichloride of mercury solution should not be employed in intra-uterine douches, as when this salt comes in contact with blood it forms an innocuous albuminate. Bumm has shown that bichloride injections penetrate the tissue to only a slight extent. The antiseptic does not remain long enough in contact with the infected tissue to exert much germicidal action. For this latter reason, and because the main object of the douche is to wash away débris which has been detached by the curette or finger, many prefer to employ for this purpose simple sterile water or salt solution.

In **gonococcal** endometritis it is better to employ no local treatment, as the majority of these cases recover without it; or at the worst are left with a chronic endometritis which can be treated to better advantage later.

Local treatment should not be persisted in when it is evident that it fails to improve the condition of the patient. In these cases all that can be done is to direct our efforts to the general improvement of the condition of the patient.

General Treatment.

These patients should receive all the food they can assimilate. The **diet** should consist chiefly of milk, eggs, and meat-juice. These should be given in large quantities, at short intervals, and if necessary should be predigested.

The depressant action of the toxins should be combated by **free stimulation**, and for this purpose our most potent remedies are alcohol and strychnine.

As much *alcohol* should be given as can be consumed without producing its physiological effects. It is surprising what a quantity of alcohol these patients can take without apparently producing any untoward result.

Strychnine should also be given in large doses, from $\frac{1}{50}$ to $\frac{1}{20}$ grain may be administered every three hours in serious cases. *Digitalis* may be combined with the strychnine when the pulse-rate is high.

To **control the temperature**, cold wet packs should be employed, as well as the ice-cap. As a rule, antipyretic drugs should be avoided on account of the depressant action they exert.

Bumm has recommended the routine employment of **ergot** in cases of puerperal endometritis, in order to secure better contraction, and thus occlude to some degree the lymphatics in the uterine wall. Fl. ext. ergotæ ($\mathfrak{M}$ x) may be given every six hours, or it may be combined with quinine (gr. v) and given in a suitable mixture.

The **bowels** should be kept active by means of a daily saline which acts favorably by draining the pelvic lymphatics.

The subcutaneous injection of large quantities of **normal** saline solution has been employed in the treatment of puerperal sepsis with marked beneficial results. It is supposed to act by diluting the blood, thus favoring the expulsion of toxic matter. The saline solution may be injected under the breasts, as recommended in the treatment of hemorrhage; or more conveniently into the bowel, in which case at least two quarts should be given at each injection.

Recently it has been suggested that nuclein be employed in the treatment of these cases with a view of producing an artificial leucocytosis. Hirst considers that this plan of treatment gives promise of practical results, and that more is to be expected of it than of serum-therapy.

Serum-therapy: When Marmorek in 1895 published the results he had obtained by the employment of antistreptococcic serum in the treatment of sepsis, brilliant results were expected to follow its use in puerperal cases. Recent statistics seem to prove that the results thus far obtained by the employment of the serum are not more favorable than those by other methods of treatment.

As many cases of puerperal infection are due to other agents than streptococci, its routine employment in all cases can only be fraught with danger. When our means of diagnosis enables us to prove in a given case that the infection is due to the streptococccus alone, then the serum should be employed, but not to the exclusion of other methods of treatment.

If care is taken to make an accurate diagnosis that the infection is due to the *streptococcus alone*, serum-therapy may be employed, especially if it is used early and in large doses.

Parametritis: This condition may be treated by either hot or cold applications, whichever prove more grateful to the patient. The ice-bag will be found to control the extension of the inflammation in many cases, while it usually relieves the local pain to a marked degree. When it is not well borne hot flaxseed poultices may be applied to the lower abdomen and hot vaginal douches given at regular intervals.

Probably most of these cases heal by resolution, but a close watch must be kept for evidences of suppuration. When fluctuation is obtained the abscess may be opened through the vaginal vault when possible; in some cases it may be necessary to make the incision through the abdominal wall.

Peritonitis: When peritonitis develops the treatment should at first be expectant, in the hope that the inflammation will become localized. Counterirritation and hot fomentations to the abdomen, combined with the free use of saline cathartics, may give good results. If the symptoms progress or do not abate within thirty-six hours, then the abdomen may be opened and the case treated according to the conditions found. Abscess, if found, should be opened and drained. Distended tubes and ovaries should be removed, and under certain conditions it may be necessary to perform hysterectomy.

The *indications for hysterectomy* are the presence of multiple abscesses in the uterine walls; and putrid endometritis which fails to yield to repeated intra-uterine irrigations and curetting.

Phlegmasia alba dolens: The patient should be kept in bed with the affected limb elevated so as to favor the return circulation. The limb should be wrapped in cotton and bandaged loosely. The *general treatment* should be supporting and stimulating.

In the cellulitic variety *suppuration* is very likely to take place in the connective tissue of the thigh. Abscesses should be watched for and promptly opened, so as to avoid burrowing.

OBSTETRIC OPERATIONS.

Episiotomy.

Definition: Episiotomy is the term applied to any incision of the external genitals to prevent extensive laceration taking place during the passage of the child at the time of birth. The operation cannot be said to be in general use in this country, but is common in Germany and Austria.

Indications: These are:

1. Threatening central rupture of the perineum.

2. Contraction of the pelvic outlet.

3. Rigidity of the perineum, especially when due to cicatricial tissue.

4. Faulty position of the advancing part of the fœtus at the outlet.

5. Undue size of the fœtal head.

Operation: Tarnier has recommended an oblique incision passing to one or other side of the anus.   The Germans prefer lateral oblique incisions directed toward the posterior commissure.   It is stated that such an incision 1 cm. ($\frac{3}{8}$ inch) in length increases the circumference of the vulvar orifice 2 cm. ($\frac{3}{4}$ inch).

The *instrument* used is a blunt-pointed scissors.   During a pain one blade of the open scissors is slipped sideways between the head and the vulva, and then turned and the tissues cut.

The **advantage** of episiotomy is the substitution of a clean cut of definite size, in a place where it can do no harm, for an irregular laceration of indefinite size which may cause permanent injury to the patient.   Also a clean incision is much more easily sutured than a jagged laceration.

IMMEDIATE REPAIR OF VAGINAL AND PERINEAL LACERATIONS.

Whether the **pelvic fascia** or the **fibres** of the levator ani muscles are the all-important structures concerned in the support of the internal pelvic structures is still a matter of debate. It is, however, certain that the wedge of tissue between the vagina and rectum composing the **perineal body** has practically nothing to do with the support of the pelvic contents.

According to Kelly, the "real supporting mechanism" of the outlet is the *anterior portion* of the *levator ani muscle*.   The more generally held opinion, however, is that the *pelvic fascia* is the supporting mechanism of the outlet, and that the sheets forming the ischioperineal layer of the rectovesical fascia are most important in this connection.

When it is considered that the **vaginal orifice**, normally 2 to 3 cm. in circumference, **is dilated** to 33 cm. at the moment of delivery to permit the passage of an ordinary sized child, it is not surprising that laceration commonly takes place.

As a matter of routine, after the conclusion of labor, the physician should **carefully examine** the vulva and vaginal orifice for lacerations.   This examination may ordinarily be made with the patient in the dorsal position, having the thighs everted.   A good light is absolutely necessary.   When an external **superficial tear** is found it may be repaired at once, as directed below.

If, however, an **extensive laceration** should be present, further examination may be delayed until preparations have been completed for a repair operation.

Injuries to the vaginal outlet the result of childbirth may be **classified** as follows:

1. External superficial tear.
2. Internal tear, or combined internal and external tear.
3. Complete tear of the rectovaginal septum.

1. External Superficial Tear.

This form of injury from parturition is the **most frequent** and also the **least important,** as it in no way affects the supporting structures of the pelvic outlet.

FIG. 137.

The tear **involves** simply the superficial portion of the wedge of lax tissue between the vagina and rectum.   It begins at the introitus vaginæ and extends backward through the skin in the median line; occasionally it may extend inward as far as the posterior column of the vagina (Fig. 137). This laceration can be inspected throughout its whole extent by merely separating the labia.

When the tear simply extends *through the fourchette* strict cleanliness until it has healed is all that is required.

When the laceration has a base 2–3 cm. ($\frac{3}{4}$ to $1\frac{1}{4}$ inches) in length it should be sutured immediately.

When possible, it is the writer's habit to suture these tears while **waiting for the detachment of the placenta,** as the patient at that time is still more or less under the influence of chloroform.   During the slight operation the nurse is placed in charge of the fundus.

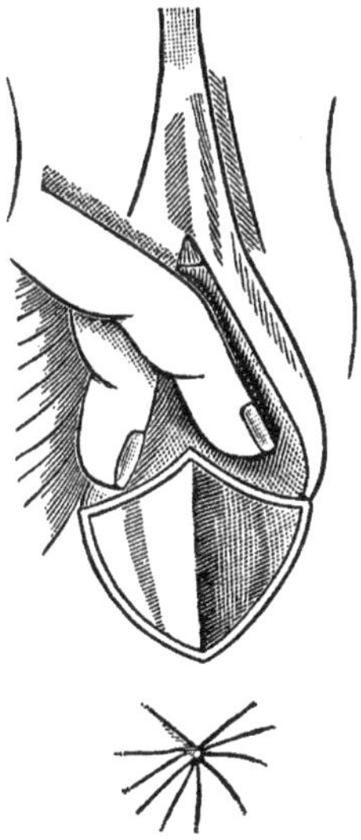

Superficial tear exposed by fingers parting labia minora.

Instead of *tying the sutures* at once, the ends may be caught in a pair of forceps and the tying completed after the delivery of the placenta.

Necessary for the operation: A couple of small curved needles, a needle-holder, three or four silkworm-gut or silk sutures, and a pair of scissors should be sterilized. Many prefer to employ an *Emmett perineum-needle* in suturing these lacerations; it consists of a needle with a large curve, mounted on a handle; the needle is passed, threaded, and then withdrawn.

The rule is to **place the patient** across the bed with the buttocks over the edge, the legs being flexed over the backs of two chairs properly arranged. In many cases it is possible to suture these simple lacerations without disturbing the patient beyond separating and everting her thighs.

Suturing: The patient being placed as most convenient, the lips of the tear are held apart by the fingers of the left hand, the threaded needle is then introduced near the upper angle of the wound about $\frac{1}{2}$ cm. ($\frac{1}{5}$ inch) from its margin, brought out at the floor, and reëntered, to emerge on the skin surface opposite the point of entrance. A similar suture is then placed near the lower angle, and both sutures tied after the wound has been cleansed.

If the approximation is not quite satisfactory, one or two **superficial sutures** may be required. The end of the sutures should be left fairly long, so that they may be easily found and prevented from causing the patient inconvenience by pricking. The sutures may be *removed* on the eighth day.

2. Internal Tear, or Combined Internal and External Tear.

Conditions: An *internal tear* when present is found to extend from the fourchette inward from one to two inches, involving one or both lateral sulci (Fig. 138). This tear always destroys the integrity of the pelvic supporting structures, and if neglected leads to serious results.

Such an internal laceration may be present *without an external wound;* but usually the external injury (already described) is to be found *associated with* the internal tear when it is present. On inspection a ragged bleeding wound will be found in the posterior vaginal wall, associated probably with more or less external laceration.

Method of Repair.

The patient should be **placed** across the bed with the buttocks over the edge, as previously described.

FIG. 138.

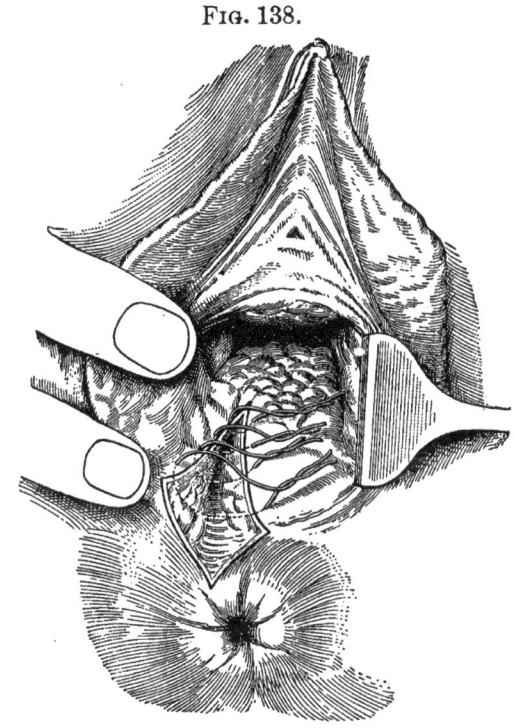

Superficial combined internal and external tear, showing portion of tear in vagina that may escape notice.

The **illumination** of the field of operation should be the best obtainable.

Unless the patient is prepared to suffer a little pain, an **anæsthetic**, preferably ether, should be administered. Throughout the operation an assistant should guard the fundus uteri to prevent relaxation.

The **instruments** required are the same as before mentioned, with the addition possibly of a couple of vaginal retractors.

24—Obst.

The **first step** in the operation is to ascertain the nature and extent of the laceration. To obtain a good view, it may be necessary to pack the upper part of the vaginal canal with sterile gauze or cotton to prevent the flow of blood from above. All ragged and badly bruised tissue should be then cut away, and the upper angle of the wound exposed by means of the fingers of the left hand or by a retractor held by an assistant.

The **suturing** should commence at the upper angle of the tear, and the sutures should be about a centimetre apart; as many should be employed as are required to bring the edges of the wound, or wounds, well together.

FIG. 140.

The **method of inserting the sutures** is of very considerable importance, as the object is to secure the union of the supporting structures of the pelvic floor (Fig. 139). The needle should be introduced on the mucous surface 0.5 cm. ($\frac{1}{5}$ inch) from the margin of

FIG. 139.

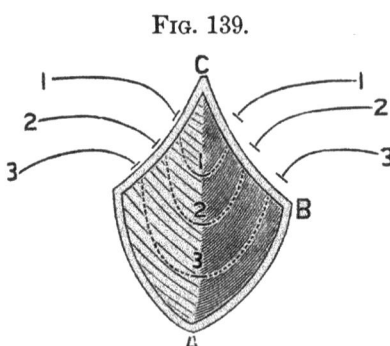

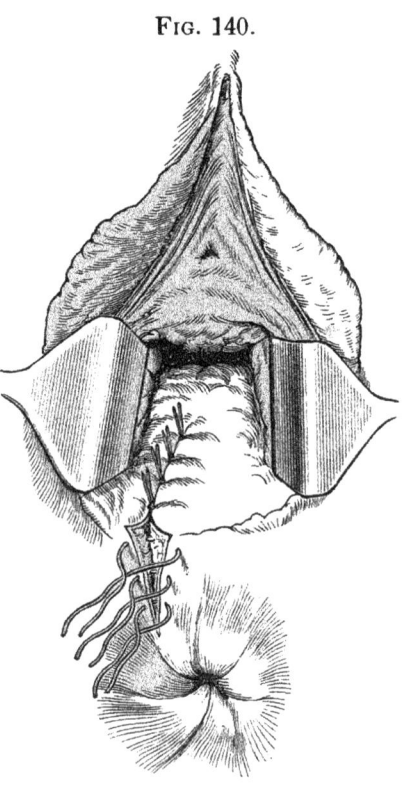

Same as Fig. 127, with internal sutures passed, ready to tie.

Internal stitches tied; external stitches in position.

the wound and directed through the tissues in the direction of the outlet, brought out at the base, then reintroduced, and directed inward and upward so as to emerge on the mucous surface at a point opposite its insertion. Thus the loop of each suture when in place is directed toward the operator (Fig. 140).

Each suture should be tied before the next is introduced. The last suture thus introduced should bring together the torn edges of remains of the hymen at the vaginal orifice.

The external wound may then be repaired by a few superficial sutures introduced from the skin surface.

Fig. 141.

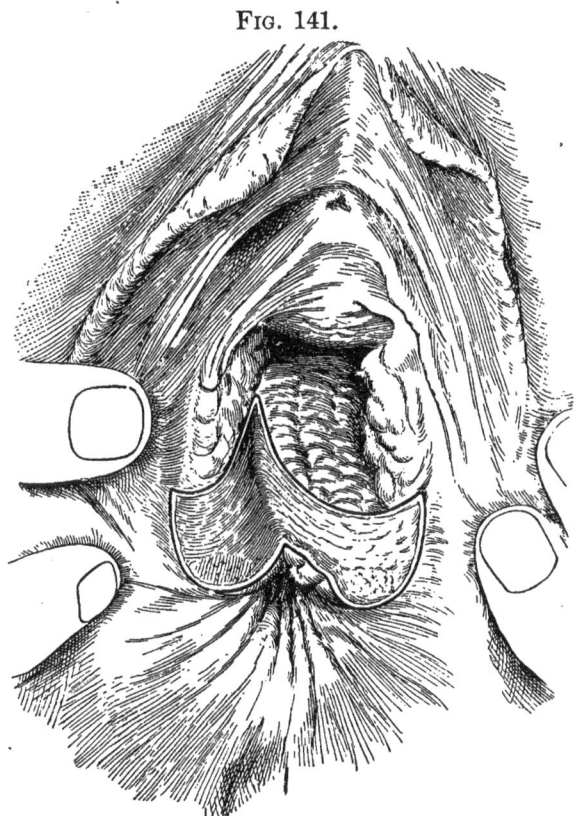

Complete tear, involving the rectovaginal septum.

Dressing: The temporary gauze tampon may then be removed and the wound dusted with an antiseptic powder before the vulvar pad is applied.

After-treatment: No special after-treatment is required. Constipation should be avoided, and the patient forbidden to strain while having a motion of the bowels. If there be much tension on the suture, catheterization may be necessary in order to relieve the bladder. The sutures may be removed on the eighth or tenth day, but the patient should be kept in bed for at least fourteen days.

3. Complete Tear.

Conditions: A complete tear of the perineum is one extending from the fourchette backward through the sphincter ani, and involving the rectovaginal septum to a greater or less

FIG. 142.

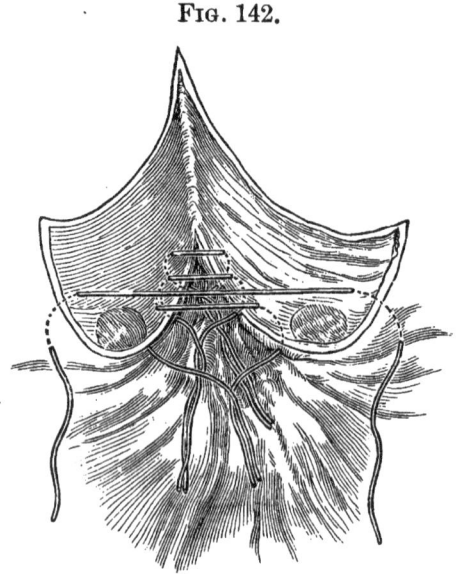

Complete tear; closing the rent in the bowel.

extent (Fig. 141). Such tears involve destruction of the function of the sphincter ani muscle, and result in incontinence of fæces and flatus. The condition of the patient thus becomes most distressing.

Operation.

Anæsthesia in this instance is imperative for the proper performance of the operation.

The **position** of the patient should be as for the previously described operation. The nature and extent of the wound should be first ascertained and the field of operation thoroughly cleansed.

The **rectum** is first repaired by means of interrupted catgut sutures introduced from the mucous surface. The ends of the sphincter must be carefully approximated by means of buried catgut sutures.

The **vaginal rent** should then be repaired as before recommended ; and, finally, the *skin surfaces* of the perineal wound must be brought together.

Fig. 143.

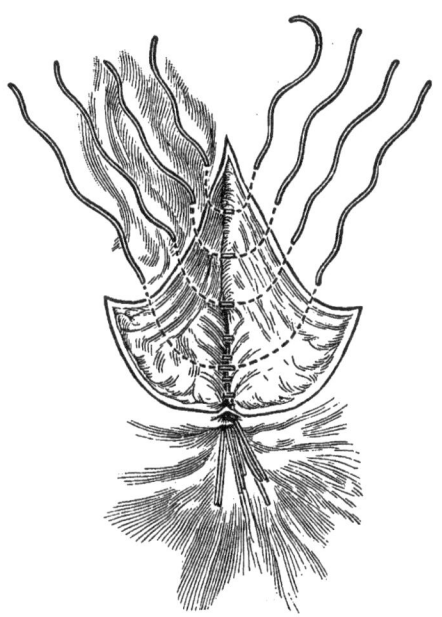

Deep interrupted lifting sutures in position.

It is well to **reinforce** the catgut sutures uniting the torn ends of the sphincter, by means of a large suture of silkworm-gut introduced on the skin surface so as to include in its loop a considerable portion of the muscle as well as of the septum above it (Figs. 142–145).

After-treatment: Constipation should be avoided, the

bowels being opened on the third day and every second day afterward. An oil enema should be given just before a movement is expected, and the edges of the wound should be supported by the nurse, the patient being warned not to strain nor force while evacuation is taking place. The wound

FIG. 144.

FIG. 145.

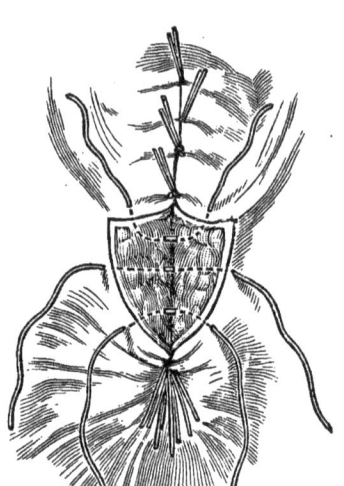

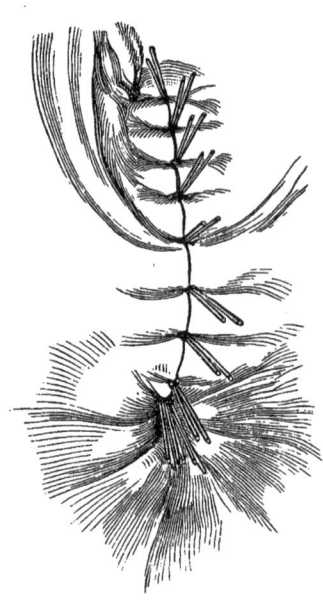

All sutures laid ; vaginal sutures tied.

Internal and external sutures tied.

should be kept well cleansed. The sutures may be removed on the tenth to the twelfth day. The patient should remain in bed for three weeks.

IMMEDIATE REPAIR OF CERVICAL LACERATIONS.

Lacerations of the cervix are **rarely repaired** unless the circular artery is involved and severe hemorrhage results.

Cervical lacerations, even when severe, frequently heal by first intention **without operation.**

Operation: The operation can usually be performed without difficulty. The patient is placed as recommended in the previous operations, the cervix is seized with a tenaculum, drawn down, and held in position for suturing.

The sutures should be placed about one inch apart, and the first should be placed at the upper angle. Silkworm-gut should be employed, and the stitches may be removed on the twenty-first day.

INDUCTION OF ABORTION.

Definition: By the induction of abortion is meant the artificial emptying of the uterus before the period of viability of the child is reached—that is, before the end of the twenty-eighth week of pregnancy. Some authors limit the term "induction of abortion" to the emptying of the uterus before the end of the sixteenth week, because the methods of operation differ before and after this period.

Indications: The occurrence of pathological conditions consequent upon pregnancy, and the aggravation of certain diseases by gestation, give rise occasionally to the necessity of emptying the uterus by artificial means at the expense of the child's life in order to save the woman. Among the conditions which may render necessary the induction of abortion the following may be mentioned:

1. *Hyperemesis gravidarum.*
2. *Renal insufficiency*, with threatened eclampsia.
3. *Death of the fœtus.*
4. Insanity, resulting from or aggravated by pregnancy.
5. Incarceration of a retroflexed uterus.
6. Presence of benign or malignant tumors which would preclude the delivery of a viable child or render Cæsarean section at term inadvisable.
7. Acute hydramnios and cystic degeneration of the chorion.
8. Certain blood diseases, as leucocythæmia and pernicious anæmia.
9. Rarely hemorrhage from placenta prævia may render necessary the termination of pregnancy before the period of the viability of the child is reached.

The attending physician should consult with a colleague before deciding the question of interference, and a full explanation of the circumstances of the case should be made to the members of the family most directly concerned.

Methods of Inducing Abortion.

The **administration of drugs** internally for the purpose of inducing abortion is only mentioned to be condemned. Their action is slow and uncertain, and their use is not infrequently attended with danger.

Up to **the end of the sixteenth week** the quickest and most certain method of terminating the pregnancy is the following:

Dilating the Cervix and Curetting the Uterine Cavity.

Advantages: The operation can be done in from ten to twenty minutes; it is certain in effect, and when properly carried out it is practically unattended with danger to the patient.

The **instruments required** for this operation are, a volsellum forceps, a Simon perineal retractor, a set of Hégar's dilators, a pair of branched dilators, such as Goodell's, an Emmet curette-forceps, a sharp curette, and a pair of long uterine dressing-forceps. Some strips of iodoform gauze (10 per cent.) for packing the uterine cavity and vagina should also be prepared.

Preliminary to operation: The patient, after being anæsthetized, is placed in the lithotomy position on a table which is in a good light, the limbs being held in position by means of a rolled sheet or by a crutch. The vagina and vulva are then scrubbed with spirits of green soap and hot water, cotton-wool swabs being employed. The parts are then disinfected by means of a douche of formalin solution (1 : 500).

The operation: The perineal retractor is placed in the vagina and the anterior lip of the cervix seized with a volsellum and drawn well down. These instruments may then be held by an assistant. The *cervix* is then *dilated* by means of Hégar's and Goodell's dilators till it easily admits the forefinger. The Emmet curette-forceps is then inserted into the uterine cavity and the ovum seized and crushed before the instrument is withdrawn with whatever may have been grasped. The fœtus and as much of the rest of the ovum as is possible should be removed by these forceps; after which the uterine walls should be carefully and systematically *curetted*, but without much force.

After operation: The uterine cavity is then douched with hot formalin solution and afterward packed with sterile gauze. The volsellum and perineal retractor are then removed and the operation is completed.

Some operators prefer **not to empty the uterus at one sitting**, but after removing the fœtus to pack the cervix with gauze and to tampon the vagina with antiseptic wool, which are left in place for twenty-four hours. On their removal, if the remainder of the ovum is not discharged from the os, the cervix being softened by the tampon, is further dilated and the uterine cavity is thoroughly curetted; and is then douched and packed with gauze as above recommended. This gauze packing should be removed in from twenty-four to thirty-six hours.

The patient should be **kept in bed** from one week to ten days after this operation.

Abortion, when induced **after the sixteenth week** is accomplished by means of the methods to be recommended for the *induction of premature labor.*

INDUCTION OF PREMATURE LABOR.

The **indications** for the induction of premature labor are much the same as those given for the induction of abortion. In addition, however, may be mentioned *contracted pelves* in which it is desired to avoid the necessity of Cæsarean operation or symphysiotomy. Placenta prævia, while a rare indication for abortion, not infrequently necessitates the induction of premature labor.

It may be necessary to induce labor prematurely in advanced heart disease and in tuberculosis.

Methods of Inducing Premature Labor.

Krause's method : This is the simplest and the most satisfactory in the vast majority of cases.   It consists in the *introduction of a bougie* into the uterine cavity between the membranes and the wall of the uterus.

One or two bougies (No. 10 or 12 English) are sterilized by
soaking for an hour in a cold solution of formalin 1 : 500.
The patient is prepared by having the vulva and vagina
washed and douched as previously described.   She is then
placed in the dorsal position across the bed with her feet on
two chairs.   The operator, after sterilizing his hands, introduces two fingers of his left hand into the vagina as far as
the external os.   A bougie anointed with carbolized vaseline
is then guided along the fingers into the cervix and pushed
steadily up until only an inch or so remains outside the external os, care being taken not to rupture the membranes.

FIG. 146.

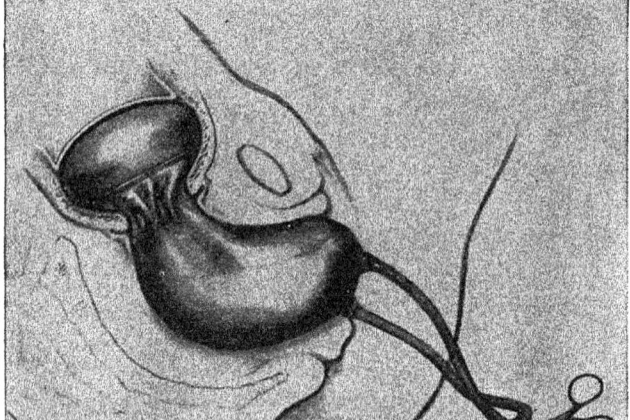

Pomeroy's bag.

Sterile gauze is then packed about the butt of the bougie, to
keep it in place and to prevent injury of the posterior vaginal
wall.   If at the end of twenty-four hours labor-pains have

not manifested themselves, the gauze and bougie should be removed, the vagina douched, and another bougie inserted.

Numerous hydrostatic bags have been devised with the object of dilating the cervix, and are employed in the induction of labor. They are generally made in two or three sizes, and are usually composed of rubber or a composition of silk and rubber. The most commonly employed are those of Tarnier, Champetier de Ribes, and Pomeroy.

If the lumen of the os does not permit the introduction of the smallest bag, the cervix is dilated to about 1.5 cm. by means of a metal dilator, and then the bag is introduced within the internal os, collapsed, and folded; it is then filled with sterile water by means of a bulb syringe attached to the tubing projecting from the lower part of the bag employed. Within a few hours it is generally expelled and a larger bag is inserted, and so on till the os is sufficiently dilated.

Bossi has invented a many-branched metal dilator, by means of which complete dilatation of the os and cervix can be obtained. It is a bulky, awkward instrument, and in unskilled hands most dangerous.

Accouchement force: In certain conditions, such as impending or actual eclampsia, concealed or accidental hemorrhage, acute edema of lungs, or rapidly failing cardiac compensation, it may be necessary to rapidly empty the uterus.

The forcible dilatation of the intact or partially dilated cervix and rapid delivery of the child is termed *accouchement)forcé.* With a firm cervix and undilated canal the operation of accouchement forcé is a difficult and frequently dangerous operation, but with the cervix soft and the os uteri partially dilated the prognosis is not serious.

MANUAL DILATATION : If the os will permit the introduction of one finger, dilatation can usually be effected by the employment of the method suggested by Harris.

The patient should be completely under the influence of an anæsthetic, and prepared as for a high forceps operation. The operator's hand, smeared with vaseline, is inserted into the vagina and the index-finger carried up into the cervix. Gradually, one finger after the other is worked into the os, until finally the thumb is introduced, and by opposing the pressure of the fingers facilitates complete dilatation of the canal.

When the os is too rigid for manual dilatation, multiple incisions of the vaginal portion of the cervix may be resorted to, as recommended originally by Dührssen.

FIG. 147.

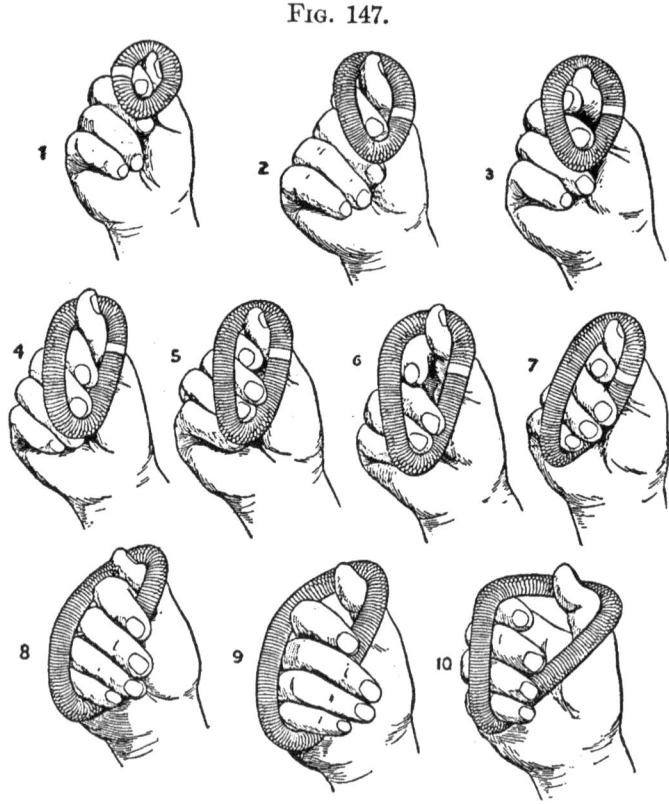

Rapid manual dilatation of os and cervix uteri by the **Harris** method.

VAGINAL CÆSAREAN SECTION : The ideal method of terminating pregnancy in cases where the cervix is undilated is by means of vaginal Cæsarean section or vaginal hysterotomy, first suggested by Dührssen in 1896.

The operation may be at times difficult, requiring surgical experience in the operator, and should only be undertaken in hospital practice.

The patient is prepared in the usual manner and placed on a table in the lithotomy position. The cervix, having been exposed by means of retractors, is seized and drawn down by means of a volsellum forceps. A large curved needle threaded with strong silk is then inserted within the external os, and passed out to the side through the cervix into the lateral fornix and drawn through. A similar suture is then inserted on the opposite side of the cervix. These, left long, then serve as traction sutures, and the volsellum is removed.

A longitudinal incision is then made through the anterior vaginal wall, from just above the meatus to the anterior lip of the cervix. The bladder is then separated from the anterior wall of the uterus by means of the tip of the forefinger, and the bladder held out of the way by means of a retractor. By this means the anterior wall of the uterus is bared as high as the retraction-ring. The anterior uterine wall and cervix are then slit by means of scissors for a distance of about 10 cm. The retractors are removed, and the hand introduced into the uterus after the rupturing of the membranes. The child is then turned and carefully delivered in the usual manner. The placenta is immediately expressed or, if it fails to come away promptly, manually extracted.

The retractors are then reintroduced and the cervix drawn down by means of the long traction sutures, when the whole wound comes into view. The edges of the wound are brought together by means of interrupted catgut sutures, beginning at the top of the wound. The vaginal incision is usually sutured by continuous catgut.

If the child is small, the anterior incision of the uterus usually permits delivery without extension of the wound. In cases at term, or where the child is large, it is better to make a posterior incision of the uterus before proceeding to cut into the anterior wall. This is done by making a transverse incision of the posterior vaginal fornix, pushing up the peritoneum, and cutting through the posterior wall of the uterus to a height of about 4 cm. The wounds are then sutured in the order they were made.

If the hemorrhage from the uterus is severe after removing the placenta, the uterine cavity should be packed with sterile gauze before proceeding to close the incisions. This gauze may be left in place for twenty-four hours.

FORCEPS.

History : It is probable that the obstetric forceps in crude form were employed before the Christian era. The instruments seem to have fallen into disuse and were practically unknown in the middle ages.

The invention of the modern instrument is generally credited to one Peter Chamberlan, the son of a French Huguenot physician, who had settled in England. The obstetric forceps remained a family secret with the Chamberlans for three generations. It was not till 1725 that the secret of the Chamberlan family leaked out in England and the obstetric forceps became public property.

These forceps had only the cephalic curve, which permitted a firm grasp of the head. Later, Smellie in England and Levret in France improved the forceps by adding a second curve, which adapted the instruments to the curvature of the pelvic cavity. The *modern* *forceps* are simply improved models of those invented by Smellie and Levret.

Description : The obstetric forceps consists of two interlocking branches or blades, each of which is provided with a handle to facilitate traction.

The *blades* are usually fenestrated, and have a double curve, a *cephalic*, adapting them to the shape of the fœtal head, and a *pelvic*, accommodating them to the shape of the pelvic canal.

The *articulation* of the blades is in the form of an open lock in the English models, while the Continental models generally have the French lock, which consists of a mortise and tenon tightened by means of a screw. The English lock, having the advantage of easy adjustment, is to be preferred to the more complicated and rigid French lock.

The *handles* of the forceps are usually serrated or grooved transversely, to give a better hold. In the better models the handles are provided with projecting shoulders to facilitate traction. A *good obstetric forceps* should be made of well-tempered steel, polished and heavily nickel-plated throughout. The edges of the blades and the fenestra should be rounded and smooth. In England and America the favorite forceps is the Simpson-Barnes. It has the Barnes blades and the Simpson handles.

The *writer* has found that for general use the most satisfactory obstetric forceps is Dr. Cameron's model of the Simpson-Barnes instrument. Dr. Cameron has modified the pelvic

FIG. 148.

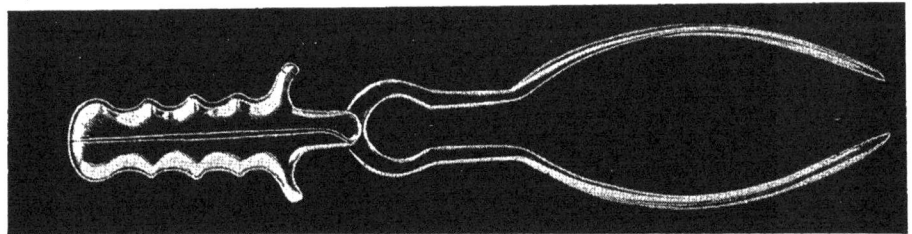

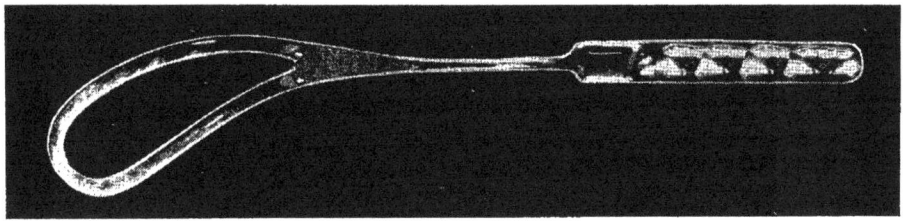

Cameron's model of Simpson-Barnes forceps.[1]

curve of the blades in such a manner as to permit a much more secure grasp of the fœtal head being obtained than is the case in other models (Fig. 148).

For **low operations** a simple, light instrument, such as Sawyer's, is very useful.

In **high operations** the line of traction must correspond as much as possible to the axis of the pelvic inlet. In such operations a great amount of traction force is lost because it is impossible to get the handles of the ordinary forceps back far enough on account of resistance offered by the perineum. This difficulty has been overcome by the invention of the *axis-traction forceps* by Tarnier, in 1877 (Fig. 149). By means of traction rods attached to the base of each blade, fitting at their lower ends into a specially curved perineal bar, to which is attached a cross-bar as a handle, the line of the traction force is brought into relationship with the axis of the brim. The Tarnier forceps is so constructed that

[1] J. H. Chapman, Montreal.

when the lower ends of the traction rods are held 1 cm. from the shanks the line of the pull will be in the axis of the birth-canal no matter what the position of the blades may be in the pelvis.

Many *other models* of axis-traction forceps have been invented, but none has proved so generally satisfactory as the Tarnier.

Fig. 149.

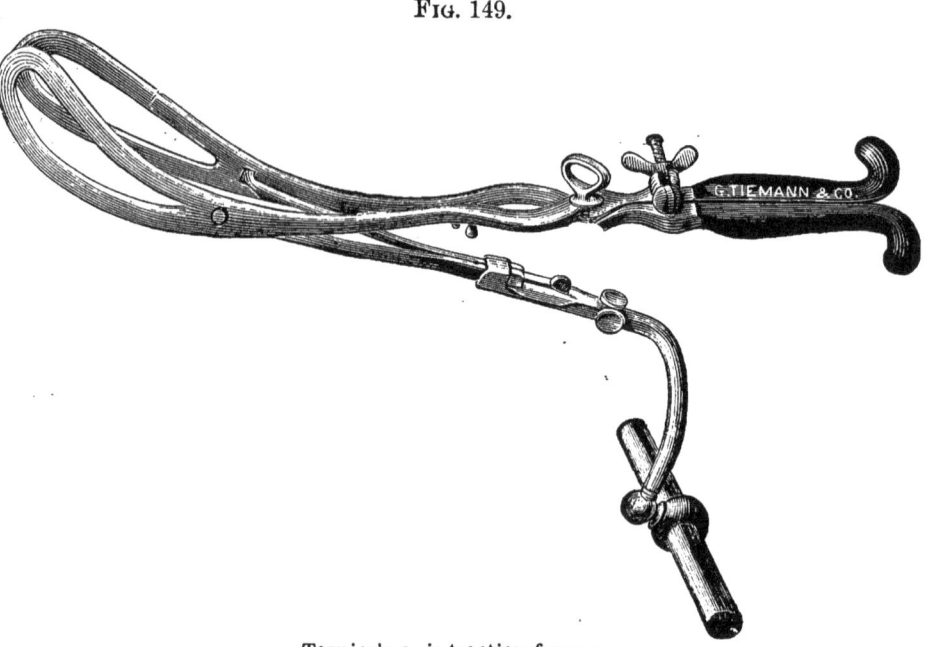

Tarnier's axis-traction forceps.

Indications for the Use of Forceps.

In **general terms** it may be stated that the failure of a woman to deliver herself, when delay in delivery will endanger the life of the mother or the child, or both, is an indication for the employment of forceps to terminate labor.

Anomalies of the mechanism of labor resulting in failure of the presenting part to advance have been fully discussed in detail.

Other indications: Insufficient expulsive power, as uterine inertia from whatever cause; increased resistance in the pelvic canal from moderate pelvic contraction or from unusual rigidity of the soft structures; over-size or undue ossification of the fœtal head; abnormal presentations or positions of the fœtal head, as face presentation and occipitoposterior positions; *accidental conditions,* such as eclampsia, placenta prævia, prolapse of the funis or of a fœtal member.

Exhaustion of the mother is evidenced by a steady increase in the rapidity of the pulse-rate, rising temperature, and a progressive failure in the force of the uterine contractions.

Danger to the child is indicated by the fœtal heart beats becoming rapid and weak or slow and feeble.

If in the course of the *second stage* of labor the **head fails to advance,** and, either because of feeble contractions or from increased resistance, **is arrested for half an hour,** the labor should be terminated by forceps.

When forceps are indicated the following **conditions must be present to render the application of the blades permissible:**

1. The os must be completely dilated or easily dilatable;

2. The membranes must be ruptured;

3. The child must be living and viable;

4. The head must be engaged in the brim; or it must be possible to crowd the head down to the pelvic inlet by external pressure;

5. The head must be of average size and consistence, or else the blades will not retain their hold;

6. The relative proportion between the head and the pelvis must be such as to make extraction possible with safety to mother and to child;

7. The position of the head must be favorable; for instance, it is practically impossible to deliver a mentoposterior position of the face.

Preparation for the Forceps Operation.

Instruments, etc.: The obstetric forceps, as well as such instruments and sutures as may be required for the repair of lacerations subsequent to delivery, should be wrapped in a clean towel and boiled for ten minutes, after which they may be placed in a basin containing cold sterile water, to cool off.

25—Obst.

Preparation of the patient : The *bladder* and *rectum* should be emptied ; after which the abdomen, thighs, and external genitals should be rendered as aseptic as possible. If there be reason to suspect contamination of the *vagina*, the internal passages should be thoroughly scrubbed and douched as for a surgical operation. The lubricity of the parts may then be restored by the application of sterilized glycerin or vaseline.

When the operation has to be done with the patient *in bed*, a Kelly pad or rubber sheet should be arranged under the patient's hips so as to conduct all discharges into a baby's bath-tub or other vessel on the floor. The *patient's limbs* should then be wrapped about with freshly laundried or sterilized sheets.

The **operator's hands** and forearms should be sterilized, and he should wear either a sterilized apron or a sheet to protect his clothing ; or a sterile linen coat and rubber gloves.

Preliminary to operation : The operator should then sit down facing the genitals of his patient. Close to his hand should be placed his instruments and a basin containing a weak formalin solution (1 : 1000), as well as some pieces of sterilized gauze or a plentiful supply of clean towels.

Before proceeding to apply the forceps the quality and frequency of the *fœtal heart-beats* should be ascertained and an exact knowledge of the *position* and *character* of the *fœtal head* obtained. For this latter it may be necessary to pass the entire hand into the uterus ; hence the patient should be anæsthetized before making this examination. Any malposition of the head should then be altered if possible before the application of the blades is attempted.

Anæsthesia : It is rarely possible to employ the obstetric forceps satisfactorily unless the patient is under the influence of an anæsthetic. For prolonged or difficult cases ether should be used in preference to chloroform, and its administration entrusted to a medical assistant.

Posture of the Patient.

The application of the obstetric forceps is possible with the patient either in the dorsal or in the left lateral position. Many consider that the application of the forceps is more difficult in the left lateral than in the dorsal position; but this difficulty is more apparent than real.

Generally speaking, the **lateral position** offers many advantages, especially if the operator lacks a skilled assistant. In this position the patient's limbs do not require to be supported. The application of both blades is accomplished with the right hand, while the fingers of the left hand placed within the vagina serve to guide both the blades into position. During traction the perineum is under constant observation, and extraction is easier and safer.

Walcher's position: On account of the increased mobility of the sacro-iliac joints in the latter months of pregnancy a certain limited amount of rotation of the sacrum is possible on a transverse axis passing through its second vertebra.

After experiments with the live subject and with the cadaver, Walcher demonstrated that by placing the woman at full term on a table in the dorsal position with the buttocks close to its edge, and the lower limbs hanging *unsupported*, the conjugate diameter is lengthened by from one half to one centimetre. This posture of the patient is known as Walcher's position. The posture may be utilized to advantage in high forceps operations or in difficult versions.

The Forceps Operation.

There are **two methods** of application of the forceps. That known as the *English method* is to apply the blades so as to correspond to the sides of the pelvis, quite regardless of the position of the head.

The *Continental method* is to apply the blades to the sides of the child's head regardless of the pelvis.

The pelvic application of the blades—*i. e.*, the English method—is on the whole safer and better, as less damage is possible to the maternal soft parts.

The cephalic application of the blades—*i. e.*, the Continental method—should only be employed by experienced and expert operators, as it is the more complicated and difficult.

The operation is **divided** into the *high*, the *medium*, and the *low*, according to the position of the head in the pelvis.

In the high operation the head is arrested at or just engaged in the pelvic brim. In the *medium* operation the head is arrested well within the pelvic cavity. In the *low* operation the head rests upon the pelvic floor.

In **high operations** the axis-traction forceps should be employed, and the patient should be placed in Walcher's position until the head has been drawn down into the pelvic cavity. As a rule, it is more convenient for the operator and better for the patient if she be placed on a table for the high forceps operation.

In **medium** and **low operations** the patient may be placed either in the left lateral or in the dorsal position, whichever is more convenient for the operator.

Forceps Operation in the Dorsal Position.

The patient having been prepared for the operation, is **placed in the dorsal** position, across the bed with the buttocks projecting slightly over the edge.

Support of the limbs : When assistants are not obtainable to hold the limbs, they may be supported as in the lithotomy position by means of a rolled sheet passed under the neck and over one shoulder, having the ends fastened at the patient's knees.

A *better method* is to place two ordinary wooden chairs a short distance apart with their backs to the edge of the bed. The patient's knees are then flexed over the backs of the chairs, folded towels being so placed as to protect the popliteal regions from injury. The operator sits facing the patient.

Introduction of the blades : Having made an internal examination and having satisfied himself as to the exact position of the fœtal head, the operator selects the *left,* or *lower, blade* of the forceps, which he grasps close to the shaft with the fingers of the *left hand,* holding the instrument as he would a pen. Two or more fingers of the *right hand* are inserted within the vagina, and if possible, within the cervix, their palmar surfaces being in contact with the child's head. The fingers are carried as high as it is possible to introduce them, and the maternal soft parts held outward away from the head.

The *left blade is then held perpendicularly* to the woman's body, and the tip is guided along the fingers of the right hand within the vulva. No force is required to introduce the blade, which is guided along the fingers of the internal hand, by slowly sweeping the handle downward along the internal surface of the mother's left thigh. This blade when in position rests between the head and the left lateral wall of the pelvis.

The *upper blade* is then held in the *right hand* in similar fashion, and is guided along the fingers of the left hand within the vagina, the handle being depressed along the mother's right thigh.

The **forceps are then locked** by depressing the handles toward the perineum and gently rotating the blades into position. Care should be taken not to include hair or a portion of the vulva in the bite of the lock. In guiding the blades into position it is important to have the fingers of the internal hand introduced as far as possible and to press the maternal tissues well to one side.

After locking the forceps a careful internal examination should be made to ascertain if a good grasp of the head has been obtained, and that nothing but the head has been included in the bite of the forceps. The *handles are then grasped* near the lock with one hand, the fingers being hooked over the projecting shoulders while the back of the hand is directed upward.

Extraction is effected by steady pulling, or, better, by exerting a slight pendulum movement at the same time.

The **line of traction** should correspond to the axis of the plane of the pelvis in which the head is engaged; thus in *high operations* the line of traction is directly backward to correspond to the axis of the brim; in *medium operations* the line of traction is directly horizontal; while in *low operations* it is upward, so that the handles are directed toward the mother's abdomen.

The tractions should be **intermittent**, like the natural pains. A good rule is to pull for one minute and then to rest for two. During the intervals it is better to *unlock the forceps*, so as to relieve the head from pressure and also to favor its rotation as it descends.

Traction, when once the **perineum begins to distend**, must be made very carefully in order to avoid the sudden descent of the head.

The *line of traction* should be pretty much horizontal until the *occiput pivots* under the pubic arch. After this has occurred *no further traction* is necessary, but the head is slowly and carefully extended by pushing the handles upward in the direction of the mother's abdomen.

When the *head can be retained in the perineum* by pressure applied from behind in the coccygeal region, the forceps may be gently removed and the head delivered without them. The

FIG. 150.

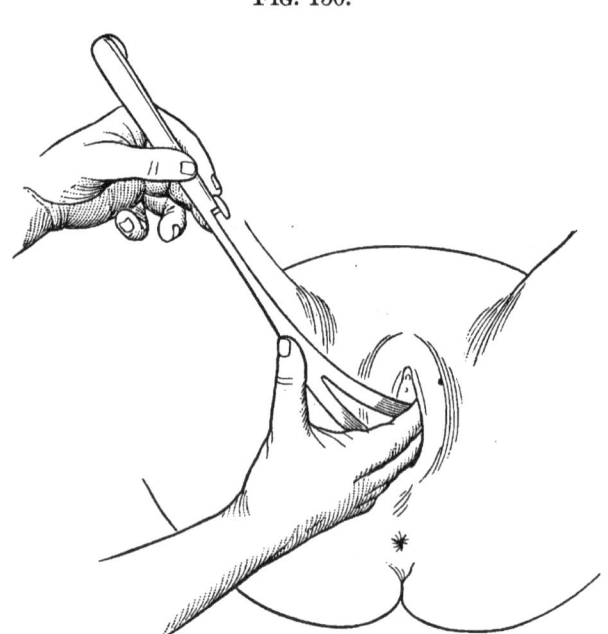

Use of forceps at outlet. Introduction of first blade. (Zweifel.)

head *is held in position* by grasping it through the perineum with the left hand. On no account should the fingers be inserted into the anus for this purpose, as it is unnecessary and dangerous to do so.

When the head *can be held in position* the **blades may be removed** in the reverse order of their application. The utmost gentleness should be employed in their removal, and no force should be exerted if any obstacle be encountered. When gentle manipulation fails to release a blade, it should be left in place until the head is delivered.

After the forceps have been removed the head can be delivered by **pressure over the perineum.**

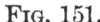

Fig. 151.

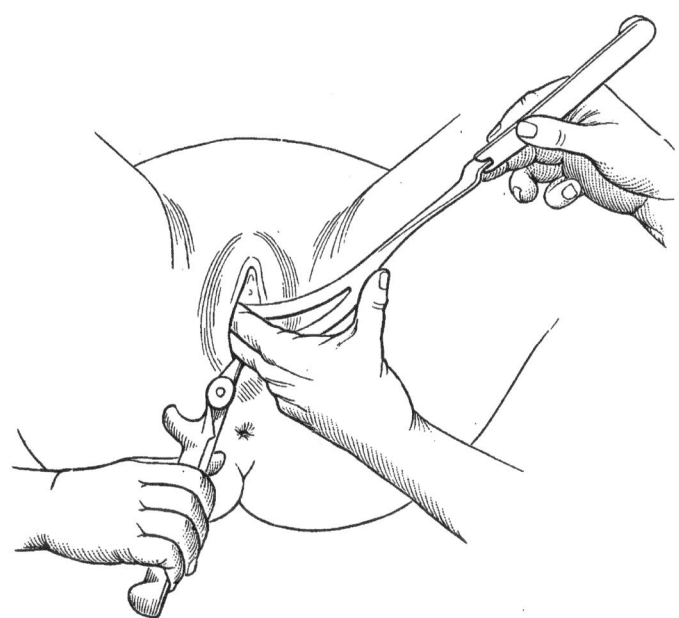

Introduction of second blade. (Zweifel.)

As a general rule, forceps operations are performed with excessive speed, hence the **frequency of lacerations** of the maternal soft parts following their employment.

Axis Traction.

In high operations **axis-traction forceps** should be used, though a certain degree of axis traction may be obtained with the ordinary forceps; as will be described later.

The patient having been placed on a table in the **dorsal position,** with the buttocks at the edge and the limbs held by assistants, or supported by chairs, the blades are inserted in the ordinary manner with the traction-bars fastened (Fig. 152). After insertion the blades are locked, and, if Tarnier's

FIG. 152.

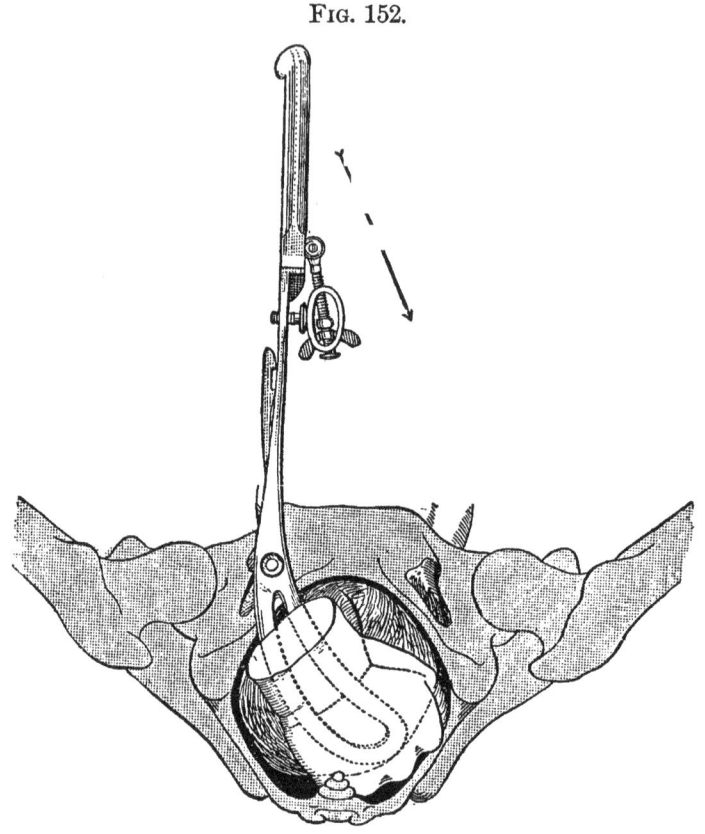

Guiding-hand and forceps blade; high application.	(Farabœuf and Varnier.)

instrument is used, the lock-pin is screwed moderately tight. The bar connecting the handles is then thrown across, locked, and the screw tightened until the blades have secured a firm but not too tight grasp of the fœtal head. The lower ends of the traction-bars under the shanks are then loosened and the perineal handle adjusted to them and locked.

After ascertaining that a proper grip of the head has been obtained and that the various screws are properly adjusted without the inclusion of portions of vulvar tissue the patient can be placed in the **Walcher position** by removing the supports from her limbs. By placing large blocks or books under the table-legs nearer the operator the table can be inclined in such a manner that the buttocks will not be pulled too far over the edge when traction is exerted. The line of traction should be downward and backward as far as possible,

FIG. 153.

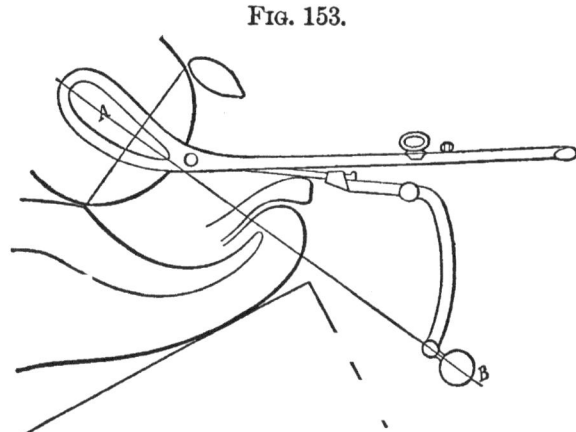

Line of pull with axis-traction forceps applied to the head.

the traction-rods being kept about a quarter of an inch from the shanks throughout the pull (Fig. 153).

Between the tractions, the connecting-bar between the handles should be unscrewed and the pin-lock loosened in order to relieve the fœtal head from continued pressure.

When the **head has been drawn down to the pelvic floor** there is no further need either for the Walcher position or for the axis-traction rods. The patient may then be placed in the ordinary position, the perineal handle may be removed, and the traction-rods fastened in their places beneath the blades, the forceps then being used as the ordinary instrument. Some operators prefer to remove the Tarnier instrument as soon as the head reaches the pelvic floor, completing the delivery by means of Sawyer's small forceps.

In high operations a certain amount of axis traction can be exerted with the **ordinary long forceps.** By Paget's or Galabin's manœuvre the line of traction can be brought to correspond fairly well with the axis of the pelvic inlet.

Thus by pressing or pulling downward with one hand placed as near the shanks as possible, and by pressing or pulling upward with the other hand on the handles, two forces are brought into action, with the effect that the resultant acts in the line of descent of the head. The forceps by this manœuvre is used as a lever, the hand grasping the shanks being the fulcrum.

In employing this manœuvre the greatest care must be exercised to prevent the blades slipping.

Forceps Operation in the Left Lateral Position.

The patient is **placed** somewhat obliquely across the bed, lying on her left side with her thighs well flexed, the hips being brought well over the right edge of the bed. A folded pillow may be placed between her knees to keep the thighs separated. The operator sits facing the patient's buttocks.

The **preparations** for the operation are otherwise the same as mentioned in dealing with the application of forceps in the dorsal position.

Insertion of the blades: Two fingers of the operator's *left hand* are inserted along the posterior wall of the vagina, through the cervix when possible and well over the presenting part, pivoting the finger-tips upon the head globe, while the cervix, the posterior vaginal wall, and the perineum are pressed back as far as possible out of the way.

The *lower blade* being held in the right hand with the pelvic curve directed backward, so that the tip of the instrument is in contact with the left hand, is thus introduced within the vagina. To facilitate the introduction of the tip of the blade in this position, the handle must be held low down, corresponding to the direction of the gluteal fold of the patient's left buttock (Fig. 154). As soon as the *tip* of the blade has been guided by the fingers of the left hand over the convexity of the head the *handle* is raised, being swept upward over the mother's right thigh, and finally backward and downward, until the shank falls behind the operator's left wrist. The handle thus sweeps through nearly three-quarters of a circle as the blade is being introduced and pushed up. This movement of the handle causes the tip of the blade to sweep around and under the head.

Fig. 154.

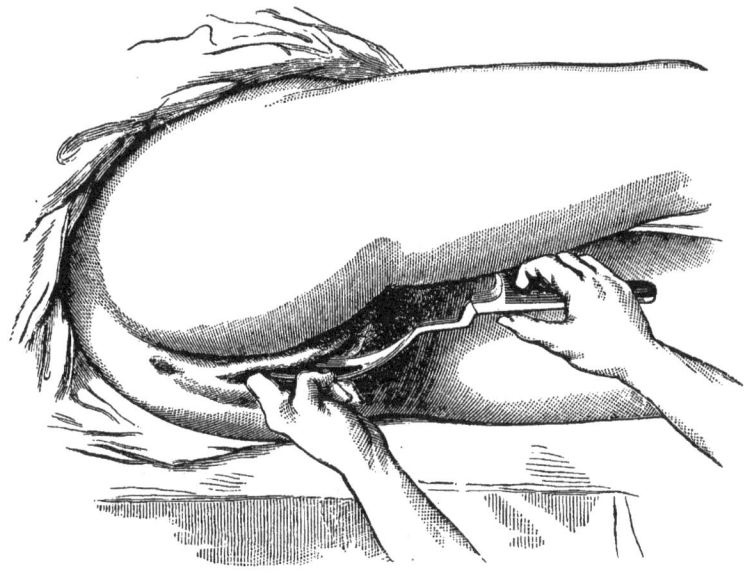

Introduction of the upper blade.   (Playfair.)

Fig. 155.

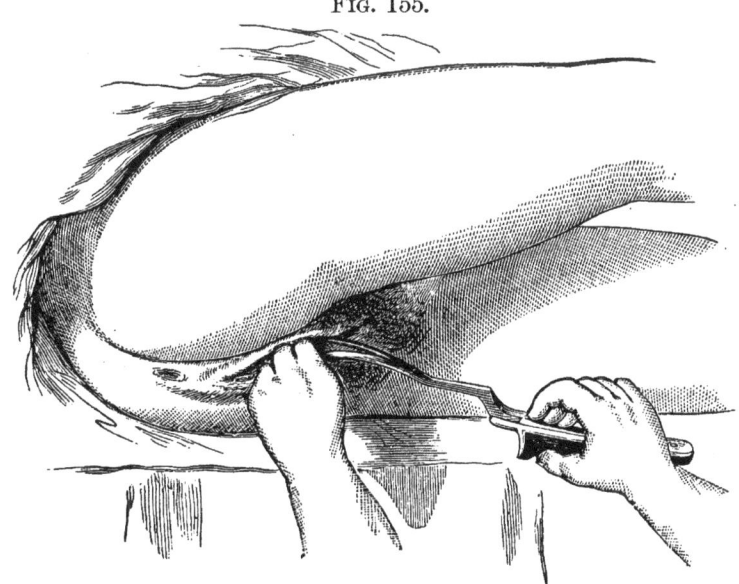

Position of patient for forceps delivery and mode of introducing lower blade.
(Playfair.)

The *fingers of the left hand* remain in contact with the head throughout the insertion of both blades, the first blade being held in position after its introduction by resting against the back of the left wrist while the second is being manipulated into position.

The *upper blade* is then grasped in the right hand and its tip introduced into the vulva above the shank of the first

FIG. 156.

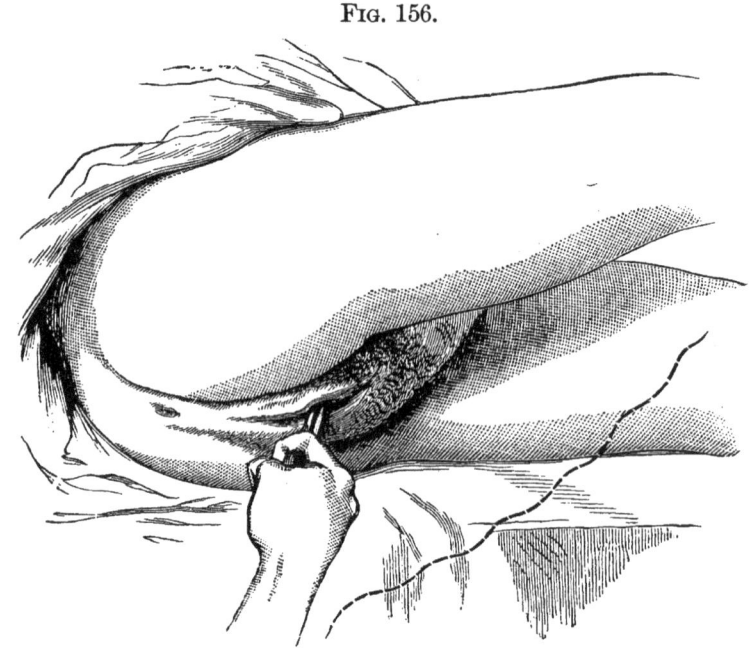

Forceps in position. Traction in the axis of the brim, downward and backward.
(Playfair.)

blade with the pelvic curve directed forward. The *tip* is guided into position over the convexity of the head by the fingers of the left hand (Fig. 155). The *handle* is then swept downward and backward along the mother's left thigh, thus causing the blade to move around the *upper* surface of the head to take its position opposite the right ilium.

The second blade, having been placed in position, is used as a guide in locking the handles. It is held steady while the first blade, which may become displaced during the introduction of the second, is manœuvred into position so as to lock (Fig. 156).

Extraction: After examination to see that all is secure, the operator, grasping the handles over the projecting shoulders with his right hand, exerts traction as far backward as possible, at the same time steadying the patient's hips with his left hand. During extraction in the lateral position the handles describe a horizontal arc from left to right.

When the head can be **retained in the distended perineum** the forceps may be gently removed and the delivery completed without them.

Forceps in Persistent Occipitoposterior Cases.

Ordinarily, when it is necessary to terminate labor by means of the forceps in posterior positions of the occiput, if the *head is well flexed* before the instruments are applied, and if the blades are disengaged completely by unlocking them after each tractive effort, the occiput will be brought in contact with the pelvic floor first, and will thus rotate to the front without special difficulty.

When **rotation forward** of the occiput **fails** to take place plenty of time should be given for proper *moulding* of the head to occur.

The normal mechanism of delivery in face to pubes cases must be borne in mind, and the forceps so used as to aid nature. The line of traction should be in the axis of the pelvic cavity—that is, horizontally—until the forehead emerges sufficiently for the glabella to pivot under the pubic arch; the handles are then raised so as to bring the occiput over the perineum, after which the face generally delivers itself by extension of the head.

Once the *glabella has pivoted* many operators prefer to remove the blades and deliver the head manually.

Forceps in Face Presentations.

In **posterior positions** of the chin in face presentations the forceps are contraindicated.

In **mento-anterior positions**, when nature's efforts are insufficient to complete delivery, the forceps may be employed. The blades should be applied to the sides of the child's head in such a way as to secure a firm grasp of the occiput. *Traction* should be made *horizontally* until the chin is brought under the pubic arch ; then by raising the handles and without pulling, the head is flexed, thus sweeping the face, vertex, and occiput successively over the perineum. This *movement of flexion* should be made with great deliberation, and when laceration of the perineum takes place and threatens to extend into the rectum a *lateral incision* should be made in order to avoid this troublesome complication.

Forceps in Breech Cases.

Indications : When in breech cases it is impossible to reach a foot or to employ a fillet or the finger to draw down the presenting part, the forceps may be used. When possible, the axis-traction forceps should be employed for this purpose.

The **grasp of the breech** may be obtained by placing the tip of the blades over each trochanter and below the iliac crests. When this hold cannot be obtained, the blades may be introduced so that one is in contact with the sacrum and one ilium of the child, while the other is in contact with the posterior surface of the opposite thigh, as recommended by Ollivier.

The **after-coming head** has occasionally to be delivered by forceps after the failure of other methods. The application of the blades is not difficult, provided the child's body is held up over the abdomen of the mother by an assistant.

The Dangers of Forceps Operations.

The forceps judiciously and skilfully used should seldom result in the production of serious injury to either mother or child.

When forceps operations are undertaken by unskilled operators and in unsuitable cases the most disastrous consequences may follow : the uterus has been perforated by the tips of the blades ; the cervix and lower uterine segment have been torn away ; the pelvic joints have been sprung apart; while most extensive vaginal lacerations are not infrequent, as the result of improperly performed forceps operations. The most common injuries are: lacerations, more or less extensive, of the perineum and vagina, and certain injuries of the child's head the result of compression of the blades. Contusions and abrasions of the face or scalp are not infrequent, and occasionally facial paralysis may follow pressure upon facial nerve-trunks. Intracranial hemorrhages are not infrequent after forceps operations. Such hemorrhage may result in rapid death of the newborn child, or, if survived, may give rise to idiocy, hemiplegia, epilepsy, etc. Occasionally the cord may be around the child's neck, and be so exposed to pressure from the tip of the blades that fatal asphyxia may ensue.

VERSIONS.

Definition: The general term *version* is applied to such obstetric operations as are designed to bring about any alteration in the relation of the long axis of the child's head to the long axis of the uterus.

Varieties: There are three varieties of versions:

Cephalic, resulting in presentation of the head;

Pelvic, of the breech; and

Podalic, of one or both feet.

Methods: There are three methods of performing version:

External version, which is accomplished by manipulation through the abdomen;

Bipolar version, accomplished by external and internal manipulations combined;

Internal version, accomplished by the introduction of the hand within the uterus.

External Version.

By means of **external version** either the head or the breech can be made to present at the pelvic brim. It is probably the simplest and safest method of turning, as there is practically no danger connected with it.

The more practised the operator is in abdominal palpation

of the pregnant uterus the more skilful will he prove in the performance of external version.

Indications: The most common indication for external version is breech presentation, when diagnosed during the latter weeks of pregnancy. While the indications for this form of version are in general the same as those that apply

FIG. 157.

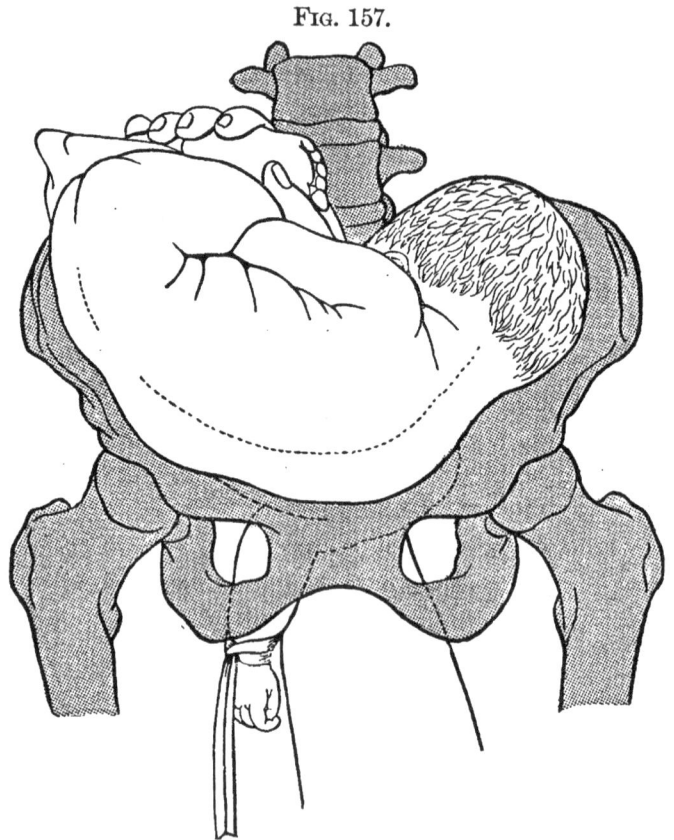

Right hand grasping feet in right shoulder (arm) presentation, dorso-anterior position. (Davis, after Faraboeuf and Varnier.)

to the other forms, the fact that it can be employed only *before* or *very early in* labor limits its availability.

Conditions for external version: The membranes should be intact or but recently ruptured. The uterine and abdominal walls should be lax and the child freely movable. These conditions are only present before the onset of labor or very early in its course, hence to these periods the operation is limited.

Preparations: The bladder and rectum should be emptied. The patient should be in the dorsal decubitus, with her thighs

FIG. 158.

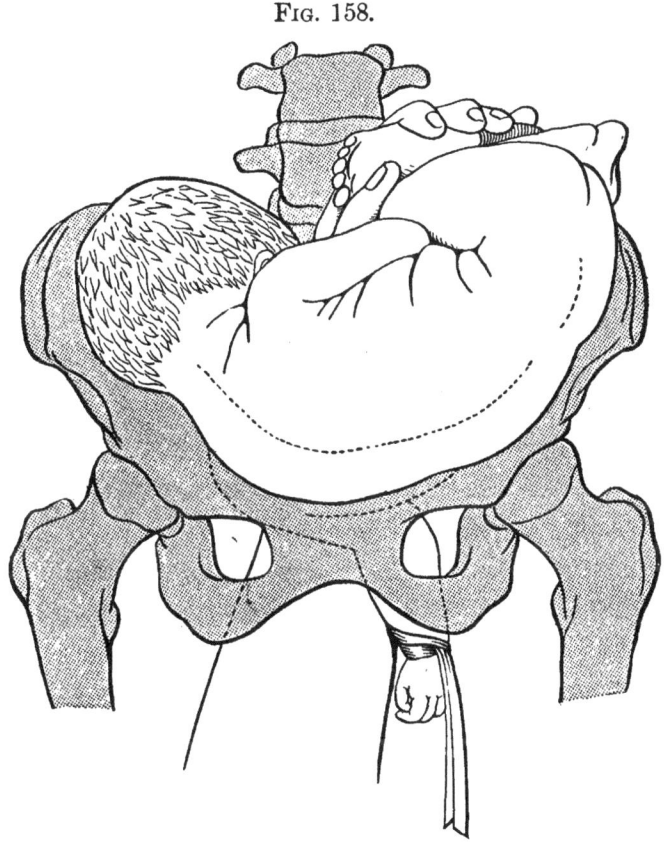

Left hand grasping feet in left shoulder (arm) presentation, dorso-anterior position.
(Davis, after Faraboeuf and Varnier.)

slightly flexed and the head and shoulders supported by pillows. The abdomen should be exposed or covered only by a sheet, under which the hands of the operator are placed. An anæsthetic is not required unless the patient is extremely nervous.

26—Obst.

Method of Operation.

The first duty of the operator is carefully to map out the position occupied by the child. This is done by palpation, supplemented by auscultation of the fœtal heart.

Fig. 159.

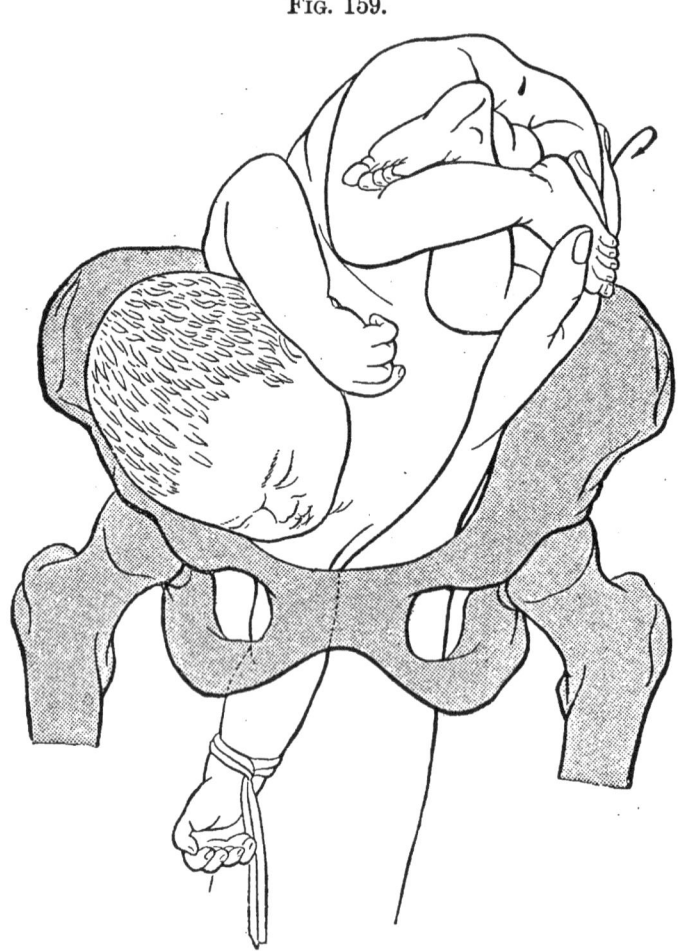

Right hand grasping feet in right shoulder presentation, dorso-posterior position. (Davis, after Farabœuf and Varnier.)

He should then **plot out** the manœuvre he wishes to accomplish from beginning to end, before attempting to displace in any way the fœtus.

In performing external version the **most important point** is to keep the fœtal ovoid intact throughout the operation.

The manœuvres: The operator places a hand on each end of the fœtal ovoid, with the palms facing and the fingers of one hand directed toward the wrist of the other. By the alternate flexion of the fingers of either hand the version is

FIG. 160.

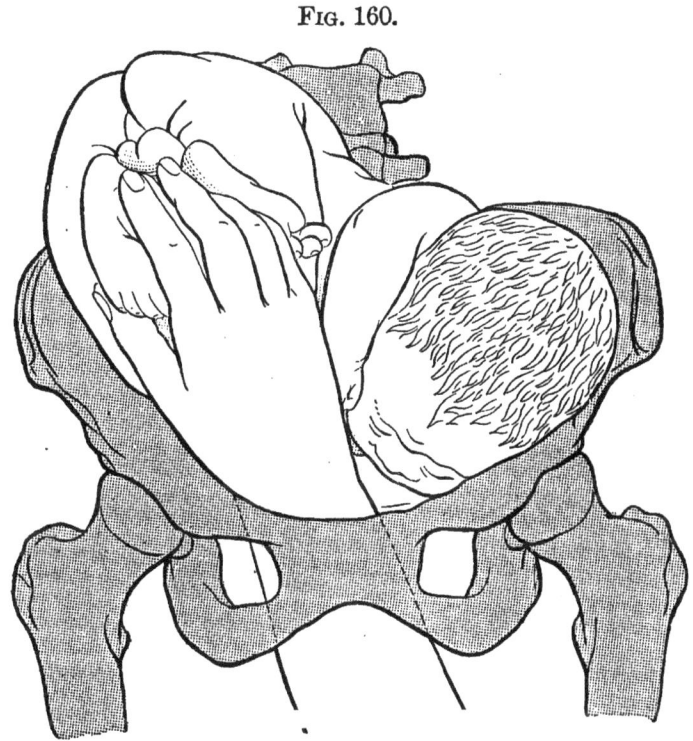

Direct method of reaching feet in dorso-posterior cases. (Davis, after Faraboeuf and Varnier.)

accomplished. One hand gives a movement of ascent and the other a movement of descent, each acting alternately.

The extremity of the fœtal ovoid it is desired to bring down is made to follow the shortest route which will bring it into proper relationship with the pelvic brim. Should **uterine contraction occur** during the manipulations, the operator must be content to hold the fœtus in the position gained until relaxation occurs, when the operation may be proceeded with.

When the fœtus has been **placed in the desired position** a vaginal examination should be made to ascertain whether the presenting part is properly over the inlet.

To *retain the foetus* in position until the presenting part has engaged, longitudinal pads composed of folded towels, may be placed on either side of the fœtus and a firm abdominal binder applied.

Occasionally, when external version has been carried out after the onset of labor, it is advisable to **rupture the membranes,** so as to favor the retention of the fœtus in its new position.

Bipolar Version.

The **chief advantage** of the bipolar method is that complete dilatation of the cervix is unnecessary, as by this method version can be accomplished as soon as *two fingers can be inserted through the os uteri.*

Bipolar version has the **disadvantage** that it fails to give the operator such control of the fœtus as is obtainable by the internal method.

This form of version is also known as the **Braxton-Hicks method.**

Indications : *Placenta prævia* with but partial dilatation of the os is given by most text-books as the chief indication for selection of this method of performing version.

In the experience of the writer, the very fact that the placenta is situated in the lower uterine segment *contraindicates* the employment of this method, as, with only two fingers through the os, the presenting part cannot be satisfactorily reached ; for the pelvic inlet is occupied more or less by the bulky placenta. For this reason in placenta prævia, when version is desirable, the internal method should be selected and the os dilated until the whole hand can be introduced into the uterus.

Other indications for this method are : abnormal presentations or positions of the head, such as face or brow presentations and prolapse of the cord, when diagnosed early in labor. It is also very useful in transverse cases, whether it is desired to bring down the breech or the head.

Conditions for bipolar version : The membranes should be intact or so recently ruptured that the child is still freely movable. The cervix should admit two fingers, and the vagina be capable of containing the operator's hand if necessary. The uterine and abdominal walls should be lax.

Preparation: The patient should be prepared as for a forceps operation. She should be placed in the dorsal position, across the bed, with her hips at the edge, the legs being supported by chairs. The operator sits between the patient's thighs. The external hand can be kept from contamination by wrapping it in a sterilized towel.

Anæsthesia is desirable, but not necessary, provided the vagina and vulva are lax and the patient not nervous.

Method of operation: *Before proceeding to operate,* the diagnosis of the position of the fœtus should be confirmed by careful external and internal examination. The details of each movement of the operation should then be planned so that the operator has clearly in mind exactly what he wishes to accomplish by his manœuvres.

In *head presentations,* in which it is desired to bring down the breech, the head should be moved in the direction in which the occiput points.

The fingers of the hand, the palm of which points in the direction in which it is desired to move the presenting part, are then introduced through the cervix. Thus, if presentation is L. O. A. and it is desired to bring down the breech, two fingers of the left hand are introduced within the cervix, while the right hand presses down the breech, through the abdominal wall. The version is accomplished by a series of alternate pushes with either hand. Care should be taken not to rupture the membranes, should they be intact, until a foot or leg is within reach of the internal fingers at the pelvic brim.

In correcting an abnormal presentation of the head by combined manipulation the fingers of the internal hand push the lowest part of the fœtal head upward and backward while the external hand, having located the occiput through the abdominal wall, endeavors to force the vertex downward and forward within the pelvic brim.

In such cases, if the membranes have not ruptured, they *should be broken* as soon as the position of the head is altered. Pressure should then be maintained upon the fundus until the vertex has become firmly engaged in the brim.

Internal Version.

This method of version is most commonly employed, as it is probably the most rapid and effectual way of securing delivery when the head is not engaged in the pelvic brim. It is the most dangerous method of version, as the hand must be placed into the uterine cavity in order to seize one or both feet.

Indications: Eclampsia, placenta prævia, threatened sudden maternal death, prolapse of the cord, and accidental hemorrhage may be mentioned as indications for this method of version, especially when rapid delivery is desired.

Other indications are transverse presentations, moderate pelvic contraction, prolapse of fœtal members, and rupture of the uterus.

Conditions for internal version : The cervix must be dilated, or dilatable ; the pelvis must be sufficiently ample to permit the passage of the after-coming head, and the uterus must not be tetanically contracted about the child. The condition of the lower uterine segment should be ascertained before version is attempted, and the position of the retraction-ring noted, if it be present. The fœtus must not be impacted in the pelvis, but should be sufficiently movable to permit the presenting part to be pushed back. The child should be viable.

Preparations: When possible the patient should be placed on a table for operation. Preparations should be made as for a forceps operation.

It is well to have at hand some sterilized bandage-material or broad tape, in case it may be necessary to pass a noose about the fœtal limbs, to facilitate extraction. The patient should be *anæsthetized,* and for this purpose chloroform is usually recommended as bringing about better uterine relaxation than ether. It is desirable that the anæsthetic should be administered by a medical assistant.

The patient should be *placed* in the lithotomy position with her hips at the edge of the bed or table. The operator, wearing sterile rubber gloves and a sterile gown, sits or stands facing the patient.

Method of operating: The *first step* in the operation is to confirm the diagnosis of the fœtal position by a combined internal and external examination. The various steps of the operation of turning the fœtus are then planned, and a decision made as to which hand shall be introduced into the uterus and which foot of the infant seized.

When the long axis of the fœtus is in the long axis of the uterus, the operator should *introduce the hand which corresponds to the side of the mother toward which the presenting part is directed.* Thus in L. O. A. or L. O. P. positions the left hand is introduced into the uterus. In such cases the anterior foot should always be seized. In case of doubt both feet may be brought down.

When the long axis of the fœtus is transverse to the axis of the uterus *the hand to be introduced is the one which corresponds to the side of the mother to which the breech is directed.* When the breech is directed to the mother's right side the operator should introduce his right hand.

In dorso-anterior positions the near foot should be seized and brought down, and in dorsoposterior positions the remote foot. Thus, when the breech is directed to the mother's right side, the operator's right hand is introduced and the right leg of the child is seized. If the breech is directed to the left side of the mother, the left hand is introduced and the child's left leg is brought down. This rule applies whether the dorsum of the child is directed anteriorly or not.

Before introduction the hand should be dipped in lysol solution or smeared with sterilized oil.

The hand, with the tips of the fingers and thumb placed together *so as to form a cone,* is then introduced through the vagina and cervix with a rotary motion. The uterus should always be entered with the palm of the hand directed toward the abdomen of the fœtus. The hand should be pushed steadily though gently upward to the fundus, where the feet are usually to be found. A common mistake of inexperienced operators is to feel about for the feet before the hand has been introduced far enough. The foot can be easily recognized by the prominence of the heel and malleoli.

The *external hand,* protected with a sterilized towel, should co-operate by making counter-pressure on the fundus, in order to steady the fœtus as well as to press the breech down, so that the feet may more easily be reached.

If the membranes be found intact, they *should be ruptured* and the hand pushed quickly up, in order that the forearm may plug the vagina and so prevent escape of the liquor amnii. *Should uterine contraction* occur, the hand with the fingers extended should be held quiet until relaxation has taken place.

If the *shoulder be found impacted* in the pelvis and an *arm prolapsed*, a noose of gauze bandage or tape should be slipped over the child's wrist, and then the impaction may be reduced by gentle upward pressure upon the body of the fœtus.

In reducing an impaction of the fœtus the same rule applies as in the reduction of an impacted hernia, "The part that has come down last should be returned first." Thus the upward pressure should first be applied to that portion of the fœtus nearest the pelvic brim, and then successively along the body until the apex of the shoulder is reached.

When *a secure grasp of the desired foot* has been obtained it is drawn steadily down toward the pelvic outlet, the external hand at the same time being employed in directing the head toward the fundus. This turning movement should only be made when the uterus is entirely relaxed.

The operation may be *considered as complete* when the child's breech is engaged in the pelvic inlet. When possible the case should then be left to nature to complete the delivery.

After the completion of version the fœtal heart should be auscultated and the general condition of the mother ascertained. Should either be at fault the case should be terminated by rapid extraction of the fœtus.

For details as to the various methods of *extraction of the breech*, the reader is referred to the section on the Management of Breech Cases.

The **dangers** of internal version are : laceration or rupture of the uterus from the employment of undue force, hemorrhage, shock, and subsequent sepsis from uncleanliness at the time of operation. In order to prevent the latter the uterine cavity should be douched with a hot antiseptic solution (formalin, 1 : 500) as soon as the placenta has been delivered.

SYMPHYSIOTOMY.

Definition: Derived from σύμφυσις, a joint, and τομή, a cutting, symphysiotomy is the term applied to the operation of section of the symphysis pubis in a woman in labor. The *object* of the operation is to increase the diameter of a contracted pelvis, and thus to permit the delivery of a living child through the natural passages.

History: The operation was first performed successfully by Sigault, in Paris, in 1777. It was comparatively popular during the early decades of the present century, but fell into disrepute by 1858.

In 1866 the operation was successfully revived by Morisani, of Naples, to whom is due the chief credit of the improved technique of the modern operation. It was reintroduced into Paris by Pinard in 1892, and was first performed in America by Jewett, on Sept. 30, 1892.

Rationale of symphysiotomy: The separation of the symphysis causes a lengthening of the diameters of the pelvis, the conjugate being the one affected most in consequence of the ends of the pubic bones moving downward as well as outward when separated. The descent of the separated ends is due to the fact that each of the sacro-iliac joints rotates upon an oblique line running from above downward and from without inward. A separation of 3 cm. (1⅕ inches) causes a descent of 2 cm. (¾ inch); still further descent being caused by the downward pressure of the fœtal head. The separation of the pubic bones also permits the anterior parietal eminence of the fœtal head to project into the interpubic space.

Thus symphysiotomy results in enlargement of the pelvic canal by the separation and descent of the ends of the pubic bones, and by permitting a prominence of the fœtal head to occupy the interpubic space.

Symphysiotomy became extremely popular for a time, but statistics soon showed that the maternal mortality ranged about 12 per cent., while the fœtal mortality ranged between 9 and 13 per cent., and, again, the convalescence was prolonged and attended with much inconvenience. These results compared with those of Cæsarean section soon led to the practical abandonment of the operation.

PUBIOTOMY OR HEBOTOMY.

Pubiotomy has replaced the operation of symphysiotomy as a means of obtaining a temporary enlargement of the pelvic diameters. The operation consists of severing the pubic bone to one side of the symphysis by means of the Gigli saw.

History: Gigli, an Italian, in 1893, impressed with the dangers of symphysiotomy, proposed that the pubic bone itself should be severed, as thus the attachments of the bladder would not be interfered with and the wound would heal more rapidly and be less liable to infection. Bonard, also an Italian, first carried out Gigli's suggestion in 1897, severing the pubic bone by means of a flexible saw invented by the latter.

Originally, the operation was performed by making a large incision, exposing the pubic bone, and passing the flexible saw up from below behind the bone.

Döderlein, in 1904, improved the method of operating by making a small incision parallel to and above the pubic bone by the method described later.

Others perform the operation entirely subcutaneously by means of a specially large curved needle inserted through the tissues at the upper part of the labium majus, and, under the guidance of the finger placed in the vagina, carrying it up behind the pubic bone so that the point emerges on the upper margin between the pubic spine and the symphysis.

Indications: Pubiotomy is an operation of considerable gravity and should not be lightly undertaken. It is preferable to Cæsarean section, in so far as it can be performed after the patient has been some hours in the second stage of labor. It comes into competition with Cæsarean section and the induction of premature labor in moderate degrees of pelvic contraction. Its advantage is that the patient may have a fair chance to deliver herself before the operative proceedings are undertaken.

It may be said to be indicated in :

1. Simple flat pelves with a conjugata vera of between 7 and 9 cm.

2. Generally contracted pelves with a conjugata vera of between 8.2 and 10 cm.

3. Impacted face or occipitoposterior presentations.

Operation: The patient is prepared in the usual manner, and placed on a table in the lithotomy position, the legs being held by assistants. An incision, sufficiently large to admit the forefinger, is then made parallel to the upper margin of the pubic bone extending inward from the pubic spine. The tissues are cut through down to and including the periosteum. The tissues are then separated from the posterior surface of

FIG. 161.

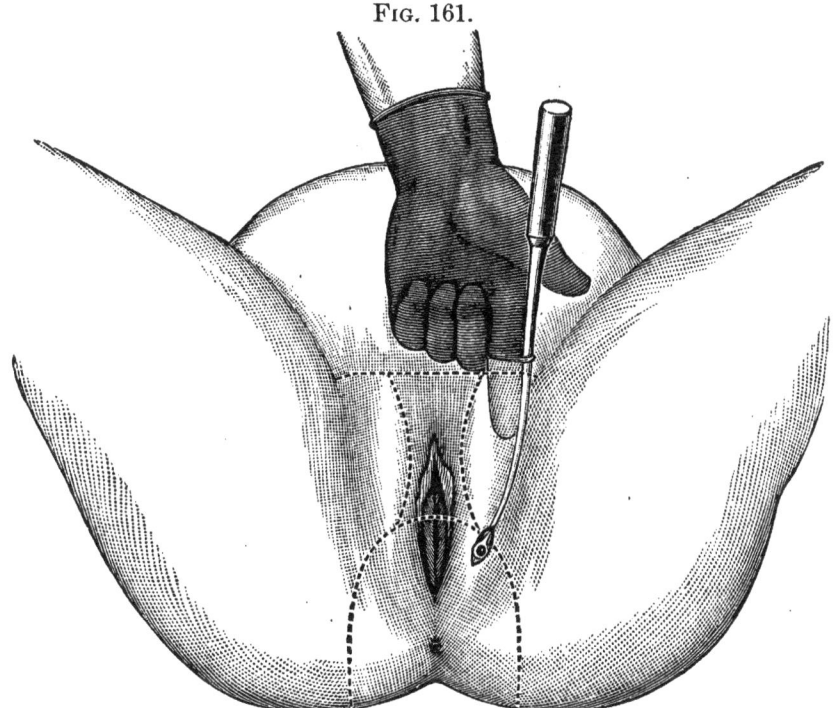

Döderlein's method of performing pubiotomy. Incision and needle in place for attachment of Gigli saw.

the bone by means of the finger thrust into the wound. A specially constructed needle (Bumm-Stoeckel or Döderlein) is passed down behind the bone until its tip can be felt through the upper part of the labium majus below. To it the saw is attached, drawn back through the wound, and brought out above. The handles are then attached to the Gigli saw, and keeping the hands well apart, to avoid breaking the saw, the bone is cut through.

The ends of the severed bone may then spring apart, but this is not the case unless the ligamentary structures have been divided; these usually give way as the child's head comes through the pelvis.

Usually on withdrawing the saw a sharp hemorrhage takes place, but is soon checked by firm pressure with gauze-packs.

The child is then delivered by means of forceps or version, though many obstetricians leave the delivery to nature.

FIG. 162.

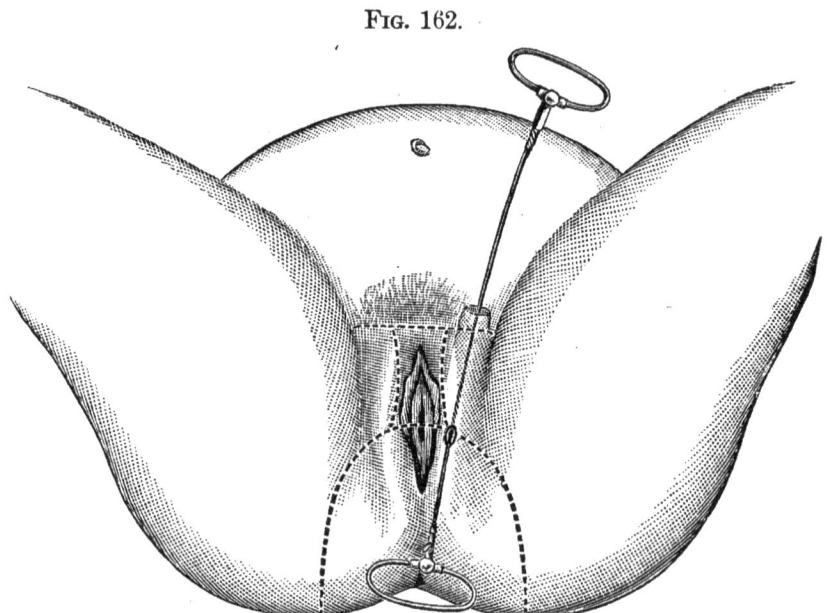

Pubiotomy: Gigli saw in position with handles attached, preparatory to sawing bone.

While the child is passing through the pelvic canal the severed ends of the bone may gape to the extent of 5 or 6 cm. Further separation should be avoided by having the assistants make firm pressure from either side.

After delivery a small drain may be inserted in the lower wound and the upper wound sutured.

Having carefully examined and repaired any lacerations if found, the patient is then cleansed, a sterile pad applied over the upper wound, and a strip of adhesive plaster 20 cm. wide is passed completely around the body so as to compress the pelvis and bring the severed ends of bone into the closest apposition.

The patient is then placed in bed on a firm, level mattress. Usually no special treatment is required, though there may be some considerable œdema of the labium, particularly on the side operated upon.

Complications: Occasionally extensive lacerations occur during extraction of the child. Less frequently the bladder may be injured. Hæmatoma have been reported in many cases, but usually give but little trouble. These conditions should be treated on general surgical principles.

CÆSAREAN SECTION.

Definition: Cæsarean section may be defined as an obstetric operation for the delivery of a mature fœtus by means of an incision through the abdominal and uterine walls.

History: The operation dates from prehistoric times. The first recorded operation was performed by a butcher in Switzerland, in 1500. Until the development of antiseptic surgery the operation was attended by enormous fatality, and was only performed as a last resort. The uterine incision was formerly left unsutured, as it was supposed that sutures would not hold on account of uterine contractions.

Sänger, of Leipsic, has done probably more than anyone else to perfect the modern operation. In 1882 he showed that the uterine incision could be sutured with safety provided the suture-material employed was sterile. Since that time the mortality attending the operation has been steadily reduced.

The **indications** for this operation may be *absolute* or *relative*:

An **absolute indication** is the presence of some condition which renders impossible any other method of delivery—*e. g.*, extreme degrees of pelvic contraction (conjugate under 6.5 cm.); marked pelvic deformity resulting from osteomalacia, kyphosis, and spondylolisthesis; foreign growths obstructing the pelvic canal; cicatricial contraction of the vagina; and carcinoma of the cervix or of the rectum.

A **relative indication** is the presence of some condition which makes doubtful the delivery of a living child by the natural passages. In some cases the question to be decided is whether Cæsarean section or one of the alternative operations (pubiotomy, forceps, version, craniotomy) will secure the best results. The individual peculiarities of each case as it arises must be studied before a decision can be made. In general, after consultation with a *confrère*, the physician should leave the decision to the woman or her husband, having explained to them the nature of the case.

The commonest relative indications are : a conjugate of 6 to 8 cm. (2½ to 3⅛ inches) ; and tumors which cause but a moderate degree of pelvic obstruction (Fig. 128).

The best **time** for operation, when this is elective, is within a week of the expected date of labor.

Preparations for Cæsarean Section.

The **patient**, if possible, should be under observation for some days before the operation is undertaken. During this period the urine should be examined, the diet restricted, and the bowels carefully regulated. General tonics, especially strychnine, should be given daily, if there be any indication.

The *evening before* the operation the patient should be given a full dose of castor oil, or half an ounce of Epsom salt in a tumblerful of water. The abdomen and pubes should be shaved and scrubbed with a soft brush, tincture of green soap, and hot water. After being thoroughly rubbed with alcohol the abdomen is to be covered with sterile gauze and a binder applied.

If the patient is nervous and unable to sleep, sulphonal (gr. x–xv) may be given in warm broth or milk. The following morning the patient may be given a cupful of broth two hours before the operation. If the bowels have not been freely moved, an enema of turpentine and soapsuds (ℨj to Oj) may be given.

Before the patient is placed on the operating-table she should be catheterized and the abdomen, vulva, and vagina finally sterilized.

After the patient is placed on the operating-table in a slightly elevated Trendelenburg position, the chests and thighs are covered with blankets protected by sterilized towels, and a large piece of sterilized gauze composed of four thicknesses is arranged so as to cover the whole body from chest to knees.

The usual *dressings* and *accessories* for an abdominal operation should be provided in addition to the following **instruments** :

2 scalpels,

1 pair of ordinary scissors.

1 dozen artery-forceps,

1 pair of retractors,

Curved and straight needles,

1 needle-holder.

Silk, silkworm-gut, and catgut for sutures and ligatures.

Four **assistants** are required—one to give the anæsthetic, one to compress the cervix and control hemorrhage, one to receive and attend to the child, and one to assist the operator throughout the operation.

The Cæsarean Operation.

The operator first cuts a slit in the **gauze** extending from the pubes to a short distance above the umbilicus.

An **incision** is then made in the linea alba extending from a point 4 cm. (1½ inches) above the pubes to a point the same distance above the umbilicus. The peritoneal cavity is then opened with the usual precautions. The uterus is then pulled up through the abdominal wound and sterile towels packed behind it to prevent contamination of the peritoneal cavity.

The uterine vessels on each side are then clasped firmly by an assistant, who at the same time steadies the uterus. A small incision is then made into the anterior wall of the uterus with a scalpel. This wound is then enlarged by scissors as may be necessary and the membranes ruptured.

Extraction of child : The operator then plunges his hand into the cavity of the uterus, pushing to one side the placenta if it be encountered, seizes the child by a foot, and extracts it as rapidly as possible. As soon as the child is extracted the uterus usually contracts When the child is withdrawn from the uterus it is given to an assistant to hold, while the operator clamps the cord in two places with artery forceps and cuts between them.

Removal of the placenta: The placenta is then grasped on its fœtal surface and loosened from its attachment by simply squeezing it. The membranes peel off from the uterine wall as the placenta is withdrawn through the incision.

Should the uterus fail to contract properly, it may be *stimulated* by the application of hot cloths and friction.

Closure of the uterine wall: After carefully examining the uterine cavity to see that no membranes or portions of placenta have been retained, the uterine wound is closed by means of silk sutures. These sutures are placed at intervals of about 1.5 cm., or about half an inch, and should include only the muscular coat. The peritoneal edges are then approximated by a second layer of interrupted silk sutures, placed at shorter intervals than the first layer. After the sutures have been tied there should be no hemorrhage either from the wound or from the needle-punctures.

Closure of abdominal wound: The abdominal cavity should then be sponged dry with cheesecloth sponges, particular attention being paid to the renal fossæ.

Having returned the uterus to the abdominal cavity and placed it in proper position, the omentum is then to be brought down and carried behind instead of in front of it, in order to avoid omental adhesions.

The abdominal incision is then closed in the usual manner and a surgical dressing applied. The vaginal gauze is then removed and a vulvar pad applied.

After-treatment: The after-treatment should be much the same as after any abdominal operation. During the first twenty-four hours it may be necessary to give a hypodermic injection of morphine for the relief of pain. The child may be put to the breast after twenty-four hours have elapsed.

Special attention should be given to the care of the vulva, in order to prevent infection of the vagina.

The abdominal sutures may be removed from the tenth to the fourteenth day, and the patient may be allowed out of bed at the end of three weeks. An abdominal support should be worn for six months after the operation.

Many operators prefer to enter the uterus by means of a transverse incision over the fundus, extending from one tubal insertion to the other, as recommended by Fritsch in 1897, who claimed that thus hemorrhage is reduced. The method has given excellent results.

SUPRASYMPHYSEAL CÆSAREAN SECTION.

In 1907 Frank, of Cologne, introduced a new method of performing Cæsarean section, particularly for cases in which there was any possibility of infection of the uterine cavity having occurred before operation.

A transverse incision is made through the anterior abdominal wall, a few centimetres above the symphysis pubis, and the peritoneum separated from the bladder and anterior surface of the lower uterine segment. The bladder is thus pushed down behind the symphysis by means of a retractor. The lower anterior uterine wall is then incised, either vertically or transversely, and the child and placenta removed. The uterine wound is then closed by catgut sutures, the peritoneum stitched to the bladder, and the abdominal wall closed in the usual manner. In this manner the whole operation is carried out without entering the peritoneal cavity.

Since that time many have modified Frank's operation in various details, but all agree in closing of the peritoneal cavity before opening the lower uterine segment.

Porro Operation.

In 1876 **Porro** suggested that the ordinary Cæsarean operation should be supplemented by the *amputation* of the uterus along with the tubes and ovaries.

After amputation of the uterus, **two methods** of treating the stump are available.

By the **extraperitoneal** method the stump is transfixed by long needles and retained in the lower angle of the wound.

By the **intraperitoneal** method the stump is sewed over in such a manner as to cover it completely with peritoneum, after which it is dropped into the abdominal cavity.

The **advantages** of the Porro operation are that it renders subsequent uterine hemorrhage or conception impossible, and decreases the risk of puerperal infection, while it adds nothing to the danger of the operation.

27—Obst.

Indications: Cœliohysterectomy, or Porro-Cæsarean section, is indicated when labor has been prolonged and manipulations have been attempted to secure delivery, but have failed and sepsis is probable; when the uterus or its appendages are so diseased as to require a subsequent operation for their removal; and when any condition is present which will make it impossible for a child to be delivered subsequently by the natural passages.

The **preparations** are the same as for Cæsarean section, except that the following *instruments* should be added to the list given previously: 1 large pedicle-scissors; 4 curved large pedicle-clamps; 2 large volsellum forceps; 2 right and 2 left aneurism-needles; and 1 right and 1 left sharp-pointed pedicle-needles.

Operation: The abdominal incision should extend from two inches above the umbilicus to just above the symphysis. The uterus is drawn up out of the abdomen, and a sterile towel is packed into the peritoneal cavity to prevent the escape of the intestines. The assistant then draws the edges of the abdominal incision close about the cervix, which he grasps firmly with both hands so as to control hemorrhage when the uterine incision is made.

The uterus is then incised and the child and placenta removed as quickly as possible. The ovarian arteries are then sought and tied, as also the arteries of the round ligaments. The broad ligaments are then clamped and cut; peritoneal flaps for covering over the stump are then prepared, the uterus amputated, and the uterine arteries tied.

The stump is then oversewn and dropped, the peritoneal cavity is washed out, and the abdominal wall closed.

GENERAL RULES GOVERNING THE SELECTION OF OBSTETRIC OPERATIONS IN CASES OF OBSTRUCTED LABOR.

Conjugate of 9.5 cm. or less: The best method is to induce labor at or about four weeks before the expected termination of pregnancy. If the condition of the pelvis is only discovered after labor has begun, the labor may be allowed to go on for twenty-four hours. Attention should be paid to the woman's general condition and the distention of the lower uterine segment. The choice of operation then lies between forceps, version, pubiotomy, and Cæsarean section.

Forceps may be applied and the patient placed in the Walcher position ; if after twenty minutes the head does not become engaged, they should be discarded. *Version* may succeed where the forceps have failed, but the risk for the child is considerable. If the danger of version is considered too great to risk, then *pubiotomy* should be done. If after the pubis has been divided the head descends to the brim, the delivery may be completed by forceps. Should the head remain high after separation of the pubes, then version offers a more favorable result to the child.

The most important *conditions affecting* the choice of operation are the size and compressibility of the fœtal head. A compressible head may pass through a pelvis that would prove an insuperable obstacle to an incompressible head of the same size.

The relative size of the head and pelvis may be *approximately determined*, by grasping the head firmly with the extended fingers placed on the abdominal wall, and pressing it down upon the pelvic brim for some time. The pressure thus exerted should be in the axis of the pelvic inlet. If the head can thus be forced within the brim, the natural forces will certainly secure the engagement.

Conjugate of 7 cm. or less: If at the thirty-sixth week the head can be forced into the brim by steady pressure from above, labor should be induced. The risk to the child of inducing labor before the thirty-sixth week is too great to afford much chance of its surviving its birth. If at this time the head is too large to engage, the case should be left till about term and Cæsarean section performed. Embryotomy should never be performed upon a living child if it possibly can be avoided. On the other hand, Cæsarean section should not be rashly undertaken by an operator unskilled and inexperienced in abdominal surgery. As before said, the final decision should be left to the patient or her nearest relations.

When the pelvic canal is obstructed by a *tumor* which cannot be dislodged or which would be subjected to dangerous pressure during the passage of the child, the safest method of delivery would be Cæsarean section or the Porro operation.

EMBRYOTOMY.

Definition: *Embryotomy* is a generic term which includes all the destructive operations by which the volume of the fœtus is reduced to permit of its extraction through the natural passages. The term thus includes *craniotomy, decapitation, evisceration,* and *amputation of the extremities.*

Indications: Embryotomy should never be performed on a *living child* when any other obstetric operation offers a reasonable chance of saving its life.

The patient and her friends may decline any conservative operation and insist on embryotomy. In such case, if the physician is of opinion that a conservative operation would offer a reasonable chance of saving the child, he is at liberty to transfer the case to some one else should he so desire. When such a course is not open to him, the physician must under protest yield to the desire of the patient and her friends, as he has no legal right to compel them to follow his judgment.

Provided the fœtus is dead, the following conditions may be mentioned as constituting the ordinary indications for embryotomy:

1. Deformity of the pelvis where forceps or version is impossible, or would expose the mother to unnecessary risk.

2. Obstruction of the parturient canal by tumors—uterine, ovarian, malignant, or osseous.

3. Impaction of the presenting part: face presentations, occipitoposterior positions, locked twins.

4. Eclampsia, or other causes demanding rapid delivery where forceps or version would be difficult or prolonged.

5. Monstrosities; hydrocephalus; the latter constitutes an indication for embryotomy on the living child, for if the condition is so marked as to prevent delivery there is no probability of the child surviving should conservative operation be performed.

Embryotomy-instruments: The object of embryotomy being to reduce the bulk of the fœtus, the presenting part has first

to be perforated and its contents evacuated. If this procedure fails to reduce the bulk of the fœtus sufficiently, it is

FIG. 163.

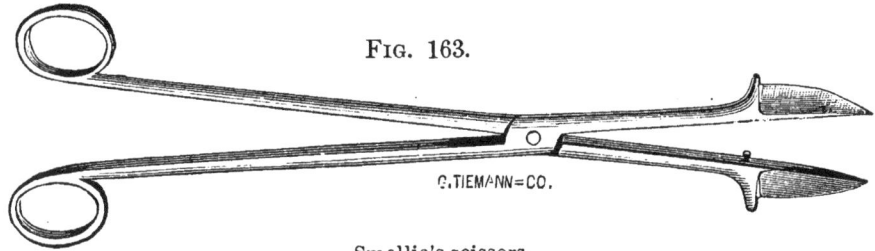

Smellie's scissors.

necessary then to crush the presenting part by means of a
powerful instrument, so that delivery may be accomplished.

Perforators : The best instruments for perforating the head

FIG. 164.

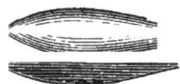

Blot's perforator.

are Smellie's scissors and Blot's perforator (Figs. 163 and 164),
though a pair of scissors with a long handle answers the pur-

FIG. 165.

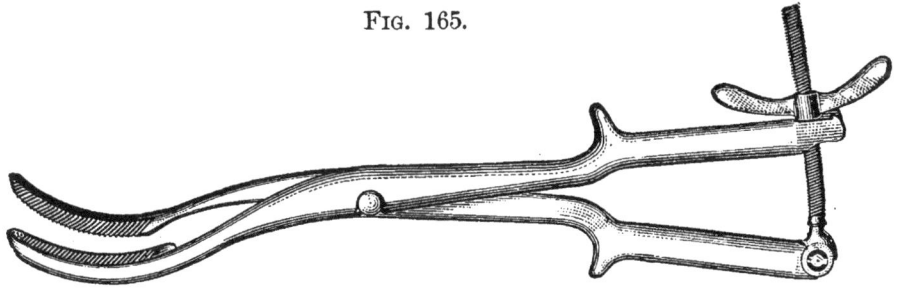

Braun's cranioclast.

pose admirably. The Germans prefer to perforate the skull
by means of a trephine with a long handle.

Cranioclast : This is a powerful instrument for seizing the head after it has been perforated (Fig. 165). It consists of two blades, one for insertion inside and the other outside the skull. At the ends of the handles there is a powerful compression screw which enables the operator to obtain a firm grip of the head.

Cephalotribe: This instrument is simply a heavy forceps specially modified for compressing the head after it has been perforated (Fig. 166). The blades are applied on either side of the head, which is then crushed by tightening a screw attached to the ends of the handles.

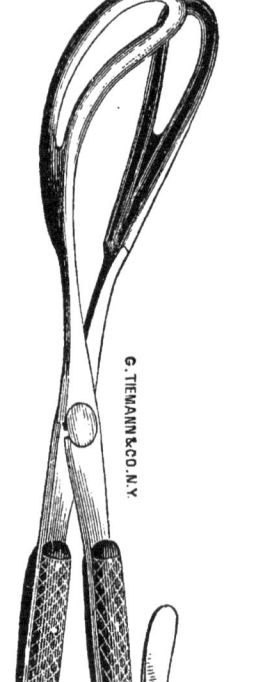

Fig. 166.

Lusk's cephalotribe.

The most perfect instrument for reducing the bulk of the fœtal head is *Tarnier's basiotribe*, which is at once a perforator, a cranioclast, and a cephalotribe (Fig. 167). This instrument is composed of a perforator, two heavy fenestrated blades of unequal length, and is provided with a powerful compression screw.

Method of use: After disarticulating the instrument the perforator is pushed through a suture or fontanelle, the short blade is then applied on the outside of the head like an ordinary forceps blade, and is then articulated with the perforator, when the compression screw is tightened until the blade is forced close to the perforator, thus crushing one side of the head.

After loosening the compression screw the long blade is applied to the opposite side of the head and its handle articulated to the handle of the short blade, when the screw is again tightened, thus completely crushing the head. Thus the base as well as the vault of the skull can be crushed and flattened to a little less than two inches (Fig. 168).

Hook and crotchet: This instrument consists of a curved metal bar terminating at one end in a blunt hook, at the other

in a crotchet tip (Fig. 169). The crotchet-tip end may be
inserted into the skull after perforation and hooked into the
foramen magnum, thus permitting the instrument to be used

FIG. 167.   FIG. 168.

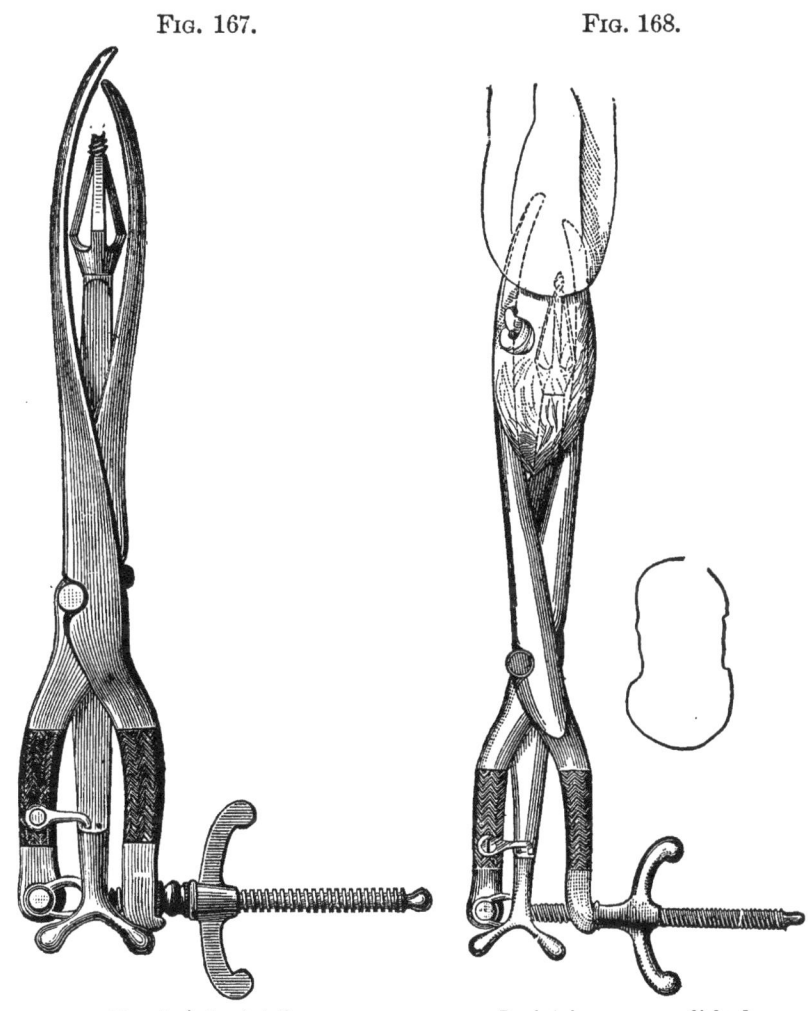

Tarnier's basiotribe.   Basiotripsy accomplished.

as an extractor. The hook may be used to pull down the
neck.

Braun's hook, which consists of a steel rod with a strong
transverse handle at one end and a sharply bent hook, tipped

with a rounded button, at the other, is employed as a decapitator.

Zweifel has devised a *decapitator* which consists practically of two Braun's hooks so arranged that by separating the handles the tips can be moved in opposite directions.

In America, where extreme degrees of pelvic contraction are rarely to be met with, embryotomy can usually be carried out with comparatively little risk to the mother, provided the operator is careful and moderately skilful, by means of a pair of **blunt-pointed scissors** with short blades and a long handle ; and an old-fashioned hook and crotchet. The writer has performed seven embryotomies with these two instruments, and

FIG. 169.

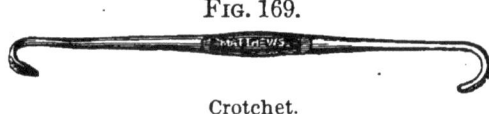

Crotchet.

in no case was there laceration or injury of the maternal soft parts, and the mothers all made uneventful recoveries.

The **time** for operation is at the conclusion of the first stage of labor.

Preparations : The patient after being anæsthetized is placed in the lithotomy position with her hips at the edge of the bed or table on which she lies. The vulva, vagina, and inner surfaces of her thighs are then scrubbed with spirits of green soap and hot water, to be followed with a douche of formalin or bichloride solution. The bladder is then catheterized. The douche-bag should be filled with sterile water and hung in a position to secure a good, forceful stream.

The **instruments** to be used in the operation are then placed in a convenient position after being sterilized.

Operation.

The operator, suitably prepared, first makes a careful **internal examination**, to ascertain the exact conditions present. If possible, the hand should be passed into the uterus till the cord can be reached, to make certain the fœtus has perished. When the head is found presenting at the brim it should be steadied from above by an assistant when possible.

The **perforator**: The operator then locates the suture or fontanelle with the tips of the index and middle fingers of his left hand placed in the vagina. The perforator held in his right hand is then guided into position between the fingers of the left hand placed on the head. The head is perforated by steady upward pressure of the instrument held in the right hand. Having penetrated the skull, the perforator is swept in every direction to break up the brain, and the opening is enlarged in every direction. The douche nozzle is inserted into the opening in the skull, and, a return flow having been provided for, a stream of water is let into the cavity to wash away the broken-up brain-substance.

If a **cranioclast** or **cephalotribe** is at hand, it should now be applied and the head carefully extracted, care being taken to guard the sharp edges of the cranial bones from cutting the maternal tissues.

When the **crotchet hook** is used, it is to be thrust into the skull and hooked into the base about the forearm magnum. After obtaining a firm hold the head is drawn down.

When **long scissors** are employed to open the skull-cavity the tips of the blades should be kept between the two fingers of the operator's left hand which are in contact with the head. The cutting is done by little snips, separating the blades as little as possible. Having cut through to the skull, the tip of the scissors with the blades closed is thrust through a fontanelle or suture. The blades are then separated as widely as possible and swept about to break up the brain-substance. The cerebral cavity is washed out and the crotchet used as described.

Sometimes after the cranial contents have been removed the child is expelled by **natural efforts**.

In most cases in which the pelvis will permit of their proper application, the **ordinary forceps** may be used as extractors of the perforated head.

Perforation of the after-coming head: When it is necessary to perforate the after-coming head, the perforator may be inserted through the quadrilateral fontanelle behind the ear, or into the foramen magnum through the mouth of the child.

Decapitation: In impacted shoulder presentation it may be necessary to sever the head from the trunk in order to effect delivery.

This may be performed by passing the hook end of the hook and crotchet over the neck to draw it down as far as possible, where it is held by an assistant. By means of a pair of long-handled scissors the operator can then cut through the neck, being careful to guard the blades between the two fingers of the left hand held in the vagina.

Evisceration : This is rarely indicated. When necessary it may be done with a pair of long-handled scissors.

In all cases after the separation of the placenta, the uterine cavity should be **douched** with hot salt solution. Lacerations of the soft tissues should then be sought, and if found sutured at once.

Dangers of embryotomy : The chief dangers of embryotomy are, lacerations of the maternal tissues by spicules of bone or by instruments ; and sepsis.

As the mother has been exhausted by prolonged and ineffectual efforts to complete labor, before embryotomy is performed, she has but little resisting power should septic infection take place ; while the bruised and lacerated condition of the soft parts favors the development of sepsis.

INDEX.

427

28

Lightning Source UK Ltd.
Milton Keynes UK
UKHW02f0739160818
327336UK00010B/706/P